Critical Reviews and Pr
Arthritis and Autoimmu

"Dr. Poehlmann covers an (
microbiology; even biofilms), diagnostic measures and treatment
methods [than her first book]....**THE encyclopedia for managing and
conquering complex, life-robbing arthritides that affect millions of
Americans**....In 2004 I specifically sought her out and recruited her as
a board member for the APF because of her unique expertise evidenced
in her first book, which has helped tens of thousands of people find
hope and relief. **[This book is] a gift to the millions afflicted with
arthritic conditions.....**"
— Richard Longland (Founder & CEO of the Arthroplasty Patient
Foundation (www.arthropatient.org) and producer of the 2012
film *Why Am I Still Sick?* (www.biofilmcommunity.org)

"You have done an outstanding job, covering an extensive number of
possible causes and treatments...**I recommend this book as a
practical, well researched presentation of both conventional and
unconventional treatments.**"
— Dr. Gabe Mirkin (Immunologist, Radio talk show
host, Author of 16 books plus hundreds of Internet
articles at www.drmirkin.com)

Critical Reviews and Praise for
Rheumatoid Arthritis: The Infection Connection

"Dr. Poehlmann has compiled **an outstanding resource** that finally
offers the lay and professional audience a long-needed contemporary
natural medicine update of Dr. Brown's pioneering low-dose antibiotic
protocol for RA...**This therapy works!**"
— Dr. Joseph Mercola, D.O. (operates the most visited
natural health website worldwide, www.mercola.com)

"**Mycoplasmas are certainly a very, very important part of not
only rheumatoid diseases, but also many other degenerative
diseases. Dr. Poehlmann has covered this aspect with great
attention to accuracy and detail.** This foundation certainly welcomes
and recommends *Rheumatoid Arthritis: The Infection Connection.*"
— Perry A. Chapdelaine, Sr. (Executive Director
of the nonprofit Arthritis Trust of America,
www.arthritistrust.org)

"...**400 information-packed pages... solid, practical advice** on how to get the most out of Dr. Brown's treatment...Dr. Poehlmann was blessed with **input and support from some of the great stalwarts of antibiotic research [Dr. Harold Clark, Dr. Garth Nicolson, Dr. Joseph Mercola]**...She couldn't be in better company. And she couldn't have written a more useful book."

—Henry Scammell (Former President of The Road Back Foundation and author of *The New Arthritis Breakthrough* and *Scleroderma: The Proven Therapy That Can Save Your Life*)

"...**written in a language easy for everyone to understand**.... helpful, important, well done! **Your book should be in the hands of every RA/Fibromyalgia/CFS/Scleroderma/Lupus patient**..."

—Shirley Bentley (President of the US Chapter of the Common Cause Medical Research Foundation, which publishes the *Journal of Degenerative Diseases*)

"...**scientifically impeccable and well documented yet highly readable**....incredibly thorough and convincing...I tell [patients and listeners] to arm themselves with your book; **hopefully it will cause a major attitude shift among rheumatologists and family practitioners.**"

—Dr. Gabe Mirkin (Immunologist, Radio Talk Show Host and owner of www.drmirkin.com)

"...**an important and ground breaking book**...a giant step in the right direction...Chapter 7...**contains some of the best nutritional and lifestyle information that I have ever read anywhere.** By itself, it is worth the price of the book ....[this book] is a tsunami in a rising tide of information that is beginning to swamp the old ideas. **It is hoped that Poehlmann's call for the medical establishment to wake up will be heard** and that there will be a major shift in research toward identifying the microbial basis of chronic disease **so that we can work toward cures instead of just treating symptoms.**"

—Dennis Littrell (science teacher and one of Amazon.com's Top 50 reviewers), five stars

"...**logical, balanced, right on target**...Your views concerning a more balanced and holistic approach to maintaining and improving good health and preventing, controlling, and reducing disease make much sense...Overall, **the issues and inconsistencies in the literature that you identified are fundamental and need to be addressed and resolved.**"   —Dr. Joel Baseman (Univ. of Texas Health Science Center at San Antonio)

Arthritis and Autoimmune Disease: The Infection Connection

Finding and Treating the Many Causes of Inflammation and Chronic Fatigue

Third updated, revised,
and expanded edition of
*Rheumatoid Arthritis:
The Infection Connection*

Katherine M. Poehlmann, PhD
with Karl F. Poehlmann

 satori press

Arthritis and Autoimmune Disease: The Infection Connection

Finding and Treating the Many Causes of Inflammation and Chronic Fatigue

by Katherine M. Poehlmann, PhD
with Karl F. Poehlmann

Publisher: Satori Press, P.O. Box 7009, Torrance, CA 90504

First edition: 1997 as doctoral dissertation
2nd edition: March 2002 (completely revised, expanded)
2nd printing: July 2002
3rd printing: February 2003
4th printing (POD Amazon ed.): Sept. 2011 and March 2012
3rd edition: April 2012 (updated, revised, expanded)
2nd printing: November 2012 (with expanded index)

Printed in the United States of America

Library of Congress Cataloging-in-Publication Data

Arthritis and autoimmune disease: the infection connection
by Katherine M. Poehlmann, PhD with Karl Poehlmann—3rd ed.

Includes appendices and an index.

ISBN-10: 1469949237
ISBN-13: 978-1469949239

Arthritis—Causes and treatments. 2. Polymicrobial infections—
Identification and treatment. 3.Chronic illness—Nutritional aspects.
4. Immune system—Improvement. 5. Chronic Fatigue. 6. Lyme
Disease. 7. Autism 8. Alzheimer's. 9. Allergies. 10. Vitamins and
supplements

0 9 8 7 6 5 4 3 2

Question to Dr. Sabat: *"If you could change one thing*
in the world, what would it be?"
His answer: *"I would eradicate ignorance."*
—Dr. Steven Sabat, psychologist at Georgetown
University, author of *Dementia* (2006) and
The *Experience of Alzheimer's Disease* (2001)

"Truth is incontrovertible. Panic may resent it.
Ignorance may deride it. Malice may distort it,
But here it is."   ---Sir Winston Churchill

"For every complex problem, there is a solution
that is clear, simple, and wrong."
—H.L. Mencken, American writer (1880-1956)

"Bugs are always figuring out ways to get around the
antibiotics we throw at them. They adapt; they come
roaring back."   —Dr. George Jacoby,
Harvard Medical School, 1992

"Absence of evidence is not evidence of absence."
—Carl Sagan, astrophysicist, in chapter 12
("The Fine Art of Baloney Detection")
in *The Demon-Haunted World* (1995)

"We humans naively believe that we are at the top of the
food chain. Pathogenic microbes would laughingly
disagree as they tie on their little bibs."
—Katherine Poehlmann

"So, Nat'ralists observe, a Flea
Hath smaller Fleas that on him prey,
And these have smaller Fleas to bite 'em,
And so proceed ad infinitum."
—Jonathan Swift, Irish author and satirist, 1720

"Messieurs, c'est les microbes qui auront le dernier mot."
(Gentlemen, it is the microbes who will have the last word.)"
— Louis Pasteur

Warning—Disclaimer

About the Author

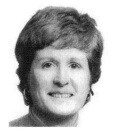

Dr. Katherine Poehlmann is a professional researcher and systems engineer with a magna cum laude degree in mathematics and an MBA. At TRW and later at the RAND Corporation she authored scientific reports on space technology, pattern recognition, defense policy analysis, and database design/management.

Her husband Karl is also a "rocket scientist" (Apollo program, Space Telescope, communications satellites). His research skills merged with Katherine's as they sought a cure for her Rheumatoid Arthritis triggered by physical trauma— badly torn ligaments in both ankles after a fall down stairs.

Disabled with RA in 1993, Katherine was unable to keep her senior research staff position at RAND. She and Karl spent months gathering information on RA from medical texts, articles, university medical libraries, and discussions with specialists. They also evaluated various alternative medicine approaches to RA. Katherine decided to make her health research pay off by pursuing a doctorate in the area of complementary medicine (Health Science).

She and Karl looked for the most benign solution possible, dubious about the usual treatment with powerful drugs and risky side effects. They were thrilled to discover Dr. Brown's impressive book *The Road Back* describing the connection between rheumatic disease and bacterial infection.

By following Dr. Brown's low-dose, long-term antibiotic protocol for eight months, Katherine progressed from being "25% disabled," as determined by four rheumatologists, to being completely ambulatory and pain-free in 1996.

Since her recovery from RA, the Poehlmanns have hiked in Chile, Central America, Tibet, U.S. National Parks, and over sections of the Great Wall of China. Katherine has lectured nationally and internationally, is a frequent guest for radio and television interviews, and gives free health talks to RA and chronic illness support groups in southern California.

Dedication

To Dr. Thomas McPherson Brown, (1906-1989), highly credentialed rheumatologist, microbiologist, and Dean of Medicine at George Washington University. Dr. Brown discovered the link between rheumatic illness and bacterial infection. His scientifically proven antibiotic protocol continues to give new hope to those suffering with Rheumatoid Arthritis. The protocol has brought thousands of patients to remission including this book's grateful author. Dr. Brown's groundbreaking contributions to medical science make him a true hero.

In Remembrance

Since the 2002 edition was published, the medical community has lost four important contributors. The authors mourn their passing.

Mr. Henry Scammell (1934-2006) co-authored *The Road Back* with Dr. Brown. Henry carried on Dr. Brown's legacy by publishing *The New Arthritis Breakthrough*, which contains the text of *The Road Back* in its entirety. He founded the nonprofit Road Back Foundation in 1993.

Dr. Harold Clark (1922-2007) was Dr. Thomas McPherson Brown's lab manager for 40 years. A mentor, friend, colleague, and fellow panelist at medical conferences, he wrote the foreword to the 2002 edition of this book.

Dr. Lida Mattman (1912-2008), whose perceptive research, lectures, and publications on cell wall-deficient forms earned her a nomination for the 1998 Nobel Prize in Medicine.

Dr. Tsuyoshi Okada (1931-2011), a dear friend and caring medical professional, reviewed the prior edition of this book and made very valuable suggestions to its content.

FOREWORD TO THE 2ND EDITION

by Dr. Harold W. Clark

This book offers both patients and health care providers an unabridged encyclopedia of information on the infectious cause and effective treatments of rheumatoid arthritis and other related chronic illnesses. Hundreds of books about arthritis have been written but few are more extensively referenced in support of both cause and treatment than this one.

The introduction of antibiotic therapy in rheumatoid and related chronic diseases by my colleague, the late Dr. Thomas McPherson Brown, was based on a mechanistic approach to an infectious cause rather than the typical symptomatic control of broad systemic illnesses. I believe that the treatment was successful because under our multi-disciplinary team approach the patient was educated and became part of the team. These patients encouraged us to document their success stories in *The Road Back* and *Why Arthritis?*.

Prior to our experiments, research was aimed at the typical viral and bacterial responses that do not fit the premise of an Infection Connection. The diverse therapeutic agents for RA, such as gold salts, hydroxyquinoline, bee venom, and the tetracycline antibiotics all inhibited Mycoplasma. These are uniquely different microbes being noncytopathic *in vitro* but are persisting viable allergens in the host.

Our target was narrowed to filterable and pleomorphic microbes that were difficult to isolate and identify. These served as the key allergens in a chronic and progressive hypersensitivity reaction. They elicit antibody responses with the formation of more pathogenic immune complexes that activate the proteolytic complement system.

The tetracyclines have several actions in the host as a result of their chelation and electron scavenging properties. These actions include: immunosuppressing, antioxidant; anti-inflammatory; blocking the immune complex formation; nucleophilic, inhibiting protein synthesis and the proteinases; and inhibiting the metalloenzymes such as collagenase. Pulse therapy (taking a tetracycline dose between meals on alternate days) can be beneficial with minimum toxicity; it limits the development of resistance while allowing cellular renewal.

The complex and ever-changing environment of infectious microbes, in turn resulting in a variety and location of symptoms, blurs the identification of these organisms as the cause of RA in their human hosts.

When these pathogenic microbes incorporate basic proteins from a variety of tissues (IgG cells, pancreas, myelin, kidney, etc.) the alteration (conformation) of attached basic cell proteins is recognized as non-self (i.e., a foreign allergen). As a result, mycoplasmas acquire the role of auto-antigens. With their insoluble lipoprotein membrane, mycoplasmas can also act as an adjuvant required in experimental autoimmune reactions. The several common strains of human mycoplasmas each have their characteristic properties that are dependent on the host tissue composition and the resulting systemic reactions.

It took me ten years after my retirement to publish *Why Arthritis?*, which perhaps in retrospect should have been titled *Why Do You Still Have Arthritis?*! I can't wait another 30 years for the medical and scientific community to remove their self-imposed cataracts to see what's on the horizon.

My hope is that this book will raise their curiosity to complete the untold story of the cause of rheumatoid disease.

H.W.C.

ACKNOWLEDGMENTS

The authors relied upon a variety of essential resources and references during the development of this book.

Human Resources

The author thanks family members, friends, and colleagues who encouraged and supported this research project and writing effort, directly or indirectly, especially Margaret Medvetz, John Medvetz, Robert Zwirn, David and Rena Aviv, Dennis Littrell, Mary Lyn Miller, Al and Carolyn Glenn, Charles Weber, Bernadette Shih, Laura and Tony Ponter, Pandora Mitchell, Dr. G. H. Kirk, Don and Virginia Fullerton, Dale Maduri, and Cheryl Ferguson.

Particular appreciation goes to Karl F. Poehlmann, whose perceptive comments, spirited discussion, analytical critique, website and IT support, provocative questions, thoughtful suggestions, unflagging support, patience, good humor, and husbandly encouragement during all phases of the production of this book were priceless. Several key write-ups, web pages, and tables appearing at www.RA-Infection-Connection.com are the result of countless hours of Karl's special topic research.

Text References

Dr. Thomas McPherson Brown's theories on myco-plasmal infection started me on my own "Road Back" to recovery, restoring my health, mobility and independence. His prescient scientific observations and rigorous testing methods make him one of the as-yet unheralded giants of medical research. The Arthritis Institute of the National Hospital in Arlington, VA, has been renamed the Thomas McPherson Brown Arthritis Institute in memory of its founder and former director.

Mr. Henry Scammell, prolific writer of popular health articles, was Dr. Brown's co-author for *The Road Back* in 1988. Henry wrote *The New Arthritis Breakthrough* in 1998 to document several double-blind studies, notably the Minocycline in Rheumatoid Arthritis (MIRA) study, which confirmed the efficacy of Dr. Brown's antibiotic protocol.

Harold W. Clark, PhD, gifted scientist, lecturer, author, and dear, personal friend was a colleague of Dr. Brown's at George Washington University since the 1950s. Dr. Clark published dozens of journal articles on his 45-year experience developing techniques for mycoplasma detection and treatment. This was during a period when the popular view of arthritis actively withheld support for the infectious mycoplasmal causes. Dr. Clark established the Mycoplasma Research Institute in Beverly Hills, Florida as a nonprofit foundation committed to the promotion of research and education aimed at understanding a wide variety of polymicrobial infectious diseases. His 1997 book *Why Arthritis?* presents an excellent overview of Dr. Brown's antibiotic regimen to combat RA. His book also deplores the politicization of arthritis research.

Dr. Lida Mattman's classic *Cell Wall Deficient Forms* was crucial to our understanding of the devious methods used by stealth pathogens and their roles in chronic illness.

Richard Longland, Founder and CEO of the nonprofit Arthroplasty Patient Foundation, along with his wife Terry, are living proof that naturopathic methods work. His perceptive comments and discussions regarding biofilms were especially informative. A talented videographer, he has produced a helpful film "Why Am I Still Sick?" that seeks to empower patients through awareness about the prevalence of chronic illnesses. Longland survived spinal disease through his own in-depth research on bacterial biofilm infections. His findings have attracted the attention of dental professionals worldwide.

Russell Farris's blog postings on www.polymicrobial.com has provided useful pointers to research breakthroughs in the U.S. and abroad. A former artificial intelligence analyst, engineer, technical writer, and researcher at the Autism Research Institute, his cogent comments and provocative speculations led us to follow intriguing paths across traditional medical boundaries. Our collegial association over the years has been fruitful in exchanging useful health information appearing in our respective publications. Mr. Farris's book (co-authored with Per Mårin), *The Potbelly Syndrome*, increased our understanding of the pivotal role of cortisol in Metabolic Syndrome. **Dr. Stan Monteith, M.D.**, has hosted a nationally syndicated radio show on Radio Liberty for many years. The information shared with the public has helped thousands of listeners. It has been an honor to be a guest on his show several times. He is the author of *AIDS: The Unnecessary Epidemic*.

Eshel Zweig—a caring, dedicated, undaunted father—battled Canada's unresponsive medical establishment for years to obtain effective treatment for his son Adrian, stricken at age 5 with Juvenile Rheumatoid Arthritis. Now in remission, Adrian as a teen excels in both academics and sports. We were honored to help the family find answers. Over the years, Eshel has sent us web pointers to new chronic illness study findings, leading us to pursue lines of exciting research. Many of those key insights appear in this book.

Electronic Media

The author recognizes the wealth of data and discussion obtained via the Internet to support our ongoing research. The excellent scientific data provided electronically by Dr. Garth Nicolson's Institute for Molecular Medicine and also through MEDLINE's Medscape by Dr. Joel B. Baseman, University of Texas Health Science Center at San Antonio, and Dr. Joseph G. Tully, retired head of the Mycoplasma Chapter of the National Institute of Allergy and Infectious Diseases demonstrate the Internet's power to educate and inform on a global scale.

The "Trends and Innovations" section of the *Investors Business Daily* offers concise leads to new medical discoveries. The online edition of this newspaper is at Investors.com.

Medical Research Resources

Dr. Joseph Mercola, D.O., operates the world's most-visited natural health Internet resource, www.mercola.com, linked to over 300,000 medical pages. The articles on his website and in his free electronic newsletter offer timely, practical, and valuable information addressing the spectrum of health issues.

He offers a conservative interpretation of controversial medical issues. His website includes an improved version of Dr. Brown's protocol, which he has used successfully to treat thousands of arthritis patients. Dr. Mercola has generously given his permission to reprint this protocol as part of Appendix II of this book. Readers who wish to try Dr. Brown's regimen are encouraged to show this particular text to their doctors, since it is the only part of this book that is intentionally prescriptive.

Dr. Garth Nicolson, PhD, is currently the President, Chief Scientific Officer, and Research Professor at the Institute for Molecular Medicine in southern California. The Institute provides diagnosis and treatment guidelines for chronic illness patients. These are reprinted in Appendix III. Much more information is available at www.immed.org. Professor Nicolson has held numerous peer-reviewed research grants. He was a founding member of the nonprofit International Lyme and Associated Diseases Society (ILADS). He serves on the Scientific Advisory Board of the Road Back Foundation.

Professor Nicolson was formally the David Bruton, Jr. Chair in Cancer Research, Professor and Chairman at the University of Texas M. D. Anderson Cancer Center in Houston, and Professor of Internal Medicine and Professor of Pathology and Laboratory Medicine at the University of Texas Medical School at Houston. Dr. Nicolson was also Adjunct Professor of Comparative Medicine at Texas A & M University.

Among the most cited scientists in the world, having published over 600 medical and scientific papers, edited 18 books, he serves on the editorial boards of 30 medical and scientific journals, including the *Journal of Chronic Fatigue Syndrome.* He is an editor emeritus of *Clinical & Experimental Metastasis* and an editor of the *Journal of Cellular Biochemistry* and the *Journal of Functional Foods in Health and Disease.*

Dr. Nicolson is a recipient of the Burroughs Wellcome Medal of the Royal Society of Medicine, the Stephen Paget Award of the Metastasis Research Society and the U. S. National Cancer Institute's Outstanding Investigator Award. He has been nominated for the Nobel Prize in cell microbiology.

"The Challenge of Emerging Infections in the 21st Century" was the theme of The Institute for Functional Medicine's April 2011 international symposium in Bellevue, WA. Dr. Nicolson's plenary session presentation was entitled "Mycoplasma and Other Chronic Infections of the 21st Century." Information and insights shared by a distinguished group of nationally and internationally renowned researchers, educators, and clinicians were invaluable to clarify, validate, and expand the contents of this book for the 3rd edition.

Dr. Tsuyoshi Okada, M.D., F.A.C.P, maintained a private practice in Southern California and served on the consulting staff of several hospitals until his untimely death in 2011. Dr. Okada authored numerous publications in the areas of Geriatric Medicine and Internal Medicine. Dr. Okada's observations on interactions between prescription drugs and herbal/vitamin supplements are much appreciated.

Dr. A. Robert Franco, M.D. heads the Arthritis Center of Riverside, CA. His success with thousands of patients over the last 25 years using a combination of nutrition and, where needed, Dr. Brown's antibiotic protocol, is noteworthy. Dr. Franco treats Scleroderma patients who have been told by other rheumatologists that their condition is hopeless. He has saved countless lives by restoring these patients' health where other doctors lack the necessary skills.

Dr. Trevor Marshall's own case of Sarcoidosis and his doctors' inability to treat him sent him on a path of research leading to the well-known and internationally recognized Marshall Protocol that uses multiple antibiotics. A PhD chemist and researcher, he asserts that microbe-produced vitamin D is pathogenic in Sarcoidosis. Dr. Marshal heads the nonprofit Autoimmunity Research Foundation, which explores the causes of chronic inflammatory diseases. The Foundation proposes therapies based on a molecular-level description of inflammatory disease biology. These treatments are often considered controversial by some medical doctors. We have studied Dr. Marshall's website (www.TrevorMarshall.com) and publications to increase our understanding of many chronic illnesses.

Arthritis and Autoimmune Disease:
The Infection Connection

Dr. Aristo Vojdani, PhD, heads the Immunosciences Laboratories in southern CA. As Cyrex Labs' chief scientific advisor, he has made considerable contributions to our understanding of Lyme disease, Gluten Syndrome, Celiac Disease, and Autism. Dr. Vojdani has written or co-authored over 120 scientific publications. See ImmunosciencesLab.com.

Dr. Jack Davis, D.D.S., maintains a dental practice in Greer, S.C. His professional advice on periodontal infections, chronic illness, and cancer provided important additions to this edition.

Dr. Gabe Mirkin, M.D., has been a practicing physician for more than 40 years and a radio talk show host for 25. Dr. Mirkin is a graduate of Harvard University and Baylor University College of Medicine. He is one of a very few doctors board-certified in four specialties: Sports Medicine, Allergy and Immunology, Pediatrics and Pediatric Immunology. He has written 16 books including *The Sports Medicine Book* and *The Healthy Heart Miracle*, offers a free emailed newsletter, and provides hundreds of Internet articles at www.DrMirkin.com. His wife Diana is a nutrition expert who writes about diet plans and ways to make healthy foods taste delicious.

The work of these dedicated professionals is quoted and referenced throughout this book.

Expert Reviewers

Special and sincere thanks go to Doctors Davis, Franco, Mercola, Mirkin, and Nicolson, and to Russell Farris for offering their valuable time and professional perspective to evaluate this edition.

CONTENTS

FIGURES AND TABLES

Figures

Tables

PHOTO GALLERY
(Mycoplasma photomicrographs taken by Dr. Harold Clark)

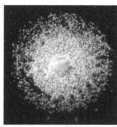

Mycoplasma hominis culture magnified 400X

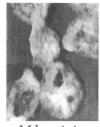

M.hominis structure details

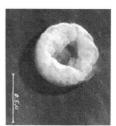

Mycoplasma ring form magnified 100,000X

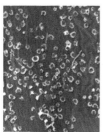

Mycoplasma culture

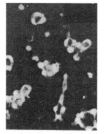

M. hominis hexoid budding forms magnified 100,000X

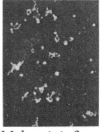

M. hominis from from RA patient various forms 20,000X

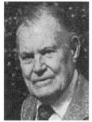

Dr. Thomas McPherson Brown, M.D.

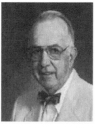

Dr. Harold W. Clark, PhD Microbiologist

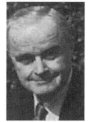

Henry Scammell Author, Founder of the Road Back Foundation

DEFINITIONS

Adaptogenic: pertaining to the natural selection of the offspring of a mutant organism better adapted to a new or changed environment, particularly applicable to drug resistant microbes.

Adjuvant: a substance that enhances the immune response stimulated by an antigen when injected with the antigen.

Absorption: the uptake of substances into or across tissues.

Adsorption: the action of a substance in attracting and holding other materials or particles on its surface.

Allergen: a substance capable of triggering an allergic state when introduced into the body. Major categories of allergens are cellular, viral, bacterial, food, chemical, and mycoplasmal. An incoming allergen produces a histamine reaction that prompts the body to generate hydrogen peroxide, which initiates the body's cell-destruction process, leading to inflammation at the site of the invasion.

Anaerobe: an organism that lives and grows in very low levels of molecular oxygen.

Anaphylaxis: a sudden, intense allergic reaction accompanied by shortness of breath, loss of consciousness, even death. Can be triggered by venom (e.g., bee, hornet, jellyfish) or foods (e.g., peanuts, shellfish).

Antibody: a soluble protein molecule with disease-fighting properties. Antibodies are produced and secreted by B-cells in response to antigenic stimulus. These molecules are capable of binding to a specific antigen, so they are shape-related to the sugar coat of the cells or microorganisms they are intended to attack.

Antigen: a substance consisting mainly of proteins (but which can also consist of carbohydrates, lipids, and sometimes nucleic acids) that is recognized as foreign and gives rise to an immune reaction, i.e., production of antibodies or immune cells. It can also be the toxin secreted by mycoplasmas.

Antigen Presenting Cells (APCs): dendritic cells that form an important bridge between the innate and adaptive immune systems.

Apoptosis: programmed cell death.

Ayurvedic: pertaining to Ayurveda, a holistic system of medicine indigenous to and widely practiced in India for more than 5,000 years. Ayurveda was first recorded in the *Vedas*, said to be the world's oldest extant Sanskrit literature.

Bacteria: any of numerous widely distributed unicellular, pleomorphic microorganisms that exhibit both animal and plant characteristics. Their three main varieties (*bacillus, coccus*, and *spirillum*) range from the harmless and beneficial to the intensely virulent and lethal.

Basophil: a granular blood leukocyte with an irregularly shaped nucleus. A basophil is also considered to be any structure, cell or histologic element staining readily with basic dyes. A high number could be an indicator of malignancy such as cancer or leukemia.

Blood/brain barrier (BBB): the biochemical partition that separates the brain and central nervous system from the blood stream so that only certain biochemicals can cross over. This complex physiologic filtering mechanism keeps many of the large molecules that circulate in the blood out of the central nervous system. The BBB blocks some drugs.

Bone Spur: an irregular calcium nodule growth produced by an infection or mineral deficiency.

Budding: the process by which microbes pull a portion of invaded cell membrane around their inner envelope and chromosomes, creating an outer protective coating and tethering the new "bud" to the parent cell.

Bursa: a pouch or sac-like cavity containing synovia and located at the points of tendon friction in the bodies of vertebrates.

Carcinogen: any cancer-causing agent or substance.

Cartilage: a fibrous elastic connective tissue forming most of the temporary skeleton of the embryo, providing a model for development of bones; also denotes a mass of such tissue, composed of collagen fibers and proteoglycans, at any particular site in the body.

Cell Wall-Deficient: see L-form.

Chelation: a medical treatment administered intravenously to bind toxic metals and minerals so they can be excreted from the body. EDTA chelation is the most common type of therapy offered, usually for vascular diseases.

Chemotactic: acting in response to chemical stimulation by initiating the inflammatory reaction, attracting leukocytes to the site of tissue damage.

Chemotherapeutic: pertains to the treatment of certain malignant diseases (e.g., cancer) by the disinfection of affected tissues through the use of chemically synthesized drugs having a specific action against certain pathogenic microorganisms.

Cholesterol: an alcohol compound ($C_{27}H_{45}O$) found in animal fats and oils, bile, blood, brain tissue, milk, egg yolk, myelin sheaths of nerve fibers, liver, kidneys, and adrenal glands.

Chondrocytes: cells that can produce cartilage by increasing the synthesis of proteoglycans.

Co-factor: an element or principle, e.g., a coenzyme, with which another element must unite in order to function. Also, a related causal element when both bacteria and viruses working together produce pathogenic symptoms. A cooperative element of a compound.

Collagen: a protein substance of the white fibers of skin, tendons, bones, cartilage, and nails.

Commensal: An organism participating in a symbiotic relationship in which one species derives some benefit while the other is believed to be unharmed.

Contractures: the chronic loss of joint motion due to structural changes in non-bony tissue.

Corticotropin-releasing hormone: A hormone produced by the hypothalamus that stimulates the anterior pituitary gland to release the adrenocorticotropic hormone.

Cytokines: chemical messengers that help regulate the immune response by mobilizing white blood cells as necessary.

Cytopathic: pertaining to pathologic (unhealthy or diseased) changes in cells.

Cytotoxic T-cells: a special category of T-cells (lymphocytes) that kill other cells infected by viruses, fungi, or certain bacteria, or cells transformed by cancer.

DNA: genetic material (deoxyribonucleic acid) that carries the directions a cell uses to perform a specific function, such as making a given protein using an RNA template made from the DNA.

Dystrophy: a degenerative disorder caused by inadequate or defective nutrition, toxins made by microbes, or drugs that block chemical pathways.

Edema: excessive fluid retention in intercellular spaces of the body.

ELISA (Enzyme Linked Immuno-Sorbant Assay): a highly accurate testing and diagnostic protocol used to identify specific antigens using IgG or IgE antibodies in a blood sample.

Endemic: a disease of tolerated morbidity present in a human or animal community at all times but clinically recognizable in only a few individuals. Lyme Disease and Dengue fever are two examples.

Endothelial cells: The cells lining the inner walls of the blood vessels.

Enzyme: an organic compound that acts as a catalyst (an element that is essential) to the change in chemical composition of a material. Certain types of enzymes are required for the proper digestion and metabolism of food in the body. Enzymes break down the agent(s) causing inflammation.

Eosinophil: a leukocyte whose cytoplasm contains coarse, round granules of uniform size. An abundance of these cells is usually associated with an allergic condition such as asthma or intestinal worms.

Epidemic: a disease of high morbidity only occasionally present in a human community, attacking many in a region at the same time and spreading rapidly. Hepatitis C is an example.

Epithelial cells: single or multiple layers of cells that line hollow organs and glands and that make up the outer surface of the body to protect or enclose organs. Most produce mucous or other secretions. Certain types of epithelial cells have tiny hairs called cilia that help remove foreign substances, e.g., from the respiratory tract.

Epitome: A localized region on the surface of an antigen that is capable of eliciting an immune response and of combining with a specific antibody to counter that response.

Etiology: a theory or description of the cause(s) of a disease.

Etiopathogenesis: the origin of the cause(s), development of cellular events, reactions and other pathologic mechanisms occurring during the progression of disease.

Exudates: materials that have escaped from blood vessels and been deposited in tissue or on tissue surfaces, usually the result of trauma or inflammation. The product is usually fluid, cells, or cellular debris.

Fastidious organism: a microorganism with unusual and/or complex nutritional and environmental requirements.

Glycoprotein: a molecule consisting of a carbohydrate plus a protein. Almost all of the key molecules involved in the immune response are glycoproteins.

Gram-negative: bacteria that lose the primary Gram stain (a violet colored chemical) and pick up a counterstain, usually carbolfuchsin or safranin.

Gram-positive: retaining the color of the gentian violet stain in Gram's method of staining.

Gram stain (Gram's method): a process developed by Danish physician Hans Gram (1853-1938) for staining bacteria; the stain used to identify broad classes of bacteria based on their cell coat or capsule's ability to pick up specific dyes.

Heme [short for hematin]: the deep red, iron-containing non-protein, component of hemoglobin and some other biological molecules.

Hematopoietic: pertaining to the formation of blood cells.

Heparin: An acidic glycosaminoglycan found especially in lung and liver tissue that prevents the clotting of blood.

Histamine: an active chemical, released from mast cells, that causes smooth muscle contraction of human bronchioles and small blood vessels, increased permeability of capillaries, and increased secretion by nasal and bronchial mucous glands.

Homeostasis: the ability or tendency of an organism or cell to maintain internal equilibrium by adjusting its physiological processes

Hydrogen Peroxide (H_2O_2): a natural chemical compound that can be generated by the histamine reaction, or by certain microorganisms when they are attacked, or by leukocytes in the process of developing killer T-cells.

In vitro: observable in a test tube or other artificial lab setting.

In vivo: within the living body.

Iatrogenic: Caused or precipitated by medical intervention.

Immunoglobulins (Ig): These antibodies are Y-shaped protein molecules produced by the B-cells. There are five important classes of immunoglobulins: IgA, IgD, IgE, IgG, and IgM.

Immunosuppressive: capable of reducing normal immune responses, e.g., drugs given to prevent transplant rejection.

Interferon: a molecule produced by cells (most often white blood cells) that can inhibit cell division and viral replication, and that has a variety of effects on the immune system.

Interstice: a small interval, space, or gap in a tissue or structure.

Jarisch-Herxheimer reaction: a short-term hypersensitivity response that is often mistakenly interpreted as antibiotic sensitivity.

Killer T-cells: see Cytotoxic.

Krebs cycle: The sequence of reactions by which most living cells generate energy during the process of aerobic respiration.

L-Form: also called the L-phase variant or CWD form; a bacterium that has partially or entirely lost its cell walls. The "L" is for the Lister Institute in France where it was first discovered. Mycobacteria and other bacteria transform to the L-form when attacked by penicillin and related antibiotics. L-forms and mycoplasmas are of similar size and usually reproduce more slowly than bacteria. L-forms can regrow their cell walls, and therefore have a means to escape attack by antibiotics and emerge later.

Leukocyte: a white or colorless blood corpuscle, constituting an important agent in protection against infectious diseases.

Lipid: any of a group of organic substances, including fatty acids, neutral fats, waxes, steroids, and phosphatides, which are insoluble in water but soluble in alcohol, chloroform, ether, and other fat solvents; lipids are a source of body fuel and an important constituent of cells.

Lipoprotein: a combination of a lipid and a protein, having the general solubility property of proteins.

Lymphocyte: white blood cells that are the smallest of the leukocytes, producing cytokines in the bone marrow and thymus, and that are essential for immune defense.

Lysis: destruction or decomposition, as of a cell or other substance, under influence of a specific agent. In context, can also mean gradual abatement of the symptoms of a disease.

Macrolide: A class of antibiotics that are produced by a species of Streptomyces, are characterized by a large lactone ring linked to one or more sugars, and act by inhibiting protein synthesis.

Macrophages: enlarged, amoeba-like cells that entrap microorganisms and particles of foreign matter by phagocytosis. They usually arrive after the neutrophils to clean up the debris of dead cells and bacteria.

Mast cells: specialized immune cells found in the skin and nasal passages and in the gastrointestinal (GI) and respiratory tracts.

Mesenteric: Any of several folds of the membrane (peritoneum) lining the abdominal and pelvic walls connecting to the intestines.

Metabolism: the sum of all the chemical and physical processes by which elements of a living organism are produced and maintained; also the transformation by which energy is made available to the organism.

Metalloenzyme: any enzyme that contains tightly bound metal atoms, e.g., the cytochromes, a class of hemoproteins that are widely distributed in plant and animal tissues and whose main function is electron transport.

Microbiome: the totality of microbes, their genetic elements (genomes), and environmental interactions within a particular environment.

Microbiota: microbial flora, the great majority of which are bacteria and fungi, harbored by normal, healthy individuals.

Microglia*: small non-neural cells forming part of the supporting structure of the central nervous system. They are migratory and act as phagocytes at sites of neural damage or inflammation.

Microorganism: a general term for protozoa, fungi, bacteria, and viruses.

Mollicutes: from the Latin for "soft" and *"skin,"* the class of cell wall-less prokaryotes to which mycoplasmas belong.

Motility: the ability to move spontaneously.

Mutagen: an agent that induces genetic mutation.

Mutate: to change a gene or unit of hereditary material that results in a new inheritable characteristic.

Mycobacteria: a slender, typically aerobic bacterium difficult to stain. Examples are tuberculosis and leprosy.

Mycoplasma: from the Latin base words for "fungus" and "fluid"; of intermediate size between bacteria and viruses; are characterized by the absence of a cell wall and pleomorphism; the smallest and simplest self-replicating organisms phylogenetically related to gram-positive bacteria, especially to mycobacteria, which have affinity for synovial tissue and cholesterol.

Myelin: the lipid substance surrounding the axis of a group of nerve fibers.

Neurogenic: originating in the nervous system, to form nervous tissue or to stimulate nervous energy.

Neuropeptide: a peptide synthesized within the body that influences neural activity or functioning.

Neutrophils: cells that migrate to the site of an injury and stick to the interior walls of the blood vessels. They then form projections that enable them to push their way into the infected tissues where they engulf and devour (phagocytize) microorganisms and other foreign particles.

Nosocomial: a secondary disorder (e.g., infection) related to a hospital that is unrelated to the patient's primary condition.

Nucleophilic: having an affinity for the nucleus of a cell.

Palliative: affording relief; also a drug that acts to do so.

Pandemic: occurring over a wide geographic area and affecting an exceptionally high proportion of the population; e.g., malaria.

Parasite: a plant or animal that lives on or within another organism, from which it derives sustenance or protection without making compensation; applies to all infectious microbes, from viruses to ringworms. Parasites can be symbiotic, i.e., adapting and providing beneficial effects on the host. Some parasites can kill the host but others evolve into forms that do not.

Pareto Chart: a method used by economists to show allocation of resources in an economic system; a histogram to illustrate comparative values in a bar chart format.

Parvovirus: a group of extremely small, morphologically similar DNA viruses resistant to fungicides and sporicides.

Peptide: any of various amides derived from two or more amino acids by combination of the amino group of one acid with the carboxyl group of another; usually obtained by partial hydrolysis of proteins.

Peyer's patches: a collection of lymphoid tissues in the intestinal tract.

Phagocyte: any cell that engulfs and ingests microorganisms or other cells and foreign particles.

Pharmacodynamic: refers to the biochemical and physiological effects of drugs on living systems (i.e., the body or microorganisms within or on the body).

Pharmacokinetic: pertains to the measurement of drug activity to determine peak concentrations that are effective under certain conditions.

Physiology: the sum of all basic processes underlying the functioning of a species or class of organism.

Phytochemicals: plant-derived chemical extracts. There are tens of thousands of these, with varying bioactivity. Some have protective and antibiotic effects, e.g., allicin obtained from garlic.

Planktonic: free-floating microorganisms whose movements are controlled by water movement (not attached to surfaces).

Plasmids: extrachromosomal circular DNA molecules capable of independent replication and carrying genetic information for a variety of different functions, such as drug resistance.

Pleomorphism: exhibiting a variety of shapes.

Polymerase Chain Reaction (PCR): an extremely sensitive means of amplifying small quantities of DNA to detect low-level bacterial infections or rapid changes in transcription at the single cell level. It can also be used in DNA sequencing, screening for genetic disorders, site-specific mutation of DNA, cloning (or sub-cloning), and forensic science applications.

Prokaryote: an organism without a true nucleus, the nuclear material being scattered in the cytoplasm of the cell, and which reproduces by cell division. A bacterium is an example.

Prophylaxis: a measure taken to maintain health and prevent the spread of disease.

Prostacyclin: A prostaglandin produced in the walls of blood vessels that acts as a vasodilator and inhibits platelet aggregation.

Prostaglandins: naturally occurring fatty acids found in various tissues that work to stimulate the contraction ability of smooth muscle, to lower blood pressure, and to affect the action of certain hormones.

Proteinase: any enzyme that catalyzes the splitting of interior peptide bonds in a protein.

Proteoglycans: the component of cartilage that gives it elasticity.

Reactive nitrogen species (RNS): a family of antimicrobial molecules derived from nitric oxide (NO) and superoxide (O_2) produced via enzymatic activity. RNS and reactive oxygen species (ROS) act together to damage cells.

Reactive oxygen species (ROS): chemically reactive molecules containing oxygen. Examples include oxygen ions and peroxides. They can be either inorganic or organic.

Retrovirus: an RNA virus that gains entry into cells, making mirror-image copies of their RNA to produce a DNA version of their genes, then exploiting vulnerable locations along the host's DNA to insert themselves, like a transposon, into the cell's genetic material.

R-factors: genetically coded Resistance Factors possessed by an organism to withstand chemical assaults by one or more chemotherapeutic agents. An example is a transferable plasmid found in many bacteria in the small intestine.

Rheumatoid factor (often called R-factor): a protein in the blood, found by tests that measure the ratio of antibody to gamma globulin. The test reveals IgM antibodies produced by some RA patients against their own IgG.

Salmonella: a gram-negative bacterium causing mild to severe gastroenteritis, occasionally leading to death,

Sclerosis: a thickening or hardening of a body part, e.g., an artery, especially from excessive formation of fibrous interstitial tissue.

Streptococcus: the genus of gram-positive bacteria, usually occurring in chains, that includes species pathogenic to humans, especially children. A typical chain would include one or more of the following: *S. pneumonia, S. synovium, S. aureus, S. hemophilia,* scarlet fever, and/or rheumatic heart disease. This initial bacterial infection could lead to production of mycoplasmal microorganisms and L-forms and in turn to rheumatic diseases.

Streptomyces: a genus of bacteria, usually soil forms, but occasionally parasitic on plants and animals.

Subacute: a condition between acute and chronic.

Synovia: pertaining to the transparent, albuminous fluid secreted by the inner layer of the synovial membrane and found in the joint cavities, bursae, and tendon sheaths where lubrication is necessary. This fluid provides nourishment to the cartilage covering the bone and contains white blood cells that battle infection.

Synovial joint: a freely moveable joint where cartilage covers the ends of the bones and the entire joint is encapsulated in a double layer of connective tissue with the joint cavity and its synovial fluid lying in-between the two layers. The outer layer of the capsule is made up of dense connective tissue holding the bones of the joint together. Some of these tissues are bundled together as ligaments. Tendons join muscles to bone. The inner layer of the capsule is made up of loose connective tissue including elastic fibers and fat.

Tetracyclines: a family of broad-spectrum antibiotics that inhibit bacterial protein synthesis; tetracycline ($C_{22}H_{24}N_2O_8$) is derived from certain species of the bacteria genus *Streptomyces*; the base and hydrochloride salt are used as an antiamoebic, antibacterial, and antirickettsial.

Tolerance Induction: A process that directly activates any of the steps required for tolerance, a physiologic state in which the immune system does not react destructively against the components of an organism that harbors it or against antigens that are introduced to it.

Transposons: genes that move from one position to another on chromosomes; at the bacterial level, movable bits of DNA that generate helpful/harmful chemicals, enzymes, or other substances that confer the ability to resist chemotherapeutic agents.

Urease: an enzyme that hydrolyzes urea, a common metabolic waste product of vertebrates that contains nitrogen and is excreted in the urine.

Vector: a carrier, usually a biting insect (tick, flea, fly, spider, chigger, mosquito) that transfers an infectious agent from one host to another.

Virulence: the capacity to injure an organism and/or produce disease by invasion of tissue and generation of internal toxins. Invasiveness and toxigenicity are measured with reference to a particular host.

Virus: any of a class of filterable, submicroscopic pathogenic agents, chiefly protein and nucleic acid in composition but often reducible to crystalline form, and typically inert except when in contact with certain living cells.

PREFACE TO THE REVISED 3RD EDITION

The 2nd edition was focused on mycoplasma infection as the primary cause of RA, and tetracycline as the drug specific to this pathogen. Our research has since made it clear that a polymicrobial zoo of harmful microbes is constantly assaulting the human immune system. Doctors try to put different labels on each type of attack, depending on the location in the body colonized by the pathogens, and/or by the symptoms manifested by the afflicted person. When the microbes act in a mutually beneficial manner, these multiple infections are very difficult to diagnose and treat. The result is a set of symptoms that lead to the label "autoimmune disease."

A common denominator to all autoimmune diseases involves two main symptoms: inflammation and chronic fatigue. The list of recognized autoimmune diseases (shown in Table 1) has grown from 59 in 2002 to 105 in 2011, with new ones (like Autism and COPD) added after consensus is reached among researchers and clinicians. Some unfortunate individuals suffer from several of these conditions.

Mycoplasmal infections have been found to be co-factors for nearly all diseases on the list. For this reason, this book presents examples of hard-to-diagnose and hard-to-treat conditions that have an infectious component that may be a combination of bacterial, viral, fungal, and other categories of opportunistic, parasitic microbes.

While Dr. Brown's groundbreaking treatment used the tetracyclines to reduce the colony of mycoplasmas, he did not fully address the important role of the patient to take charge of his/her own health. We view immune system strengthening as an essential part of recovery. This book offers many suggested approaches to achieving a robust immune system through lifestyle adjustments including diet, nutrition, exercise, stress management, and specific vitamins/supplements.

This third edition contains many of the insights and research findings presented at the 2011 International Symposium sponsored by the Institute for Functional Medicine in Bellevue, WA, entitled "The Challenge of Emerging Infections in the 21ˢᵗ Century." What we learned there added to our ongoing chronic infectious disease research over the past fifteen years. Dozens of articles and hot links can be found on our website: www.RA-Infection-Connection.com. The integrative, functional medicine approach and methods suggested in this book are intended to help *all* individuals with chronic illnesses—not just RA sufferers—who seek to improve their health and strengthen their immune systems. There is no pretense to suggest a one-size-fits-all approach or magic bullet to achieve remission from chronic illness. However, certain well-documented, scientifically proven methods—conventional as well as alternative—have been found to improve the health of thousands of individuals. Those are presented here.

Treating symptoms has not just become acceptable and commonplace; it has become big business worth billions of dollars. In this book, fellow researcher Karl Poehlmann and I suggest many benign methods to achieve pain relief and a return to health without harmful or expensive drugs, and at little or no cost.

Our hope is that the evidence presented regarding the insidious actions of pathogenic microorganisms as a growing public health hazard will inspire concerned scientists to investigate further. To that end, we are donating profits from the sale of this book to foster research directed toward the etiology, testing, and treatment of polymicrobial infections that cause chronic illness.

As a result of the recognition the prior edition has received, my ongoing intensive research, and public health outreach activities, I now serve on the Board of Directors for two nonprofit organizations: the Road Back Foundation (www.RoadBack.org) and the Arthroplasty Patient Foundation (www.ArthroPatient.org).

K.M.P

INTRODUCTION TO THE REVISED 3RD EDITION

The extraordinary complexity of the human immune system has not been well understood until very recently. Noteworthy, credible research only began in the early 1980s. Prior to the 1990s, there was no discipline of microbial ecology dedicated to studies of the behavior of microbes in the human body. At that time, investigation into the causes of disease, particularly AIDS, in immunosuppressed people became highly politicized on moral rather than medical grounds and as a result was seriously under-funded. Today AIDS is finally recognized as a growing threat with global implications. A special department of the National Institutes of Health has been established to study allergy and infectious diseases (NIAID).

During the last dozen years there has been a revolution in microbiology and immunology, launched in part by the international Human Genome Project and the ongoing Human Microbiome Project. Scientists are able to unravel not only the mysteries of human genetics but also the DNA structures and characteristics of microbes that coexist with us. Puzzling fatiguing conditions that were often dismissed as "all in your head" or impossible to test for and diagnose are now traceable to specific infectious microorganisms. Although for decades researchers have proposed poly-microbial causes for so-called "autoimmune diseases," new tools and testing methods are now able to prove these hypotheses definitively.

Dr. Homer F. Swift theorized in 1928 that rheumatic fever was caused by hypersensitivity to a bacterium after isolating streptococcal bacteria from a patient with tonsillitis. At that time, tonsillitis was a known precursor to rheumatic fever. This beta-hemolytic Streptococcus is a common cause of "strep throat" but not all cases lead to rheumatic fever. Dr. Thomas McPherson Brown, as a young resident physician in

1937, studied with Swift to find the allergic response link to the pleomorphic remnants (L-forms) of this bacterium that remain as latent parasitic infections. In the 1940s, Dr. Brown first proposed his theory that bacterial infection was the primary cause of Rheumatoid Arthritis (RA). He described the effectiveness of tetracycline in RA at the 7th International Rheumatology Congress (1949) and in the *Journal of Laboratory and Clinical Medicine.* Over the next two decades at the Rockefeller Institute, Johns Hopkins Hospital, and the George Washington University School of Medicine in Washington, D.C., Dr. Brown conducted detailed, fully documented scientific tests to prove his theory. Use of the tetracycline family of antibiotics for connective tissue diseases was also endorsed by Dr. Albert Sabin, the developer of the polio vaccine.

What has become of Dr. Brown's work? For over sixty years his successful treatment has been largely ignored by the medical community because physicians have not assiduously sought to test for the mysterious microorganisms Dr. Brown identified. There are a few noteworthy exceptions.

In the 1980s, a group of doctors and scientists exploring a variety of infectious causes and alternative treatments for rheumatic diseases established the nonprofit Arthritis Trust of America. The foundation offers free practical information, references to scientific papers, and practitioner referrals on their website, www.arthritistrust.org.

In 1993, the Road Back Foundation, a nonprofit corporation run by dedicated volunteers among the thousands of patients who found relief from RA using Dr. Brown's protocol, began a campaign to make the public aware of his effective long-term, low-dose antibiotic treatment. Under the direction of Henry Scammell, co-author of *The Road Back* with Dr. Brown, they established the www.roadback.org website. The late Mr. Scammell served as the Road Back Foundation's president from 1993-2006. At this writing, the president is Ms. Cheryl Ferguson.

In the late 1990s the website www.rheumatic.org was created to provide detailed information on a wide range of rheumatic diseases, case studies, and a suggested regimen based on Dr. Brown's findings, with links to other credible and helpful Internet resources.

Dr. Joseph Mercola has successfully treated over 3,000 RA patients since the mid-1990's using his updated version of Dr. Brown's protocol emphasizing a diet and nutrition modification program described at www.mercola.com.

The Whitaker Wellness Institute, America's largest alternative medicine clinic directed by Dr. Julian Whitaker, located in Newport Beach, CA addresses the patient's overall health as well as underlying disease mechanisms. See www.WhitakerWellness.com. Holistic treatments include Dr. Brown's antibiotic protocol in parallel with immune system enhancements, dietary adjustments, and non-invasive, nontoxic pain-relieving therapies.

Dr. A. Robert Franco heads the Arthritis Center of Riverside, CA. (www.TheArthritisCenter.com). He employs a variety of patient-tailored complementary medicine techniques including supplements and antibiotics as needed. He reports that Dr. Brown's regimen for RA has a 30-40% probability of complete remission and a 70-80% probability of significant reduction of symptoms.

Professor Garth Nicolson's Institute for Molecular Medicine (www.immed.org) continues to sponsor innovative mycoplasma research and to develop unique testing methods for a wide variety of pathogens. Some of these micro-organisms, such as the virus HHV-6, are found to be common to seemingly unrelated conditions such as Chronic Fatigue Syndrome and several types of cancer.

It is appropriate to start with fundamentals before discussing chronic infections in detail. Chapter 1 describes the various types of arthritis and currently accepted treatments, both traditional and alternative, with special attention given to Hyperbaric Oxygen Therapies, because many pathogenic microbes are anaerobic (oxygen-sensitive).

Chapter 2 gives a brief overview of the functions and components of the immune system. Chapter 3 presents the basics of how infection works, with particular attention to the various methods to suppress mycoplasmas, cell wall-deficient forms of various pathogens, and the Jarisch-Herxheimer effect. Inflammation is the common denominator to all chronic infectious diseases. One important source of inflammation is intestinal imbalance. This chapter presents new research in the impact of organisms like *Clostridium difficile* on the microbiota in the gut.

Chronic infections that are linked to cell wall-deficient pathogens other than mycoplasmas present their own set of problems for diagnosis, testing, and treatment. Chapter 4 is devoted to the serious and growing public health concern regarding antibiotic-resistant, opportunistic pathogens. Emerging epidemics and blood-borne infections are discussed in detail in Chapter 5, with several examples including Lyme Disease, Tuberculosis, HIV, and Hepatitis. The frightening statistics regarding Autism lead us to devote a detailed discussion to this diagnostic challenge.

Major advances in microbiology are possible through improved tools to culture, test, investigate, and diagnose infectious diseases before they emerge as global threats. Chapter 6 discusses a variety of diagnostic tests for poly-microbial infections and allergies, including specific tests for Juvenile RA. Knowing which tests to request and what indicators to look for helps the patient work with the doctor to obtain a definitive diagnosis. Allergic reactions can mimic RA symptoms of pain, fatigue, and joint inflammation leading to misdiagnosis. We encourage testing for mycoplasmal infection, since it figures so prominently in dozens of chronic illnesses.

Because the immune system must be robust enough to fend off attacks by aggressive pathogens, Chapter 7 is devoted to natural methods to revitalize the immune system through diet adjustments and various exercise regimens. Exciting trends and future directions in infection research are described in Chapter 8, followed by final thoughts on research methodology in Chapter 9, and conclusions in Chapter 10.

The number of grassroots advocates for more research funding for chronic infectious illnesses such as RA, Lyme Disease (LD), Fibromyalgia, Alzheimer's, Gulf War Illness, and many other debilitating conditions is growing. The list of recognized autoimmune diseases has nearly doubled over the last decade, with more additions every year as researchers find and present evidence. It is unacceptable for our government and the scientific and medical community to downplay or ignore a complex, fatiguing illness like LD, which may become the most serious global scourge since AIDS.

Determined scientists, clinicians, and innovators who embark on privately funded research, unwilling to wait for government action, are producing important breakthroughs and often startling test results. One noteworthy example is the Institute for Functional Medicine. Their website is www.FunctionalMedicine.org. They offer medical courses for credit and host several conferences annually, bringing together highly motivated and superbly qualified individuals from all facets of the health and wellness community worldwide.

This book covers a broad range of topics, representing over 15 years of infectious disease investigation that began with the authors' search for a cure for RA. As career systems engineers, skilled in rigorous analysis, the challenge was to build on work done by scientists and medical professionals.

The authors have no access to a laboratory and have no formal medical school credentials. What is presented in this book are connections and conclusions drawn from a vast collection of publications available through MedLine, PubMed, the CDC, National Institutes of Health, libraries of universities associated with teaching hospitals, books and articles on alternative medicine, web searches via Scholar.Google.com, medical textbooks, and personal interactions with topic experts.

With thousands of medical research articles published each year, a sizable body of important work by diligent scientists may be overlooked. The authors' efforts at synthesizing across the usual defined categories of medical study, ignoring traditional boundary lines and mindsets, may bring those findings to light and thus reveal and inspire new directions for future research.

The 2nd edition of this book was lauded as "cutting edge" by medical reviewers, infectious disease specialists, and clinicians. This 3rd edition text is also well supported by credible documentation and citations. However, not every reader is interested in these 1,000+ references.

Rather than devote many pages to footnotes at the end of each chapter, these citations are easily accessible on our website, www.RA-Infection-Connection.com. This approach allows the inclusion of Internet "hot links" to useful health articles, support groups, practitioners, medical resources, and the authors' continuing exploratory research into the etiology, prevention, and treatment of polymicrobial infections, autoimmune diseases, and chronic inflammatory illness.

1. ARTHRITIS AND ITS TREATMENTS

The word arthritis originates from the Greek *arth*, meaning "joint" and *itis*, meaning "inflammation." Arthritis has been found in the bones of mammals since prehistoric times. Egyptian mummies show evidence of treatment for the disease. Hippocrates offered the first description of arthritis in the fourth century B.C. using the term *rheums*, meaning, "migrating between joints."[1] Although there are claimed to be over one hundred various kinds of arthritis, this may just reflect the complexity and severity of combinations of categories of symptoms. Yet, it was only comparatively recently, within the last century, that other factors besides the joints were considered to play a role in arthritis.

Two main categories of the disease afflict millions of Americans: Rheumatoid Arthritis and Osteoarthritis. Medical texts identify several subforms of arthritis but they are all characterized by inflammation. The difference seems to be the location in the body and severity of the symptoms. For example, Ankylosing Spondylitis (AS) occurs when inflammation afflicts areas where ligament attaches to bone in the spine.[2] Psoriatic arthritis affects both the skin and the joints. Scleroderma is both a rheumatic disease and a connective tissue disease affecting the skin, blood vessels, muscles, and internal organs.[3]

Two important subforms stemming from inflammation can cause cell destruction and can lead to more serious conditions: reactive arthritis and septic arthritis. Both are caused by a bacterial, viral, or fungal infection (usually in combination). Reactive arthritis may involve physical trauma and/or allergy as a trigger. There are many polymicrobial causes of reactive arthritis, which may be severe or subclinical, and may include their pleomorphic L-forms. This is a partial list: [4]

- *Campylobacter jejuni*
- Hepatitis A, B, and C
- Human Herpes Virus (HHV-6)
- Human Immunodeficiency Virus (HIV Infection)
- Lyme Disease (all infectious forms)
- Mycoplasma (*M. fermentans, M. pneumoniae,* and many other strains)
- Paramyxovirus (mumps)
- Parvovirus B19 (*Erythema infectiosum*)
- Rubella (German measles)
- Streptococcus (*S. pneumonia, S. pyogenes*)
- Urinary tract infections such as Chlamydia, Ureaplasma, and Mycoplasma
- Varicella Zoster Virus (Chicken Pox)
- Xenotropic murine leukemia virus-related virus (XMRV)

Like reactive arthritis, septic arthritis is caused by polymicrobial infections (bacterial, viral, or fungal). There is some overlap with the types of reactive arthritis listed above:[5]

- Coxsackie virus (all forms)
- *Escherichia coli*
- Fungi (*C. albicans,* Histoplasma, Blastomyces, etc.)
- Hepatitis A, B, and C
- Human Herpes Viruses (all forms)
- Human T-cell Lymphotropic Virus (HTLV)
- Lyme Disease (spirochete form)
- *Mycobacterium tuberculosis*
- Parvovirus B19 (*Erythema infectiosum*)
- Salmonella (all forms)
- *Staphylococcus aureus*

The chronic fatigue experienced by arthritics is the sign of a body weakened by a persistent battle with the infectious cause(s) of the disease. Mitochondrial energy loss is linked to intracellular infections.

In Rheumatoid Arthritis (RA), infection leads to a buildup of calcium nodules that wall off and surround the infecting organism. The same process occurs with cancer cells. This may be the result of the body's attempt to keep the organism from spreading. If these nodules are present in the feet, they may be mistaken for the needle-shaped uric acid crystals that characterize gout, another subform of arthritis. These RA nodules are painless, hard, round or oval masses that appear under the skin, usually on pressure points such as the elbow or Achilles tendon, and often in the small joints of the hands. Nodules are present in about 20% of RA cases.[6] Occasionally they are found in the eye where they can cause inflammation (conjunctivitis).

In this book, the word "arthritis" is intended to refer to Rheumatoid Arthritis, although inflammation associated with other arthritis categories may also be the result of some type of infection plus a rheumatoid component.

TWO MAIN TYPES OF ARTHRITIS

Although physicians like to categorize arthritis, at least one of the following symptoms are experienced by all arthritis sufferers:

- swelling, redness, warmth, pain/tenderness or irritation in one or more joints;
- stiffness around the joints, usually upon awakening and lasting about an hour; or
- difficulty or pain in normal movement of the joint(s).

At this writing, the Centers for Disease Control (CDC) in Atlanta, GA, estimates that some form of arthritis afflicts an estimated 50 million American adults. They project that by 2030, sixty-seven million persons in the United States may be afflicted with arthritis, and the activities of 21 million persons may be physically limited by arthritis symptoms.[7]

Rheumatoid Arthritis (RA)

Many rheumatoid diseases are assumed to be the result of normal aging or wear and tear, so there has been little motivation to find a cause or cure. However, RA is a chronic disease afflicting both the young and the old, male and female, and all races. Rheumatoid disease is a systemic inflammation with joint involvement, so it is understandable why investigations into the causes and cures have baffled medical specialists. With hundreds of symptomatic variations and various stages, zeroing in on probable cause(s) is a daunting prospect. Compounding the problem are each individual's unique biochemical makeup, varying lifestyle habits, particular environmental influences, and possible co-infections (active and latent).

Every cell in the body uses substances supplied by the blood, lymph system, and surrounding cells. These substances are either acquired topically or ingested. The old saying we "are what we eat" is not completely true; we are what we *assimilate*. The health of every tissue and organ depends on thousands of delicately balanced chemical reactions that occur continuously within our bodies. Rheumatic diseases exhibit inflammatory destruction of collagen proteins that hold cells together as connective synovial tissue, blood vessels, tendons, and skin.

Rheumatoid Arthritis is actually a family of similar chronic diseases characterized by persistent or cyclic bouts of inflammation of the joint membrane. In general, localized, short-term inflammation is a good thing, because it shows that the body is actively dealing with an invader, as the white blood cells (leukocytes) fight the infection. In RA, however, inflammation is not short-term nor does it have any known beneficial effect. The inflammation occurs in the layers of tissue (the synovia) lining the joint, causing pain, swelling, and stiffness when the joint is moved.

Inflammation around a joint space that looks and feels normal can be detected using a highly sensitive radioisotopic scan or magnetic resonance imaging (MRI). The characteristic early morning joint and muscle stiffness reported by individuals with rheumatic disease does not necessarily indicate a lack of lubricating oils (synovial fluid) in the joints. In fact, there may be an excessive amount of fluid in the joints that inhibits flexibility, building up pressure on the joint and causing pain. The temporary stiffness indicates inadequate blood supply circulating through the tendons and muscle tissue surrounding the joints.[8]

As we age, fluids circulate more slowly. Natural blood thinners[9] (cod liver oil, vitamin E) and enzyme therapy (serrapeptase,[10] Co-enzyme Q_{10}[11]) could help. A physician and/or nutritionist should be consulted on this matter.

Morning joint stiffness also correlates with overnight body temperature drop caused by lower blood pressure and decreased circulation. Joint fluid becomes more viscous and stiff until increased activity through exercise or applied warmth (water, heating pad, massage, topical creams containing stimulants) raises body temperature.

In addition, the supply of nutrients and metabolites normally carried by the blood to the joints may be diverted and depleted as the body attends to the gastrointestinal problems sometimes associated with RA. Adequate daily water intake and healthy fats in the diet (e.g., olive oil, coconut oil) can offset these gut problems.[12] Fats and oils are discussed in Chapter 7.

When a joint becomes inflamed or degenerates, the muscles surrounding it tighten in a protective spasm. This reflex is designed to prevent further injury but often leads to restricted movement and pain due to friction within the joint.

Whether the bulk is fluid or inflamed tissue or muscle spasm, the effect is the same: painful pressure on the swollen joint. Tendons, connecting the muscles that supply force to operate joints, may also be affected as the sheath containing the tendons becomes inflamed. This sheath is the same type of tissue as the synovium. Scar tissue may form between the tendon and its sheath, causing tendon operation to become stiff. Damage to the tendon itself may result, with the loss of the use of the hands or limbs. Deformities characteristic of RA may be seen in the sideways displacement of fingers or toes. Calcium nodules may also cause these bumps around joints. A notional drawing of a joint capsule and surrounding tissue is shown in Figure 1.

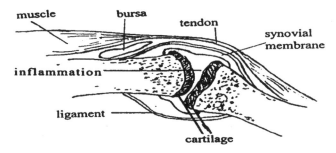

Figure 1. Joint Capsule

Although any joint can be affected, RA is first noticed in the small peripheral joints, such as those in the fingers or wrist. Figure 2 shows the web-like pattern of synovial membranes in the hand. These tissues are thin layers between bone surfaces that would otherwise rub together.

The synovial membrane of the knee joint is the largest and most extensive in the body. Joints are often affected symmetrically, so arthritis sufferers will usually have pain in both knees, elbows, shoulders, and/or hands. Other symptoms of RA include the presence in the blood of a protein called the rheumatoid factor or R-factor, found by tests that measure the ratio of antibody to gamma globulin. After several months, pits or erosions in the joints can be observed using x-rays. Tests are discussed in detail in Chapter 6.

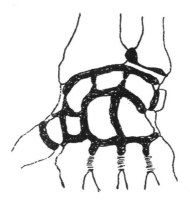

Figure 2. Synovial Tissue (shaded) in the Hand

According to 2008 CDC statistics, RA afflicts nearly 2 million Americans of all ages, occurring three times as often in women as in men. The prevalence of RA appears to be decreasing only because of a more restrictive definition of the disease.[13] Estimates show that 1 in 250 children under age 18 have been diagnosed with arthritis or another rheumatologic condition.

Most RA patients have a progressive disability. Some disability occurs in 50-70% of RA patients within five years after onset of the disease, and half will stop working within ten years. The CDC reported in 2003 that arthritis and other rheumatic conditions cost the United States $127.8 billion ($80.8 billion in medical care expenditures and $47 billion in lost earnings). A 2012 update to these statistics is pending.

Common to all cases of RA is the systemic inflammation that the immune system cannot suppress and dispel as a transient problem. The invasion and compromising of T-cells by pathogens make it impossible for the immune system to distinguish between friend and foe. This topic will be discussed in detail in Chapter 3.

RA can occur at any age, even in babies, but it usually begins to affect people in their forties and older as the immune system begins to deteriorate as part of the aging process. A contributing factor is the malfunctioning of the immune system after years of stress, poor diet, allergies, and indiscriminate medication with immunosuppressing drugs. For the most part, RA strikes when people are active and vigorous. However, the elderly have a range of other disorders not seen in young patients, including endocrine, metabolic, neurological, and vascular disorders that can lead to degenerative joint disease.

Thus, clinicians are faced with the difficult task of diagnosing multiple overlapping causes, without an effective treatment strategy. For example, arthritis symptoms might result from a pre-existing thyroid dysfunction[14] or perhaps by malabsorption as part of a gastrointestinal condition. The latter could be brought about by prescription medications. Recent studies have examined latent infections contracted early in life and developing slowly over the years that lead to chronic illness. Some examples are presented in Chapter 3.

No race or genetic type is spared rheumatic disease. Despite the United States' reputation for high quality medical care, our country has some of the most severe and crippling forms of arthritis. Rheumatic disease itself is not considered to be contagious, but as this text will assert, there are linkages to an initial infection with the onset of RA and the persistence of symptoms. E.g., RA's infectious organisms can be passed from mother to unborn child, or between adults through exchange of body fluids, or via blood transfusion or vaccines.

This assertion runs counter to the prevailing medical establishment's stance that the body's own defense systems attack healthy cells in the synovial membrane by mistake. They call this process an "autoimmune reaction."[15]

It seems counterintuitive that the body would suddenly attack itself. This book will show that so-called autoimmune reactions are triggered by a dysfunctional immune system's inability to cope with a colony of cell-invading microbes, allergies, stress, vitamin deficiencies, accrued toxins, trauma, an imbalance of the microbiota in the gut, and other factors. A partial list of most common of over 100 recognized autoimmune diseases (as of 2011) appears in Table 1.[16]

Table 1. Recognized (Named) Autoimmune Diseases

Aseptic Meningitis
Ankylosing Spondylitis
Autism Spectrum Disorders (ASD)
Autoimmune Addison's Disease
Autoimmune Hemolytic Anemia
Autoimmune Hepatitis
Cardiomyopathy
Celiac Sprue-Dermatitis (gluten-sensitive
    enteropathy)
Chronic Fatigue Syndrome (CFS) [also called
    Chronic Fatigue Immune Dysfunction
    Syndrome (CFIDS)]
Chronic obstructive pulmonary disease (COPD)
Coxsackie myocarditis
Crohn's Disease
Dermatitis herpetiformis
Discoid Lupus
Endometriosis
Graves' Disease
Guillain-Barré Syndrome
Hashimoto's Thyroiditis
Fibromyalgia – Fibromyositis
Insulin-dependent Diabetes (Type 1)
Interstitial cystitis
Juvenile Rheumatoid Arthritis (JRA)
Lupus (Systemic Lupus Erthematosus or SLE)
Lyme Disease, chronic
Meniere's Disease

Multiple Sclerosis
Myasthenia Gravis
Myositis (including Polymyositis)
Peripheral Neuropathy
Pernicious Anemia
Polymyalgia Rheumatica
Postmyocardial Infarction Syndrome
Primary Biliary Cirrhosis
Psoriasis (including Psoriatic Arthritis)
Raynaud's Phenomenon
Reflex Sympathetic Dystrophy (RSD)
Reiter's Syndrome
Restless Leg Syndrome
Rheumatic Fever
Rheumatoid Arthritis
Sarcoidosis
Scleroderma
Sjögren's Syndrome
Ulcerative Colitis
Vasculitis

Carpal Tunnel Syndrome (CTS) is curiously absent from this list. Increasing and widespread instances of CTS (tendonitis or synovitis) are possibly caused by *Mycoplasma synoviae*. PCR testing can prove or disprove this theory.

CTS has been found to be either caused by or exacerbated by a vitamin B_6 deficiency.[17] Since all vitamins in the B-complex typically work together, a B_6 deficiency probably points to other diet deficiencies. A lack of adequate B_6 weakens the body's ability to synthesize collagen and elastin fibrils that bind tissues together. This condition makes tissues more vulnerable to injury and/or infection. Decreased collagen production takes its toll on cartilage throughout the body, but especially in the weak, continually stressed CTS area where arthritis may develop. Vitamin C is an excellent collagen stabilizer. The many benefits of vitamin C are described in Appendix V.

To call RA—and perhaps many other chronic diseases listed in Table 1—an "autoimmune disorder" is not precisely true. The immune system is indeed attacking the body's own cells, but they have been infiltrated by insidious pathogens which use the healthy cells to cloak themselves. As with many chronic illnesses on that list, Lupus is difficult to diagnose because there is no uniform pattern of symptoms. Lupus involves chronic inflammation affecting many parts of the body including heart, lungs, skin, joints, muscles, kidneys, and the nervous system. The nonprofit Lupus Foundation of America provides details on symptoms, tests, and treatments www.Lupus.org.

Osteoarthritis (OA)

Often called the "wear and tear" disease because it involves cartilage degeneration over time, OA occurs much more often than RA. According to CDC and the U.S. Agency for Healthcare Research and Quality, OA afflicts about 27 million Americans, mostly women. It is cited as the main reason for nearly 543,000 knee and 230,00 hip replacement surgeries every year.[18]

Dr. Gabriel Cousens, M.D., has treated hundreds of patients since 1993 at his Arizona clinic.[19] His therapy is a combination of exercise, massage, diet, and meditation. Dr. Cousens is a psychiatrist, family therapist, researcher, and holistic physician. He has concluded that OA is caused by faulty nutrition, overindulgence in junk foods, and lack of gentle aerobic exercise. The toxins trapped in the joints are a result of poor circulation, improper digestion, and sluggish organs unable to clear those toxins. His detoxification program has a 95% improvement record for OA patients.[20]

The non-stop inflammation of RA destroys cartilage much faster than OA's wear and tear. Until bone scanning techniques were invented, it was common for doctors to assert that the patient had either OA or RA, but never both. About half of human OA cases also display some degree of RA symptoms.[21] Tetracycline can be used as a benign probe for infection, as discussed in Chapter 6. Methods to prevent and/or retard joint damage are shown in the next sections.

CARTILAGE DEGENERATION

Connective tissue makes up one-third of our body weight, most of it in the form of collagen. Tightly interlaced collagen fibrils form better than half of human cartilage, giving it its compressible and elastic characteristics. These fibrils act as resilient "springs" to confine and compress the water-binding proteoglycan molecules in a cartilage matrix that can bind up to 1,000 times its weight in water. This matrix is constrained by the collagen network, creating an intrinsic pressure ranging from 2.5 to 5 atmospheres. Lubrication is maintained by compression and by the intact nature of the cartilage matrix.[22] Cartilage is an essential structural substance found throughout the body and is of four types, shown as shaded areas in the drawing in Figure 3:

Fibrocartilage, notable for tensile strength (the ability to resist breakage), found primarily between the vertebrae but also in some interarticular areas of the joints. It contains numerous thick bundles of collagen fibers;

Articular, which is found in the joints, has the resilience to rebound from compression, and enables bones to slip over one another smoothly;

Elastic, found at the front of the rib cage, allowing expansion with breathing action; and

Morphological, e.g., found in the nose and ears.

Destructive enzymes, in particular proteoglycanase and hyaluronidase, attack and break down the cartilage matrix. Some bacteria, such as *Staphylococcus aureus, Streptococcus pyogenes, and Clostridium perfringens,* produce hyaluronidase as a means of using hyaluronan as a carbon source. [23] With this damage, the matrix's water-binding capability is decreased and absorption of nutrients is diminished. As cartilage erodes, its collagen fibers are exposed to wear, and the cushioning effect is lost. The exposed fibril ends act as irritants within the joint capsule.

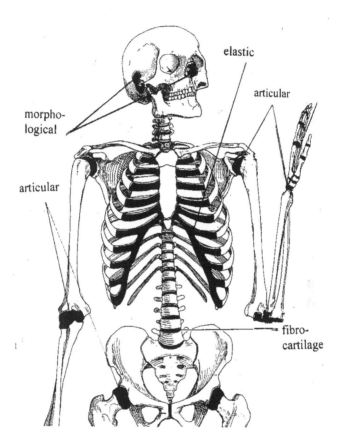

Figure 3. Human Body Cartilage (shaded)

As the immune system responds, the result is a release of chemicals and heat that promote reddening, swelling, and pain in the surrounding nerves and tissues. What follows is the destruction of collagen proteins that hold the cells together as functional connective tissues—synovia, blood vessels, and skin. Arthritics typically look older than their chronological age because their skin is deficient in collagen. Vitamin C as a collagen stabilizer can retard this destruction by protecting hyaluronic acid (HA), which is a major component of the synovial fluid that lubricates the joint. If HA-generating cells are lost, stem cell therapy may be useful to regrow them.[24]

Scar tissue and bone gradually replace the eroded joint regions, causing irregularly shaped articulating surfaces. Age, weight-bearing stresses, and other external forces on joints over time contribute to the ultimate degeneration of cartilage, especially in the hips and knees.

Cartilage is highly susceptible to stress but the under-lying (subchondral) bone bears much of the brunt of compressive forces. Exposed to repeated mechanical stress, such as jogging, this bone can become unusually stiff by a series of healed and calcified microfractures over time. The stiffer this bone, the more the nearby softer cartilage degenerates. Thus, care of one's bones is as important as cartilage health for arthritic individuals.[25, 26]

Cartilage erosion can be caused through what is called "chronic tension," the effect of sustained isometric muscle contraction of any of the numerous joints of the body. For example, sustained compression of intervertebral cartilage in the cervical spine and disks.[27, 28] Bone health is discussed later in this chapter.

In the case of OA, cartilage continues to erode and then to grow back. Irregular regrowth masses can eventually cover the entire joint. This accounts for the swelling visible from the exterior side of the skin as well as contraction and alignment problems. In advanced cases, the load-bearing cartilage of the joint becomes rough and pitted, damaged to the point where bone rubs against bone, and more severe pain occurs. A life-threatening joint complication can occur when the cervical spine becomes unstable through cartilage and bone erosion. Bone friction and destruction is the characteristic feature of Osteoarthritis. The same joints may be affected as with RA, but OA is a localized problem while RA joint pain can move to various sites in the body. Typically, OA is directly related to unusual wear or damage to the joints, or to loss of lubricating fluid between the joints, typically associated with the aging process. In both RA and OA, joints can wear abnormally for a variety of reasons:

- trauma damages cartilage, causing the immune system to go into tear-down mode to remove the injured tissues and cells;

- circulation is impaired, so lubrication material is not transferred effectively to the joint or sheath area to rebuild injured cells;

- poor nutrition does not provide strong skeletal material during childhood development or after injury;

- pain inhibits joint motion and lymph fluid transport of harmful enzymes out of the injured area is impeded;

- muscles do not adequately support the joint, or they spasm so motion is limited;

- constant application of misdirected mechanical forces puts excessive stress on the cartilage in a particular joint; and/or

- improper (or extreme) physical therapy and/or exercise can literally wear out the joint(s).

As the body tries to repair itself, cartilage may grow abnormally, seen as knobs under the skin and protruding from the area around the joint. Since there are no pain nerves within cartilage, deterioration generally goes unnoticed until pain and swelling occur. When the surface of the cartilage becomes abraded, the body sends antibodies to attack the exudates of debris that should have been removed by the white blood cells of a robustly functioning immune system. The antibodies' interaction with these sloughed-off bits results in pain and inflammation.

OA can affect either or both load-bearing joints of the knees, hips, and ankles as well as non-load-bearing joints of the fingers, elbows, and hands. OA is also characterized by calcium deposits, which can accumulate like bony spurs on pressure points and impinge on nerves. The pain and inflammation symptoms are similar to RA, but OA is considered by many unmotivated medical practitioners to be a noninflammatory form of arthritis that is hereditary and incurable.

However, several significant studies indicate otherwise. E.g., in 2003 Indiana University researchers showed that the tetracycline-family antibiotic doxycycline helps prevent OA knee damage by inhibiting harmful enzymes that break down joint cartilage. Doxycycline was found to lessen OA pain in damaged knees and to improve cartilage in normal knees.[29]

Another large double-blind study done in 2005[30] with 431 participants was not reported in the media until 2011.[31] The results showed a slowing of OA progression as indicated by measuring joint space narrowing at the outset of the study and again after 30 months of doxycycline treatment. Dr. Kenneth D. Brandt, M.D., lead author of the study, concludes, "Our findings indicate that Osteoarthritis is a disease whose natural history can be modified by pharmacologic therapy."

Pets afflicted with OA and/or RA respond well to an improved diet and glycosaminaglycan or hyaluronic acid supplements, which fortify cartilage in diseased joints. Acupuncture, chiropractic adjustments, and certain popular herbs such as boswellia, and spices such as turmeric (curcumin), also assist in relieving pain in arthritic animals. Antioxidant vitamins can help reduce pathologic inflammation.[32] Chapter 7 discusses these supplements.

Prolotherapy [33]

A non-surgical approach to chronic pain in the joints that has been applied since 400 BC is a technique called Prolotherapy (<u>prol</u>iferation therapy). Hippocrates first used it on Olympic athletes with torn ligaments and on soldiers with dislocated shoulder joints. Dr. George Hackett, M.D. popularized Prolotherapy in 1939, when it found favor with osteopathic physicians.

Prolotherapy uses a non-pharmacological solution, usually dextrose-based, which is injected into the ligament or tendon where it attaches to the bone. This action results in a localized inflammation that increases the blood supply and flow of nutrients into the injured area, and in turn stimulates the tissue to repair itself. Response varies depending on the extent of the injury and the person's healing ability. Four to six treatments are the average needed. [34]

There are three classes of proliferant solutions used to initiate inflammation: chemical irritants (e.g. phenol), osmotic shock agents (e.g. hypertonic dextrose and glycerin), and chemotactic agents (e.g. morrhuate sodium, a fatty acid derivative of cod liver oil). Injections are intended to mimic the natural healing process by causing an influx of fibroblasts that synthesize collagen at the injection site, leading to the formation of new ligament and tendon tissue. The newly produced collagen is intended to support the injured or loosened ligaments, creating a more stable and strong muscle base in the process, alleviating pain. Prolotherapy is sometimes used as an alternative to arthroscopic surgery.

Prolotherapy is useful for many different types of musculoskeletal pain, including arthritis, back pain, neck pain, fibromyalgia, sports injuries, unresolved whiplash injuries, carpal tunnel syndrome, chronic tendonitis, partially torn tendons, ligaments and cartilage, degenerated or herniated discs, sciatica, and pain in the jaw joint (TMJ).

Sadly, at this writing, despite thousands of successful treatments, most insurance companies and Medicare do not yet cover Prolotherapy. They should, since HA injections and acupuncture, which provide temporary relief, are allowed. A revolutionary new treatment for Osteoarthritis is said to be noninvasive, safe, and painless. According to Dr. V.G. Vasishta, Sequentially Programmed Magnetic Field (SPMF) therapy™ or what is popularly known as Quantum Magnetic Resonance (QMR) Therapy not only stops the progress of disease but also reverses the process of disease by cartilage regeneration. He has treated over 2500 cases of OA successfully since 2006 at his Bangalore, India, healthcare center. QMR is also a cancer treatment regime.[35]

BONE HEALTH

The human skeleton is a surprisingly active structure of active metabolic tissue that changes continually throughout one's life. Bone modeling occurs in our youth when 100% of the bone surface is active. Adult bones undergo bone remodeling at a rate of 20% surface activity where older bone tissue is cyclically destroyed and replaced by new tissue.

The bone loss associated with OA indicates that destruction occurs at a faster rate than formation. Study subjects with age-related Osteoarthritis (and/or Osteoporosis) who took omega-3 polyunsaturated fatty acids as fish oil supplements showed an increase in serum calcium, osteocalcin, and collagen. The study also found that evening primrose oil potentiates the beneficial effects of fish oil supplements.[36, 37]

Bone disease often signals an imbalance of the body's required essential minerals such as calcium. Eating a balanced diet with enough calcium and vitamin D is key to preventing osteoporosis. The best source of calcium is food rich in this nutrient, such as yogurt, rhubarb, tofu, and salmon. The body more efficiently and easily absorbs small portions consumed throughout the day. Calcium intake of 1,000 mg per day (combined food and supplements) can restore some lost bone mass at any age. Too much calcium (over 2,500 mg per day) may cause absorption problems.[38] Calcium is never found free in nature because it readily combines with carbon and oxygen to make calcium carbonate, which is sold as a supplement. The term "elemental" designates the percentage of the substance that is pure calcium. The recommended dose refers to the amount of elemental calcium, so the 100% daily value is equal to 1,000 mg of elemental calcium. We should get enough daily calcium from food sources, but supplements may be needed in some cases.

These are typical contents of calcium supplements: [39]

- Calcium carbonate (e.g., Caltrate®, and Os-Cal®): 40% (2.5 tablets = 100%)
- Calcium phosphate: 38% (2.5 tablets = 100%)
- Calcium citrate (e.g., Citracal® and Solgar®): 21% (5 tablets = 100%)
- Lactate calcium: 13% (7-8 tablets = 100%)
- Calcium ascorbate: 10% (10 tablets = 100%)

Calcium citrate is the best absorbed because it does not require additional stomach acid. Coral calcium is simply calcium carbonate with no proven health benefits. Always read labels on commercial supplements to be sure of the calcium source. E.g., lead may be found in dolomite, oyster shell, and bone meal products. Aluminum, mainly found in antacids that are also sold as calcium supplements, is also harmful. Lead, aluminum, and zinc inhibit absorption of calcium.[40]

High, continuous doses of cortisone-like drugs (e.g., prednisone) or thyroid medication can increase the risk of bone loss. A dysfunctional or overworked immune system may be linked to a calcium deficiency and bone loss. When a pathogenic organism invades the body, the immune system's response includes building a calcium nodule around the invader to protect the healthy cells from harm. Failing to find adequate calcium in the bloodstream, the immune system will steal calcium from bones. A bone density scan is a useful test to determine whether the body is under attack by infection and unable to defend itself adequately.

Bone Marrow

Bone marrow is the spongy, fatty tissue that contains stem cells, located in certain large bones. These stem cells are transformed into white and red blood cells and platelets, essential for immunity and circulation. Bone marrow tissue, as part of the lymphatic system, fights pathogens like fungi, bacteria, and viruses. Anemia and lymphoma cancers like leukemia can compromise the resilience of bone marrow.[41] Bone marrow transplants are a treatment for these lymphatic system conditions that are otherwise incurable. High doses of certain drugs can cause bone marrow damage (e.g., aspirin, acetaminophen, sulfasalazine, cancer treatment drugs).[42]

COMMON CONVENTIONAL TREATMENTS

There are hundreds of remedies and formulations for arthritis relief, ranging from ancient herbs to highly sophisticated pharmaceuticals based on the premise that the disease is a metabolic disorder of unknown origin. Some of our present-day drugs are derived from proven herbal remedies or mineral salts such as gold and copper, but they may be concentrated to near-toxic strength.

Conventional RA treatment often consists of simply prescribing drugs that relieve pain in the short term but this does not address the root cause of the problem. Naturopathic practitioners suggest herbs, diets, and purges that are not effective in the long term. Both groups are endeavoring to solve a highly complex problem with extremely limited tools. Consider the incredible diversity of the polymicrobial zoo and the human immune system that has evolved assorted mechanisms to combat the constant assaults of shape-changing and adaptive invaders.

The way in which these two groups (physicians and naturopaths) approach the problem of disease is philosophically the same. Both try to restore the body to an undefined ideal called "balance." However, the body is not a static entity—pathogenic microbes continue to evolve and adapt to their changing *in vivo* environment—so there is no single prescription drug or herbal substance that will provide a balanced solution. That said, orthomolecular deficiencies could be overcome through vitamins and supplements. Probiotic microbes can be added to body flora. Vaccines can train the immune system to recognize and combat harmful microbes. Infectious pathogens can be attacked and possibly eliminated (or at least controlled) with specific drugs.

The body's dynamic collective and interacting mechanisms typify the ultimate control theory problem, as discussed in Chapter 3. There is much to be learned through cooperation and sharing, rather than the adversarial relationship that exists, sometimes overtly, between conventional medical doctors and practitioners of alternative or complementary medicine.

Several celebrities, notably Doctors Joseph Mercola, Andrew Weil, and Gabe Mirkin have shown that medical doctors can and should seek out information from any source that will help heal their patients. By practicing what they call "integrative" or "functional" medicine, they are taking a holistic view of their patients, rejecting the us-versus-them relationship that has stifled progress in the treatment of chronic disease. The Institute for Functional Medicine (www.functionalmedicine.org) advocates patient-centered health care based on understanding the biofunctional interactions among genetic, environmental, and lifestyle factors influencing health; complex, chronic diseases; and immune system reactivity.

Prescription Drugs [43]

A patient reporting arthritis symptoms of pain and swelling in the joints to a physician will usually be given a prescription for one of the nonsteroidal anti-inflammatory drugs (NSAIDs) such as ibuprofen (Advil, Motrin, others) and naproxen (Aleve). Stronger NSAIDs are available by prescription. Side effects may include ringing in the ears, stomach irritation, heart problems, liver damage, and kidney damage. These drugs relieve inflammation symptoms but do not change the overall progression of the disease.[44] NSAIDs also deplete potassium and vitamin C.

A physician will usually prescribe NSAIDs first, and then move to disease-modifying antirheumatic drugs (DMARDs)[45] like leflunomide (Arava), hydroxychloroquine (Plaquenil), sulfasalazine (Azulfidine), and minocycline (Dynacin, Minocin, etc.). Side effects vary but may include liver damage, bone marrow suppression and severe lung infections.[46] In persistent cases, the doctor may prescribe immunosuppressants such as azathioprine (Imuran, Azasan), cyclophosphamide (Cytoxan), or cyclosporine (Sandimmune Neoral, Gengraf). Note that by inhibiting immune system actions, these drugs increase susceptibility to infection.[47]

Another category of powerful drugs designed to reduce pain and swelling is TNF-alpha inhibitors such as etanercept (Enbrel), infliximab (Remicade), adalimumab (Humira), golimumab (Simponi) and certolizumab (Cimzia).[48] Potential side effects include increased risk of serious infections, congestive heart failure and certain cancers.[49]

Corticosteroid drugs like prednisone reduce acute inflammation and pain and slow joint damage. Side effects may include osteoporosis, diabetes, cataracts, or weight gain.

In the 1950's and 1960's, one potential serious side effect of prednisone was gastric ulcers after long-term use.[50] In 1994 the National Institutes of Health (NIH) reviewed numerous medical studies and concluded that a bacterium called *Helicobacter pylori* was the root cause of chronic gastritis leading to peptic ulcers. The process of sloughing off necrotic inflammatory tissue creates the ulcers in the stomach and duodenum. This conclusion had been announced over a decade earlier when two Australian scientists, Doctors J. Robin Warren and Barry Marshall, conducted meticulous experiments and proved this fact. Their research showed that *H. pylori* is a common bacterial agent colonizing an estimated 30-50% of the world's population. Prednisone was not the direct cause of ulcers—the drug had been depressing patients' immune systems, allowing the *H. pylori* infection to flourish.

Drs. Warren and Marshall won the 2005 Nobel Prize in medicine for their *H. pylori* discovery. However, at the time (1982), they were ridiculed and their findings deliberately refuted by a pharmaceutical/medical industry in the United States that had strong economic motives for keeping standard treatment of ulcers as a chronic disease in place. At stake was an $8 billion antacid market, and recurring ulcers mean regular visits to gastroenterologists.[51]

Good clinical evidence of efficacy has been provided for several triple or quadruple antibiotic therapies[52] given to eradicate the *H. pylori* bacteria, but this treatment does not affect the recurring ulcers that are shown to be one of the side effects of NSAIDs and DMARDs. About 30% of stomach ulcers are caused by the corrosive effects of aspirin-type drugs, not by *H. pylori*. Because the two types of ulcer causes are unrelated, treatment for one type won't help the other.[53] The *Helicobacter pylori* Foundation provides details on the wide variety of *H. pylori* symptoms, tests, related diseases, and suggested treatments.[54]

Natural herbal antibiotics can be effective for ulcers: the berberine compound found in both goldenseal (*Hydrastis canadensis*) and Oregon grape (*Berberis aquifolium*) kills a variety of harmful bacteria, including *H. pylori*. Herbalists recommend taking licorice root extract (*Glycyrrhiza glabra*) with berberines. Licorice is an antibacterial, and also increases production of protective mucous in the stomach. Deglycyrrhizinated (DGL) licorice is preferred to avoid water retention and high blood pressure.[55] One should discuss specific dosage with a qualified health care advisor.

Sulfasalazine

In the 1930s, when some doctors began to suspect that RA might be an infectious disease, sulfasalazine (an antibiotic compound composed of sulfapyridine and aspirin) was administered. In the 1950s, the infection theory fell out of favor with the medical community, who adopted the autoimmune theory as the standard teaching that prevails to this day. Perhaps Dr. Brown's RA infection hypothesis was abandoned because mycoplasmal and cell wall-deficient forms of bacteria were so hard to detect with methods available at that time.

Sulfasalazine is now used successfully for ulcerative colitis, called Inflammatory Bowel Disease (IBD), aka Irritable Bowel Syndrome (IBS).[56] Studies dating from the 1980s have shown sulfasalazine to be as effective as gold salts or penicillamine.[57]

The antibacterial component of sulfasalazine enters the bloodstream where it is free to move to any site of infection and to suppress bacterial activity. The positive action of this component may indicate the role of bacterial infections of the intestine in the pathogenic origin of rheumatoid diseases.

Although sulfasalazine has some immunosuppressive effects, these study results should prompt consideration of the polymicrobial infection hypothesis.[58]

Children under eight with Juvenile RA may benefit from sulfasalazine as a substitute for tetracycline, which has particular side effects for that age group, including permanent staining of the teeth.[59]

Caution: A diet high in sugar while taking sulfasalazine can result in seizures linked to glycogen imbalance and vitamin deficiencies.

Gold Salts

Sometimes injections of gold salts are prescribed to help control the inflammation of RA and to halt progression of the disease. Until recently it was not fully understood how gold slows the progression of RA but studies have shown that gold reduces vascular permeability, lowering the number of white blood cells, slowing these cells' response to antigens, and thus diminishing the inflammatory response.[60] Improvement may last only two to three years. If the RA returns, the physician usually prescribes another medication such as Methotrexate. Gold is used less frequently now than it was decades ago because of its side effects.

In 2007, researchers examined the role of a high mobility group 1 protein (HMGB1) and its impact on the immune system. HMGB1 figures in a wide range of immune-mediated diseases. This inflammation-causing protein signals specific immune system cells (e.g., T-cells) that kill infected cells and facilitate antibody production. Gold salts prevent white blood cells from releasing HMGB1. There is increased interest in how HMGB1 may be blocked in Lupus to reduce inflammatory symptoms, but it is doubtful that gold salts will be used except as an indicator of the molecular pathway that gold acts on, so that less toxic blockers can be developed.[61]

Arthroscopic Surgery

Either an orthopedic surgeon or a rheumatologist trained in arthroscopy can perform the procedure. An MRI examination is usually given prior to the surgery. The arthroscopic probe, when used along with other tests and a complete medical history, can be a valuable diagnostic tool. A dime-sized incision allows the arthroscope, a thin tube tipped with a small, lighted camera lens, to magnify and illuminate areas within the joint capsule. The examining physician is able to view and diagnose problems such as synovitis, cartilage damage, tendon and ligament tears, and loose fragments causing irritation.

The actual surgery uses specialized instruments, a miniature camera, and perhaps a laser to repair torn ligaments or cartilage, remove loose pieces of bone or cartilage, or remove inflamed joint linings. A new technique called quadriceps-sparing knee replacement uses an incision that is typically only 3-4" in length. Recovery time is much quicker, and the less traumatic nature of this approach may decrease both post-operative pain and the need for the normal rehab required after traditional surgery.[62]

An operation called arthrodesis, or joint fusion, permanently bonds the bones together, essentially removing the joint. Synovectomy is a surgical procedure to remove the synovial membrane. For back pain, arthroscopic probes and lasers cauterize nerve endings in the spine so that arthritics suffering from low back pain are afforded some relief.

These procedures do not necessarily remove the pain and do not remove the cause of the disease, so deterioration continues. Joint replacement substitutes artificial materials for joints worn away, and is usually done on the hips, wrists, elbows, shoulders, knees, and fingers. Be aware that complications after any surgery may include infections, blood clots, and damage to blood vessels or nerves. Biofilms may develop on implanted prosthetic devices.

Non-prescription Drugs

Over-the-counter (OTC) drugs such as aspirin, acetaminophen, and ibuprofen are usually suggested by doctors to alleviate joint pain for mild cases of arthritis, but even these less powerful chemicals have their own assorted side effects, depending on the individual and the duration of use: stomach pain, nausea, vomiting, low-level bleeding in the bowel, anxiety, depression, dizziness, heartburn, drowsiness, ulcers, skin rash, prolonged clotting time, and tinnitus (ringing in the ears). These drugs are discussed in Chapter 7.

Stem Cell Therapy

Adult stem cells are derived from a number of biological sources such as: blood, bone marrow, muscle, fat, placenta, umbilical cords, breast milk, dental pulp, and other sources. Stem cell therapy has been used since the 1960s in the treatment of cancer, and research has shown that it has also been effective in the treatment of over 130 other diseases such as multiple sclerosis, autism, diabetes, and many other diseases and ailments. [63]

Our skull, sternum, ribs, pelvis, and femur bones all contain bone marrow, but other smaller bones do not. Inside this special tissue, immature stems cells reside, along with extra iron. While they are undifferentiated, the stem cells wait until unhealthy, weakened, or damaged cells need to be replaced. A stem cell can turn itself into a platelet, a white blood cell like a T-cell, or a red blood cell. This is the only way such cells are replaced to keep our body healthy. Stem cell therapy has been used successfully with horses. [64]

A Swedish research team made a major breakthrough in stem cell culturing in 2010. Scientists can now produce human stem cells entirely without the use of other cells or substances from animals. Instead, the cells are cultured on a matrix of a single human protein: laminin-511. [65]

"Now, for the first time, we can produce large quantities of human embryonic stem cells in an environment that is completely chemically defined," says professor Karl Tryggvason, the study leader. "This opens up new opportunities for developing different types of cell which can then be tested for the treatment of disease."

In 2011, the first trial in humans to use the heart's own stem cells to battle heart failure has produced promising results.[66] The latest medical news, therapies, videos, and research on stem cells can be found at www.stemcell.com.[67]

COMMON ALTERNATIVE TREATMENTS [68]

Because there are many herbs that strengthen the immune system, many others that improve circulation, and still others that relieve symptoms of inflammation, pain, and swelling, a comprehensive list is beyond the scope of this book. Appendix I lists those referenced consistently in texts dealing with naturopathic treatment for arthritis and related rheumatic ailments.

The most powerful and safest anti-inflammatory agent is superoxide dismutase, an enzyme produced naturally by red blood cells. This enzyme is contained in several vegetables, as are vitamins A (betacarotene), E (alphatocopherol) and C (ascorbic acid). The potency of these vitamins is increased when combined with MSM (methylsulfonylmethane—a DMSO derivative described below), copper, zinc, and selenium. While a vitamin or dietary deficiency has not been proven to cause arthritis directly, deficiencies and allergies to certain foods or substances can affect the development and severity of a wide range of chronic diseases, including arthritis.[69]

The vitamins and supplements described in this book as immune system enhancers are given as examples of substances a doctor or nutritionist may deem important to include in a specific profile based on a particular individual's needs. In some cases, a commonly available, widely used, and otherwise benign vitamin or supplement might be contra-indicated because a pre-existing health problem or conflict with prescription medications could make it harmful.

Herbal medications may actually interfere with and complicate surgical procedures before an operation. Eight herbal substances pose some degree of risk during the perioperative (pre-surgery) period. These are echinacea, ephedra, garlic, ginkgo, ginseng, kava, St. John's wort, and valerian. These eight herbs account for more than half of all single herb preparations sold in the United States. Negative reactions include: bleeding from garlic, ginkgo, and ginseng; cardiovascular instability from ephedra; and hypoglycemia from ginseng. Use of St. John's wort leads to increased metabolism of perioperative drugs, but some nonherbal dietary supplements such as glucosamine and chondroitin appear to be safe for perioperative patients.[70] There is a risk for adverse herb/drug interactions between anesthetics and kava and valerian. These herbs seem to increase the sedative effect of the drugs.

At present, information on adverse reactions is required at varying levels of detail at health care facilities across the United States. However, there is no mandate to capture data on the exact nature or extent of problems unless the patient reports evidence proactively.

Three factors contributing to under-reporting of adverse events are (1) physicians' failing to obtain a detailed history of non-prescribed medications from their patients; (2) patients' unwillingness to admit using herbal remedies to their doctors; and (3) patients' reluctance to report and seek treatment for adverse reactions. One study[71] found that the lack of disclosure and reporting is the patient's belief either that the doctor is not knowledgeable about herbal substances or that s/he may be prejudiced against unconventional therapies.

Even if the data were to be reported, there are no mechanisms in place for logging, processing, interpretation, evaluation, or dissemination. Perhaps some day, technology will allow biochip readouts and instant sample analysis of patients' data to be transmitted directly to a central database. Until then, the quality of reported data is questionable, since herb/drug reactions experienced will be somewhat subjective and will vary among individuals.

Physicians should carefully interview patients who are candidates for surgery regarding their history of herbal medication usage and then take steps to prevent, recognize, and treat potentially serious interaction problems before surgery is performed. Both doctor and patient should be aware of pharmacodynamic or pharmacokinetic risks.

Although in most cases, patients may be advised to avoid herbal medications for 2-3 weeks before surgery, in others, abrupt withdrawal from herbal substances may be detrimental.[72] Doctor and patient must work together to determine the optimal course of action before surgery.

Homeopathic Remedies [73]

Homeopathic philosophy is consistent with ideas about vaccination and immunization, namely, that "like heals like," according to the Law of Similars, the basic principle of homeopathy. This fundamental tenet states that a substance that causes a set of symptoms in a healthy person acts as a curative medicine when given to sick people who have similar symptoms. Thus, a minuscule amount of the toxin is given to the individual to acquaint the body with the invader in order to train it to ward off future assaults.

The medicine is designed to make the patients feel worse before they feel better. It forces the immune system to react vigorously to the invading organism, thus training it thoroughly in resistance, unlike antihistamines, antibiotics, and cold medicines, which suppress the immune reaction and do not challenge the system to learn to repel the invaders. Homeopathic approaches that involve a cyclic alteration of repeated immune stimulation and gentle immune suppression facilitate transport of natural antibiotics to hidden sites of pathogenic organisms. This action is consistent with the Jarisch-Herxheimer reaction described in Chapter 3.

Specific homeopathic remedies have been found to be useful in relieving arthritis symptoms under the following conditions: [74]

- worse in warm weather, inflamed joints, intolerant of touch, and ill humored: *Colchicum* 6c.

- worse during stormy/changeable weather: *Rhododendron* 6c.

- when symptoms include pain and stiffness, made worse after rest, and in cold, damp weather, symptoms improve with continued motion: *Rhus toxicondendron* 6c.

- stitching pain, made worse by any motion, eased by rest: *Bryonia* 6c.

- joint pain, fatigue, weakness, tearing pain from wrist to elbow, pain that feels sprained, twitching, and stiffness: *Calcarea Carbonica* 30c.

- for sprains, soreness, muscle ache, backache, swelling, arthritis joint pain: *Arnica Montana* 30x.

The amounts in homeopathic compounds are very carefully measured and diluted. Medicines diluted one part to 99 parts are called *centesimal* potencies and are labeled 6c, 30c, and so on. Sometimes the dilution factor is one part medicine to nine parts liquid and these *decimal* potencies are labeled 6x, 30x, and so on. Medicines diluted 15 times or less (15c, 15x, or lower) are referred to as low potencies, while those diluted 30c, 30x or higher are considered high potencies. The ingredients in an OTC homeopathic remedy for yeast infection that includes *Candida albicans* 30x illustrate the immunization principle of the Law of Similars.

When taking a homeopathic remedy, avoid all products containing mint (including jelly, candy, flavored toothpaste, mouthwash, tea, and gum) during treatment. Other substances that affect homeopathic regimens adversely are camphor and caffeine. A physician trained in both homeopathic and conventional medicine should be able to advise the patient on these kinds of interactions. Some skeptics quickly dismiss homeopathy as quackery. However, many veterinarians report success with their animal patients. If a homeopathic remedy (*Calcarea fluorica* 6x) can dissolve bone spurs and calcium deposits in horses' joints, proven by before-and-after x-rays, it is clearly not a placebo.[75]

Chinese Herbal Medicine

Since the 1950s, Chinese medicine, as taught at Chinese universities, uses most of the modern scientific ideas and methods published in the Western world blended with traditional knowledge of medicinal herbs, diet and nutrition, acupuncture, massage, and exercise. The Chinese equivalent of the *Compendium of Materia Medica* is *Bencao Gangmu* (6 volumes in English). Containing about 1800 drugs, it was compiled over a period of 27 years by the 16th century genius Li Shizhen—physician, herbalist, and scientist—during the Ming Dynasty. Chinese medical practitioners[76] recommend natural substances such as bupleuri root, pubescent angelica root, ledebouriellua root, licorice, cinnamon twigs, and Chinese skullcap for their anti-inflammatory effects.[77]

Acupuncture has been used in Asia for centuries to stimulate endorphins in specific brain regions. Skilled acupuncturists use detailed charts to map external stimulus points to brain areas of responsibility for a variety of regions/organs where injury or disease is present. This ancient Chinese method of healing has been scientifically analyzed using an electronic probe to test the instant effects of acupuncture on calcium (Ca) and sodium (Na) ions of normal and injured muscles *in vitro*. It was found that in normal muscles after acupuncture, Ca content of the plasma membrane measurably increased, while Na content tended to decrease. At ten minutes after acupuncture, Ca content resumed to normal but Na content increased three-fold. The results indicated that acupuncture could increase the penetrability of *normal* muscle membrane to Ca and the penetrability of *injured* muscle membrane to Na. This might be the vital mechanism of changing Na-Ca exchange of cell membrane and adjusting plasma Ca content.[78, 79]

Ayurvedic Medicine

Ayurveda is Sanskrit for "science of longevity." The first records date to about 1500 BC. Two comprehensive encyclopedias of Ayurvedic medicine were compiled from about 500 BC to 500 AD. Today the Indian-sourced English language *Materia Medica* is still in print and some websites permit lookup access to part of this complex, hard-to-interpret catalog of plants and their medical properties.[80] The Indian government created a web-accessible database of traditional knowledge that includes medical formulations, so that much of the traditional medicine recipes are now in the public domain with access to a representative collection of 1200 Ayurvedic, Unani, and Siddha formulations.[81]

DMSO

DMSO (dimethyl sulfoxide), a solvent used in the wood pulp and paper manufacturing process, was hailed in the early 1960s as a "miracle drug" to relieve inflammation but the FDA quickly suppressed its use. It was not until 1978 that DMSO was approved for treatment of interstitial cystitis, a bladder inflammation, but the FDA has not yet approved its use in the treatment of a variety of other conditions, such as arthritis, Scleroderma, reflex sympathetic dystrophy (RSD), cancer, Fibromyalgia, and stroke.[82]

In 2007, the FDA granted "fast track" designation on clinical studies of DMSO's use in reducing brain tissue swelling following traumatic brain injury, but has been slow to act on recognizing results or granting approval.[83] There is great potential of DMSO in treating brain trauma injuries that afflict more than 50,000 Americans each year. Brain injuries are the most common trauma suffered by soldiers in battle. Dr. Stanley Jacob has conducted research on DMSO since the early 1960s. He notes that in Holland, a physician is breaking the law if s/he does *not* prescribe topical DMSO for RSD.[84] To date, there have been over 10,000 studies focused on DMSO for medical use.[85] Preliminary clinical trials of DMSO on traumatic brain injury patients in Europe show an 80% survival rate. About 70% of the patients experience a favorable outcome (far higher than the 10% historical rate.[86]

The chemical formulation of DMSO consists of two methyls bound to sulfur plus oxygen. When oxidized, DMSO becomes di-methylsulfoxone, a sulfur-based antibacterial known as MSM (methylsulfonylmethane). MSM is sold in health food stores in capsule form as a dietary supplement to be taken orally.

DMSO also may bind to pain source nerve sites in the area of injury, reducing the stimulation capacity. DMSO facilitates the transfer of dissolved substances into the body. Through hydroscopic action, DMSO also facilitates fluid transport from the trauma site, reducing swelling and speeding elimination of waste tissue remnants. DMSO's reputation for relieving symptoms of swelling comes from this desiccating capability. A joint filled with excess fluid will respond quickly to DMSO as the fluid is drawn out from the affected area and the pressure is relieved. DMSO is widely used topically by veterinarians on pets and by ranchers to treat horses with sprains.

Since DMSO usage is still discouraged for human use by the FDA, it would be very difficult to formulate and sell a patch that transports some other useful substance "X" into the body through the many layers of skin and tissue. However, a combination of DMSO + X could be useful. X could be copper or gold salts, but this poses some danger if too high a concentration is used. X could be tetracycline or erythromycin or minocycline. LivDerma, Inc., based in Canada, is developing a topical delivery system for medications that for whatever reason cannot be taken orally. Clinical trials are needed to be sure the dosage is correct and effective.[87] DMSO should <u>only</u> be used topically as a gel or liquid. Care should be taken in the application of DMSO. Since it is a powerful transport medium, anything that touches the solvent should be extremely clean—the area to be treated as well as the hands or device applying the solvent—lest toxins or bacteria be introduced through the skin. Washing the hands immediately after applying DMSO is strongly recommended.

<u>Warning</u>: liquid DMSO should <u>never</u> be ingested except under controlled medical circumstances. It has been touted as home remedy to dissolve cancer tumors or a clot causing a stroke.[88] However, DMSO is highly reactive with pure oxygen given by emergency room staff, releasing toxic fumes that can kill the patient and others in the room.[89]

Ultraviolet Light Treatment (Photopheresis)

Dr. Gordon Josephs, D.O. belongs to IOMA, the International Oxidative Medical Association,[90] a nonprofit group of doctors who utilize a variety of alternative therapies. Ultraviolet Blood Irradiation (UVBI) is one such treatment designed to kill viruses, bacteria, and fungi often with dramatic results.[91] UVBI therapy was once mainstream, used extensively and with excellent results during the 1930s to 1950s for the treatment of a wide variety of conditions.[92] However, when new wonder drugs like cortisone and penicillin were introduced in the 1950s, this technique was abandoned. IOMA and the Foundation for Blood Irradiation are working to renew interest in this therapy.[93]

Dr. Keith Scott-Mumby describes UVBI as a "massive whole-body antibiotic." Researchers in Russia have used this process to treat HIV with impressive results.[94] If the gut is a reservoir for HIV infection, UVBI will be only temporary. Other treatments can effectively eliminate these reservoirs by repopulating the gut with a probiotic mix of beneficial microbes. This method is described in Chapter 3.

A fundamental effect of UVBI is to "energize" the biochemical and physiological defenses of the body by the introduction of ultraviolet energy into the bloodstream that may, in part, be effective by producing small amounts of ozone from the oxygen circulating in the blood.[95] There are published reports on its use in bacterial diseases, including septicemias, pneumonias, peritonitis, wound infections; viral infections including acute and chronic hepatitis, atypical pneumonias, poliomyelitis, encephalitis, mumps, measles, mononucleosis, and herpes; circulatory conditions including thrombophlebitis, peripheral vascular arterial disease, and diabetic ulcer; overwhelming toxemias, non-healing wounds and delayed union of fractures, RA, and many others.[96] UV topical skin treatments are well known and accepted in medical dermatology.[97]

UVBI treatment is low/no risk, is non-toxic, has FDA approval, and results are observable within five weeks. Any risk might come from the use of unsterile apparatus leading to infection, but the treatment has much lower risk probability than, say, dialysis. However, a serious drawback is the treatment's high cost for up to 20 sessions required. On the bright side for patients, hospitals can usually get reimbursed from third-party payers because photopheresis is 1/2 to 1/3 less the cost of other therapies (e.g., stem cell or bone marrow transplants) and the response rate for photopheresis is much higher.[98, 99]

UVBI can be tried on any chronic illness such as RA, CFS, Lyme Disease, Fibromyalgia—that is, any disorder where a hidden pathogen like Mycoplasma could be the cause. Dr. Josephs admits that there must be some unknown infectious microorganism at work to cause RA, otherwise minocycline would not be effective. However, he notes that some patients may not be able to follow a long-term antibiotic regimen, so UVBI could be tried as an adjunct to the antibiotic protocol for faster results.

Photopheresis is currently undergoing clinical trials[100] at more than 100 centers around the county for the treatment of graft-versus-host disease, Lupus, MS, systemic sclerosis, myasthenia gravis, RA, HIV-associated disease, pemphigus vulgaris, and autoimmune insulin-dependent diabetes. At the Yale Cancer Center,[101] Dr. Richard L. Edelson developed a highly successful method of fighting Cutaneous T-Cell Lymphoma (CTCL) using a variation on UVBI.[102] He called his version Transimmunization. His group has applied photopheresis to the immunobiology of normal and diseased skin and conditions involving T-cell physiology.[103] CTCL was found to be a cancer of "cutaneous T cells" that migrate to and infiltrate the skin.

The procedure does not remove the cause of the disease but has some temporary benefit by depleting infected white blood cells (WBCs) that cause inflammation and destructive enzyme action. After the UV-treated WBCs are returned to the body, the immune system recognizes the dying abnormal cells and begins to produce healthy lymphocytes to fight against those cells. Infected WBCs gradually regenerate, so the procedure must be repeated.[104, 105]

UV has long been known to inactivate viruses while preserving their ability to be used as antigens in the preparation of vaccines. The theory is that the viral genome is more sensitive to UV damage than viral surface antigens. Thus, the virus can be killed by damage to its nucleic acids while at the same time leaving antigenic surface components (proteins, glycoproteins, and/or fatty acids) relatively intact. Viral illnesses remain a major challenge for medicine, since there are very few antiviral drugs and those are met with strong resistance *in vivo*.

Immune system dysfunctions are increasingly recognized as playing a major co-factor role in many disease processes, including cancer. Given the range of applications of UVBI therapy and its proven effectiveness, rediscovery and widespread use of photopheresis therapy is warranted.[106]

THE WD-40 MYTH [107]

A popular myth has grown around the use of WD-40 as a joint lubricant and pain reliever for arthritis. In theory, the liquid is sprayed on the painful joint much as one would fix a squeaky mechanical hinge. To date, no credible scientific studies have shown any benefit from the use of WD-40 for arthritis. In fact, there may be cumulative harmful effects. The manufacturer's warning indicates that contact with skin and vapors is harmful. WD-40 contains petroleum distillates, as do gasoline and oil. Problems ranging from mild skin rash to severe allergic reactions have been reported. Prolonged exposure can cause cancer and other serious health problems.

WD-40 has a documented dangerous synergism with insecticides, notably pyrethrin, the active ingredient in head lice medication.[108] Pyrethrin is made from dried, concentrated powder of flowers from the chrysanthemum family. Both the natural pyrethrin and synthetic pyrethroid insecticides mimic the hormone estrogen, which causes cell proliferation. Misuse of these chemicals can cause growth of breast cancer cells, endocrine disruption, kidney problems, and nerve damage.[109]

Proponents of WD-40 may be experiencing a placebo effect or may realize some temporary benefit from increased blood circulation in the affected area as the substance is massaged into the skin. Breathing the vapor may have a temporary pain-killing effect, but delicate linings in the nose, throat, mouth, and lungs may be damaged.

OXYGEN THERAPIES [110]

Oxygen treatments have been shown to be beneficial in cases of viral or bacterial infection.[111] Most bacteria associated with RA are anaerobic or borderline anaerobic. Thus they would be expected to respond to oxygen therapy. Furthermore, there is a synergy between oxygen and antibiotics. However, the FDA is currently discouraging oxygen treatments for valid reasons: the therapy has a very narrow safe dosage range and requires precision in the amount administered.[112] There are several types of oxygen therapies, described in the following subsections.

Hyperbaric Oxygen Therapy (HBOT)

Hyperbaric treatment with pure oxygen (O_2) at two atmospheres has been used to treat AIDS, arthritis, diabetes, mononucleosis, Chronic Fatigue Syndrome (CFS), Multiple Sclerosis, and infections with anaerobic bacteria. The chamber works by forcing oxygen into compromised cells and tissue, thus allowing the normal infection-fighting function of white blood cells to proceed. Hyperbaric oxygen therapy (HBOT) is believed to enhance the antimicrobial effects of antibiotics. It is commonly used to treat deep-sea divers who have "the bends." This treatment is commonly used in Europe, lasting 1-2 hours in the chamber 2-3 times/week for several months.

HBOT provides oxygen to promote angiogenesis (new vessel growth), collagen production, and wound healing in the ischemic or infected wound. Adequate supply of oxygen is key in the treatment of osteomyelitis. Be aware that HBOT can lower blood sugar, so eating a protein snack before treatment is helpful. Some clinicians suggest 400 IU of vitamin E to prevent oxygen toxicity. The treatment can increase blood pressure and induce a Jarisch-Herxheimer flare (discussed in Chapter 3). In a study to determine whether HBOT is effective for Lyme Disease, 84.8% of those treated showed significant decrease or elimination of symptoms. All except one of the 91 subjects developed a severe Herxheimer reaction, which for some participants continued for nearly a month after the treatments ended. Most subjects then began to show major improvement.[113]

Non-healing wounds in the leg and feet are a serious complication of Type 2 diabetes[114] and an excellent example of the type of wound that would respond well to HBOT. Half of all amputations performed each year are related to diabetic wounds. Most insurance companies and Medicare cover hyperbaric oxygen therapy for certain conditions.[115] However, doctors may not be taught about HBOT in medical school, so if they are not aware of a therapy they will not prescribe it.

HBOT has been used in cases of "flesh-eating" (necrotizing) bacteria." The *Streptococcus A* bacterium is a mutated strain of the microbe that causes strep throat, a common childhood disease. The bacterium isn't precisely "flesh-eating" but it has same effect—it produces toxins that deprive the cells of oxygen until they die. These bacteria may originate within the body, in deep traumatic wounds, or around foreign matter. Methicillin-Resistant *Staphylococcus Aureus* (MRSA), an increasingly troublesome and often lethal nosocomial (hospital-acquired, or secondary) infection, is another cause of necrotizing disease.[116]

Recent studies suggest that a low oxygen state prevails in cases of stroke, severe burns, skin grafts, radiation therapy, cerebral palsy, autism, or chronic viral infections. HBOT may be helpful in these cases.[117]

Migraine Headaches

HBOT can treat severe migraines and cluster headaches effectively. However, HBOT is costly, the treatment does not prevent future attacks, and the special equipment is not widely available. Migraines, which afflict over 300 million people worldwide, used to be considered a vascular one, but recent research finds it to be neurological, related to a sudden wave of nerve cell activity that sweeps across the brain. The root cause of migraines may be brain stem malfunctioning. Triggers are linked to intake of certain foods, especially wheat, dairy, sugar, chemical additives, cured or processed meats, artificial preservatives, alcohol, aspartame, caffeine, and/or MSG.[118] These are discussed in Chapter 7. The EFT type of Energy Psychology (also in Chapter 7) can achieve relief 50-80% of the time and results are often permanent.

Ozone Therapy

Ozone (O_3) by inhalation or ingestion must be done very carefully as ozone inhaled directly is poisonous. Ozone generators sold commercially as home appliances to clean the air pose a potential hazard since improper use can burn the lungs. Ozone dissolved in water forms hydrogen peroxide (H_2O_2), which stimulates inflammation in joint tissues, so this treatment is not advised for arthritics. However, controlled H_2O_2 therapies can be helpful for detoxing.

H_2O_2 Treatments

H_2O_2 is an effective and non-toxic topical antiseptic. It is included in toothpaste and mouthwash formulas to prevent gingivitis. The molecule is unstable and when warmed, degrades into water and oxygen. H_2O_2 at 10% in water is actively virucidal and sporicidal. A 3% solution is often used to cleanse and disinfect wounds, since anaerobic bacteria are particularly sensitive to oxygen. Dilute H_2O_2 injections or infusions seem to facilitate the immune response and disable some pathogenic organisms. Some cells of the immune system generate H_2O_2 while other *in vitro* enzymes act to suppress H_2O_2.[119, 120] This treatment is considerably less expensive than hyperbaric treatment, but it still involves some degree of risk if administered intravenously. Very few doctors are skilled in administering H_2O_2 treatment.[121]

Hydrogen peroxide is produced naturally in the body as part of the histamine reaction and subsequent inflammation. An element of the cell called "peroxisome" has the job to produce H_2O_2 to destroy invading viruses, bacteria, and other contaminating substances that try to attack the cell. Peroxides must be administered with extreme caution since misuse can produce anaphylactic reactions in hypersensitive individuals. Treatments can be effective if a diluted, low dose is tried first, then very gradually building up to a stronger solution. Similarly, ozone should be dissolved in a saline solution and slowly infused, gradually increased to the optimal level. A safer alternative to H_2O_2 is intravenous ascorbic acid, which oxidizes, then delivers H_2O_2 to the interior of infected cells systemically. Ascorbic acid (vitamin C) taken orally will counter natural H_2O_2 and the histamine reaction.[122]

Some invading pathogens also can generate H_2O_2 that in some unknown way must benefit the invader. Clues might be found in 2011 research into the behavior of Kaposi's sarcoma-associated herpes virus (KSHV) that establishes a latent infection in the host following an acute infection. H_2O_2 induces KSHV reactivation from latency through signaling the immune system to respond. KSHV spontaneous replication and reactivation can be mediated by H_2O_2.[123]

Endnotes and continuing research on topics in Chapter 1 can be found at www.RA-Infection-Connection.com

2. HOW THE IMMUNE SYSTEM WORKS

Observing pathogenic microorganisms, one is tempted to assign an almost human intelligence to their actions. They seem to strategize, cunningly evade detection, make allies, and skillfully organize to wage war to overcome opposing elements of the immune system. This is a fallacy, of course, but for ease of explaining the infection connection to a general audience, this book will characterize interactions between pathogens and the immune system's defenses in familiar military combat terms.

Microorganisms have no capability to think or reason. They are simply able to adapt at higher rates of selection, to mutate rapidly, and to react to specific stimuli. During their short life cycles within their own microbiome,[1] most die early, but the survivors select out and replicate with new imprinting.

Similarly, coordination among elements of the immune system appears to be intelligently orchestrated by the participating cells and organs, but it is really an example of nature's evolved design of the human biosphere.

In-depth research into the complex functions of the immune system has only been performed since the 1970s. Before that time, immune system status was used only as an indicator of one's general health. For instance, white blood cell counts were tested; a high count indicated that the body was trying to fight an infection. Antibiotics were then usually prescribed as heavy artillery to destroy the infection. Corticosteroids (cortisone compounds), NSAIDs, and/or DMARDs were then given to combat the inflammation and to stop some viral replication. Unfortunately, these drugs also suppress the immune system.[2]

The greatest risk of death following any surgery is a nosocomial (secondary) infection contracted during recovery at the hospital. This is because the drugs associated with nearly all surgeries depress the immune system to some extent, leaving the body vulnerable to infection.

Not all aspects of the immune system are fully known because it is so pervasive and interrelated with all parts of the body. What we do know is that the medical community tends to view afflictions like cancer as a local, specific disease. However, it may be that cancer is merely a symptom of a larger problem—a malfunctioning immune system coupled with a dysfunctional gut. Conventional medicine is focused on treating symptoms in the short term rather than seeking the root causes of chronic illness. Naturopaths and clinicians who practice integrative medicine take a holistic, long-term view.

Our Western science is mechanistic (i.e., must be demonstrable by double-blind studies) and materialistic (if it is not readily observable, it doesn't exist). This strictly evidence-based, logical approach cannot explain why the methods of Chinese medicine work so well, so even highly successful outcomes are dismissed as "anecdotal." This shortsighted Western view is not very satisfying to the patient who has a complex condition that can't be properly diagnosed or treated, but who is aware of alternative, benign therapies that could perhaps help.

Medical specialists in other body systems—digestive, circulatory, nervous, respiratory, and so forth—see these systems as easily described and can observe their physical connections. By contrast, immune system connectivity is on the molecular level. Moreover, it almost seems to have its own primitive intelligence, acting on the principle of action/reaction, i.e., stimulus/response.

Infections are the most common causes of human disease, produced by bacteria, viruses, parasites, and fungi. Before reaching the infection stage, the invader must run a gauntlet of immune system defenses.

The immune system can be considered to have two lines of defense. The first (innate system) represents a non-specific, rapid response to invading pathogens that attack the entry points of the body. Entry points can be outer (skin, mucosal surfaces, cilia lining the trachea, etc.) or inner (gut, organ surfaces, etc). Innate immunity depends on the genetic constitution of the individual. All living things have innate immunity to respond to polymicrobial attacks.

The second (adaptive system) is highly specific with a finely tuned memory of foreign invaders it has encountered before, and capable of a potent response on subsequent exposures. The adaptive immune system frequently incorporates cells and molecules (called "complement") of the innate system to be better prepared to fight against returning harmful pathogens. Complement molecules may be activated by antibodies (molecules of the adaptive system) that add to the adaptive system's arsenal.

In the following sections, a brief overview of the inner workings of the immune system is presented in layman's terms in order to set the stage for the chapters to follow.[3]

THE LYMPHATIC SYSTEM [4]

The collection of the immune system's physical elements is called the lymphatic system, though the entire immune system is much more comprehensive than that. Certain types of cells and molecules can create chemicals to aid in the defense of the entire system.

A healthy, uncompromised, functioning lymphatic system protects the bloodstream from malignant cells of all kinds, and also from particulate matter in the form of spores. The lymphatic system acts as a filtration unit. Lymph nodes are small ovoid structures located in various places in the body along a network of lymphatic capillaries and trunks. These 600-700 nodes trap antigens and filter them out of the lymph fluid through the network to the lymph nodes for cleaning and subsequent return to the blood stream.

In nearly every type of trauma, lymph flow is increased from the injured tissue, helping to reduce pressure by removing fluid. The lymph flow also carries away cell debris and other chemical exudates that might lead to further inflammation if they remained at the trauma site. About 90% of this fluid moves from the blood into and around injured tissues to reenter the cardiovascular system. The remaining 10% enters the dead-ended lymphatic capillaries. From there, the lymph fluid flows through a series of progressively larger vessels to two large lymphatic vessels that resemble veins.

The lymphatic system consists of two parts: the primary and secondary organs.

Primary Organs

These are the thymus gland and, collectively, the bone marrow. The thymus is the most powerful organ of the immune system, residing just beneath the breastbone near the heart. The thymus has two functions: (1) produces hormones that stimulate T- and B-cells to develop some measure of immunity against microbes and tumors by prompting interferon production to fight infection, and (2) as an endocrine system organ, produces hormones to regulate metabolism, growth, and sexual development. The endocrine system is discussed later in this chapter.

Bone marrow is the soft tissue located in large bone cavities where stem cells are produced that become leukocytes and lymphocytes. Leukocytes travel through the blood stream on sentry duty, on the alert for invaders. Lymphocytes are sent to the thymus gland where the hormone thymosin helps them mature into T-cells. From there, the T-cells travel to the secondary lymph system organs and into the blood stream. These cells are discussed in subsections below.

Secondary organs

The main organs in this class are the lymph nodes, spleen, adenoids, tonsils, liver, Peyer's patches in the small intestines, skin, and appendix. These are locations where the molecular elements of the immune system begin their work to combat bacteria, viruses, fungi, parasites, and allergens. The spleen is an important organ that filters the blood. Fever and swelling of lymph glands indicate that immune cells are multiplying in an effort to fight off foreign invaders.

In the 1940s and 1950s, it was common practice to remove swollen tonsils in cases of childhood throat infections. We know now that routine tonsillectomies were a contributing factor in the poliomyelitis epidemic of the 1950s because the operation removed lymph nodes essential to a fully functional immune system's first line of defense against disease. The medical community thus unwittingly brought about this iatrogenic (physician-caused) epidemic. Immunologists now insist that the tonsils should be removed *only* under highly serious circumstances. Yet every year more than a million tonsillectomies are performed. Some doctors still do not understand or appreciate the role of the tonsils in immune function.[5]

Incidental (i.e., nonessential) appendectomies are often done when the lower abdomen is opened for other surgery. The operation is done to avoid cost if the patient might possibly develop appendicitis in the future.[6] Appendectomy is the most common emergency surgery performed by U.S. pediatric surgeons. Appendicitis occurs in four out of 1,000 children, and 5-6% of the general population. It is most often misdiagnosed as gastroenteritis or respiratory infection. Up to 20% of appendectomies are performed on infants and children with a normal appendix.[7]

This long-considered "useless' organ is finally being recognized as a useful element of the body, a repository for beneficial gut bacteria as a biofilm colony. Appendectomy increases the risk for Crohn's disease.[8]

CELLS AND MOLECULES OF THE INNATE IMMUNE SYSTEM

The Innate (or Non-specific) Immune System is designed to protect the host against many extracellular organisms. However, it is unable to deal with all protozoa, viruses, and bacteria (intracellular organisms), so it works synergistically with the Adaptive Immune System, discussed later in this chapter.

On or within our bodies we have trillions of microbes of normal resident flora, mainly bacteria, which fight off competing microbial invaders for that same "real estate." The first physical barrier to pathogens' attacks is the skin, which is impenetrable except through an existing opening (scratch, cut, burn, or other damaged area).

Elsewhere in and on the body, protective hair-like cilia move harmful invading microorganisms out from the lungs; coughing and sneezing force both harmful and benign material from the respiratory system; sloughed-off skin takes away potential invaders; the flushing action of tears, saliva, nasal secretions, perspiration, and urine expels pathogens; acidic skin secretions inhibit bacterial growth. Internally, mucous in the respiratory and tracts traps microorganisms. The stomach is a formidable barrier since its hydrochloric acid and protein-digesting enzymes are deadly to many pathogens.

The following sections describe the specific elements of the Innate Immune System.

Mast Cells and Basophils

Both mast cells and basophils contain electron-dense granules in their cell makeup. Mast cells are present in close proximity to blood vessels in connective tissue, but basophils are in circulation. Both cell types help initiate the acute inflammatory response by cross-linking with the IgE antibody, resulting in both the release of histamine and various cytokines and also in the attraction of neutrophils and eosinophils.

Phagocytes (Leucocytes)

The three main types of phagocytes (also called leukocytes) are neutrophils, macrophages, and dendritic cells. All are white blood cells. Their job is to engulf and ingest other cells, microbes, and foreign particles in a process called "phagocytosis." These cells move through the bloodstream to the site of an injury where they either destroy the invader themselves or produce antibodies that can. Phagocytes cannot destroy viruses.

There are four major steps in phagocytosis:

1. Chemotaxis: become aware of the target and move toward it. Vitamin C enhances motility, but excess zinc levels can suppress it;
2. Opsonization: adhere to the target;
3. Engulfment: ingest the target;
4. Cidal (killing) capacity: destroy the target.

In some cases, e.g., yeast overgrowth, phagocytes can only perform the first three steps, but not the fourth.[9] This is because phagocytosis capability correlates closely with the content and quality of certain proteins that are markers of specific granules released by the neutrophil.[10, 11] A vitamin B_{12} deficiency can seriously reduce phagocytosis efficiency.[12]

The actual destruction of a phagocyte's target uses released free radicals like hydrogen peroxide and superoxide anion. The phagocyte must contain enough antioxidants to protect itself against its release of free radicals (oxidants), or each attack will be suicidal. Phagocytes store the antioxidants vitamin C and the amino acid glutathione to protect themselves. However, in some scenarios, too much vitamin C can suppress phagocytes' cidal (killing) capacity, since the free radicals released to destroy a pathogen are quickly cleaned up before they can do their job. Thus, the phagocyte must regulate its own generation of antioxidants and free radicals to enable it to function efficiently.

In Rheumatoid Arthritis, reactive oxygen intermediate molecules and other toxic molecules made by overproductive macrophages and neutrophils invade the joints, contributing to inflammation.

The many types of phagocytes belong to two groups: myeloid cells (granulocytes) and monocytes. Granulocytes are cells filled with granules of toxic chemicals that digest the invaders. Examples are basophils, neutrophils, eosinophils, and mast cells. Monocytes are short-lived phagocytes that can move quickly to infection sites to become macrophages and dendritic cells. Half of them are stored in the spleen.

Neutrophils

These cells play a key role in the process of acute inflammation. Neutrophils are in the granulocyte category. Their granules contain acidic and alkaline phosphatases, defensins, and peroxidase—all lethal to invading microbes.

Macrophages

Macrophages are long-lived cells that figure in the chronic inflammation process. They can perform phago-cytosis. These cells are associated with specific tissues and are subdivided according to location: monocytes are found in the bloodstream, alveolar macrophages in the lungs, Kupffer cells in the liver, and sinus macrophages in the lymph nodes and spleen. Acute phase proteins are synthesized by hepatocytes in the liver and are produced in high numbers in response to cytokines released from macrophages. Macrophages require the amino acid L-arginine to create the nitric oxide they use to destroy bacteria and viruses. Cancer tumors protect themselves by producing the enzyme arginase that breaks down L-arginine; supplementing a cancer diet with L-arginine, according to studies in England, seems to be helpful.[13] Macrophages eventually die (after surrounding the pathogens) producing the mucous and pus we find as the result of an infection. The effluvia of a cold (e.g., coughed-up phlegm) is a mass of macrophages.

Dendritic cells

Dendritic cells form an important bridge between the innate and adaptive immune systems. They are known as antigen presenting cells (APCs). The types of dendritic cells depend on their location: Langerhans cells are found in the cornea and skin; interdigitating cells are found in the T-cell areas of the lymph nodes and spleen. Dendritic cells engulf external, incoming pathogens, such as bacteria, parasites, or toxins in the tissues and then migrate to the lymph nodes. On their way, as they mature, dendritic cells lose most of their ability to engulf other pathogens but they develop an ability to communicate with T-cells. The dendritic cell uses enzymes to fragment the pathogen into small pieces called antigens. In the lymph node, the dendritic cell displays these "non-self" antigens on its surface by coupling them to a "self"-receptor called the major histocompatibility complex (MHC). This MHC-antigen complex is recognized by T-cells passing through the lymph node. The antigens activate CD4+ helper T-cells.

Eosinophils

Eosinophils are granulocytes having phagocytic properties. Although they represent only 2-5 % of the total leukocyte population, eosinophils are essential to combat parasites that are too big to be phagocytosed. Eosinophils are attracted to cells coated with complement C3b, where they release caustic proteins and metabolites that work together to burn holes in cells and helminths (worms).

A lab test showing a high eosinophil count (>350 cells/mL) is usually associated with autoimmune diseases, allergic diseases (eczema, asthma, hay fever), leukemia, and parasitic infections. A lower-than-normal eosinophil count may indicate alcohol intoxication or an excess of certain steroids, e.g., cortisol.

Natural Killer (NK) Cells

Also known as "large granular lymphocytes," NK cells represent between 5-11% of total lymphocytes in circulation. NK cells possess receptors for immunoglobulins type G (IgG). They also contain two unique cell surface elements: a killer activation receptor and a killer inhibition receptor. The former initiates cytokine (warning) molecules. The latter inhibits this warning from being sent.

NK cells attack and destroy virally-infected cells and certain tumor cells by releasing performing and granyzymes from its granules, which induce apoptosis (programmed cell death). NK cells are also able to secrete interferon-γ (IFN-γ), which serves two purposes: (1) prevents healthy host cells from becoming infected by a virus; (2) augments the T-cell response to other virally-infected cells.

NK cell activity is a vitally important indicator of the strength and health of the adaptive immune system. NK cells deal with any invaders that have passed the sentries in the mucous membranes and the tonsils. Each NK cell contains several small granules that act like explosive charges. E.g., when a cancer cell is recognized, the NK cell attaches itself to it and injects the granules into the cancer cell where they explode. Destruction takes less than five minutes. The NK cell then moves on to another invader. Healthy NK cells can attack two or more invaders or infected cells simultaneously.

Individuals having illnesses characterized by chronic fatigue, autoimmune diseases, cancerous tumors, and viral infections are likely to have low NK cell activity. They should request the 4-hour 51Chromium release assay test for NK cell activity. Chapter 6 discusses this test.

Complement

The complement system represents a large group of independent, complex blood proteins secreted by liver cells called hepatocytes, and by monocytes. Although these proteins maybe activated by both the innate and adaptive immune systems, the name refers to the fact that these proteins help or "complement" the antibody response.

In the innate system, activation of complement is via the invading microbe itself. The adaptive system requires the interaction of antibody with a specific antigen. When activated, complements attack in order, C1-C9. They pierce the enemy invader's cell wall, rupturing the cell and spilling out the contents. They then signal the macrophages and neutrophils to come and clean up the mess. Complements can bind to certain immunoglobulins and B-cells.

The functions of the complement system are: opsonisation (binding), lysis (destruction of a cell through damage/rupture of plasma membrane), chemotaxis, and activation of mast cells to initiate inflammation. C3 (Complement 3) is the most important serum protein of the complement system. Binding of the antigen to C3 results in its enzymatic conversion to C3b. The bacterial cell wall can either remain bound to C3b and become opsonised by phagocytes or act as target for other complement proteins (C5 through 9) that form the membrane attack complex (MAC) to induce cellular lysis. Regulatory proteins, found on the surface of the host cells, protect healthy cells from damage and/or destruction.

Proteins and Enzymes

When the immune system detects a harmful foreign invader, mast cells release the protein histamine into nearby cells. The histamine causes small blood vessels to expand and the surrounding skin to swell, starting the inflammation process. The expansion of the blood vessels causes an increased number of infection-fighting leucocytes to be sent to the inflammation site. The swelling of the surrounding skin makes it harder for an infection to spread to other parts of the body. The histamine reaction can also affect the nerves in the skin, making the skin feel itchy. It can also cause constriction of smooth muscle tissue.

An allergic reaction is an immune response that should not happen because the triggering substance(s) should not be dangerous to us. In the case of severe allergic reaction, e.g., to peanuts, life-threatening trachea closure and anaphylaxis can occur.[14] Epinephrine injection is the usual emergency treatment.[15]

Histamine poisoning can result from the ingestion of foods containing unusually high levels of histamine. Fish (usually tuna and makerel) and shellfish (usually shrimp and crab) are most commonly involved in such incidents, although cheese has also been implicated.[16] Symptoms resemble those associated with allergic reactions. Studies with asthmatic children showed that histamine overload can be counteracted with specific enzymes.[17]

Antihistamines, steroids, and decongestants can interfere with and weaken the immune system. Vitamin C deficiency can dramatically elevate blood levels of histamine. As a natural antihistamine, vitamin C keeps the immune system from making too many histamines at the start of an allergic reaction, and can detoxify the excess histamine released. Vitamin C reduces the severity with which histamines can attack. Those prone to allergies should keep vitamin C levels high and avoid deficiency. See Appendix V for details.

Collagen is a structural protein that is a component of almost every tissue in the body. For those with rheumatic diseases, the collagen of the blood vessels is destroyed as well as the connective joint tissues. The enzyme collagenase is stored primarily in white cell granules called lysosomes. When an irritant attaches to tissue cells, white cells rush to the site, releasing lysosomes of collagenase and other digestive enzymes designed to destroy the foreign invader causing the irritation. If excessive collagenase is released because there are too many localized white blood cells, the result is the destruction of surrounding tissues as well as the invader. This is how cartilage, a collagen matrix, is destroyed in inflamed joints.

A palliative solution is either to remove the surplus white blood cells or to chemically inhibit the enzymes they produce. Most NSAIDs work to limit lysosomal enzyme action.[18] While these methods will temporarily stop the inflammation, they may leave the irritant in place and do not stop the progress of the disease.

CELLS AND MOLECULES OF THE ADAPTIVE IMMUNE SYSTEM

Sometimes called the Acquired Immune System, the Adaptive System forms the body's second line of defense, developing a memory of past encounters with foreign invaders via lymphocytes (white blood cells), antibodies, immunoglobulins, barrier surfaces (e.g., mucosal surfaces, gut lining), or interleukins. Adaptive immunity depends on the strength and efficiency of APCs that coordinate antigen-specific defense mechanisms. Examples of APCs are dendritic cells, macrophages, and B-lymphocytes (B-cells).

Antigens [19]

Exogenous antigens are molecules that enter the body from the outside environment. These can be inhaled (e.g., pollen triggering an asthma attack), ingested (e.g., peanuts or shellfish prompting an allergic reaction), or introduced under the skin (e.g., a splinter or an injected substance). Exogenous antigen presentation stimulates T-cells to become either cytotoxic CD8+ cells or helper CD4+ cells.

Endogenous antigens are generated within a cell. They can be produced by viruses that replicate within a host cell or by mutated genes (e.g., cancer cells). The host cell uses enzymes to digest virally-associated proteins, and displays (presents) these pieces on its surface to T-cells by coupling them to MHC. Endogenous antigens activate cytotoxic CD8+ T-cells.

Lymphocytes

Lymphocytes are small white cells found in the secondary organs of the lymph system and also in the blood, sent there by the lymph nodes. There are two types of lymphocytes: T-cells and B-cells.

T-cells

T-cells are the master regulators of the immune system. These cells (T is for "thymus") begin development in the bone marrow before maturing in the thymus and accounting for approximately 70-80% of all lymphocytes.

There are various types of T-cells, each with a distinct function:

- Helper T-cells activate macrophages to destroy phagocytosed material; they initiate the immune response to foreign antigens immediately. They also help B-cells make a second, more long-range defense called the humoral antibody. Their quantity is measured as a CD4 protein count;

- Inducer T-cells are a subset of helper T-cells that "induce" development of T_{reg} cells in the thymus;

- Effector or cytotoxic T-cells kill infected cells and tumor cells by binding highly specific receptors on their surface to antigens, breaking them apart. They learn to recognize invaders by previous exposure to macrophages. Some of these T-cells (natural killer or NK cells) are naturally cytotoxic without prior imprinting in the lymphoid organs;

- Memory T-cells persist long after the infection has been resolved, providing the immune system with a "memory" capability to fight future infections;

- Regulatory T-cells (T_{reg} cells) limit the immune response after helper (CD4) T-cells have successfully fought off the invaders. Their quantity is measured as a CD8 count. There are usually about twice as many helper T-cells as T_{reg} cells. CD4 cells recognize antigen fragments on the cell surface and release cytokines to control development of the immune response. CD8 cells then recognize virally-infected cells and kill them. In immune system-impaired diseases like AIDS, the CD4 to CD8 ratio is seriously out of balance, making the body extremely vulnerable to opportunistic infection.

More detailed discussion of T_{reg} cells is warranted because they have such a profound effect on our health. These cells may influence the outcome of infection, autoimmunity, transplantation, cancer, and allergy. T_{reg} cell activity is context-dependent, either playing an important role in the initial stages of many chronic infectious diseases by being manipulated by the microorganism to escape from the immune system's counterattack, or being induced by the host to reduce inflammatory damage. This control function is not static, but rather a process of dynamic interaction with the aim of achieving balance and efficiency in the body. Prevailing wisdom and research suggests that T_{reg} cells are at the hub of this process.[20]

Epithelial cells are one of the four major tissue types found in the human body. (The others are connective, muscle, and nervous tissue). Epithelial cells line the cavities in the body and also cover flat surfaces.[21] The cross-talk between human intestinal epithelial cells and dendritic cells (DCs) helps maintain gut immune balance. Intestinal DCs actively participate in antigen capture across the intestinal epithelia by extending protrusions directly into the inner space of the intestine for antigen sampling.[22] These specialized DCs have been shown to drive the development of T_{reg} cells, teaching them to recognize specific food molecule shapes as harmless. Gut inflammation of epithelia interferes with this T_{reg} learning. Epithelial dysfunction thus contributes to chronic conditions such as Crohn's Disease.[23]

Certain substances like vitamin A are vital to T_{reg} cell activity within the intestinal tract. Research reveals that vitamin A metabolites are essential for multiple physiological processes, ranging from vision to embryonic development.[24] Vitamins A and D are distinct from other vitamins in that their respective bioactive metabolites have hormone-like properties.[25] A synergy between vitamins A and D, zinc, and fiber has been proposed to benefit patients with asthma.[26]

Vitamin D[27] plays an important antimicrobial role in protecting against infection in the brain. Vitamin D is also an important antioxidant; suppresses inflammatory cytokines; enhances neurotrophins (a nerve growth factor), and increases hippocampal density.[28] The hippocampus is an important brain structure that plays a role in autism.[29] Clinical disorders such as depression, Post Traumatic Stress Disorder (PTSD), and attachment insecurity are shown to be linked with reduced hippocampal cell density.[30]

Chronic illness is characterized by inflammation and oxidative stress. Dr. Michael Ash recommends specific supplements shown below in Table 2.

All offer vital immune system support, but note that some have both anti-inflammatory and antioxidant effects. Dr. Ash notes that routinely consuming foods with inadequate fiber has a significant negative impact on immune system balance. Major alterations in the microbiota composition of the gut predispose the body to infection and inflammatory diseases.[31] Dr. Mercola has made similar observations.

Some parasites (e.g., helminths, or parasitic worms) can induce regulatory immune responses to modulate parasite-specific immunity in the host and thus allow their own long-term survival and successful transmission. This symbiotic balancing activity benefits the host by modulating the overall immune system activity. Several helminth-derived molecules have been shown to interact with critical immune system cells and either suppress responses or stimulate T_{reg} cells. Research is ongoing to assess helminthic therapy for treatment of IBD, Crohn's disease, allergies, asthma, and autism.

SUPPLEMENT	ANTI-OXIDANT	FREE RADICAL SCAVENGER	INFLAM-MATION CONTROL
Vitamin A	X		
Vitamin C	X	X	X
Vitamin D			X
Vitamin E	X	X	X
Zinc	X		
Glutathione	X	X	X
N-Acetyl-Cysteine (NAC)	X	X	
Ginseng	X	X	X
Grapeseed	X	X	
Green tea	X	X	
Omega 3/6			X
L-carnitine	X	X	X
Fiber			X
Curcumin (turmeric)			X

Table 2: Dr. Ash's Recommendations [32]

B-cells

After several decades, scientists are rediscovering bacteriotherapy (fecal transplantation) to combat *C. difficile* infections and other gut-related diseases like ulcerative colitis.[33] Success rate is an amazing 90%.[34, 35]

About 12% of total lymphocytes are B-cells. Their job is to produce immunoglobulins after they become plasma cells, prevent blood-borne infections, neutralize toxins, and prevent pus-generating bacteria. B-cells can recognize an antigen through surface IgG but usually require the help of T-cells to respond to it, usually through complement. The response(s) are antigen-specific, but the effects may not be.

B-cells are responsible for the development of antibody-mediated immunity known as humoral mediated immunity. When activated by foreign antigen(s), B-cells proliferate and mature into plasma cells (found in the lymph nodes and spleen) that confer their ability to secrete antibodies (as soluble proteins). Not all proliferating B-cells develop into plasma cells. A significant number become memory B-cells through a process known as "clonal selection." This process is vital in eliminating the antigen should the body become re-exposed to it in the future. Some T-cells are also clonally selected to be memory T-cells. Although T- and B-cells behave differently, both are able to recirculate around the body migrating from blood to tissue and vice versa. This migratory capability (motility) increases the efficiency of the immune system to track and destroy the invading antigen(s).

B-cells have a relatively short life span compared to T-cells. Once the B-cells have created a specific antibody to attack a specific pathogen, their primitive intelligence remembers this information and will know it later should they run up against the same pathogen. This is called "building resistance."

Antibodies

There are two types of immune response: (1) cell-mediated and (2) humoral antibody response. The first is characterized by the production of cells that recognize and bind antigens on the surface of foreign cells. This binding action kills cells in the case of viral infections and induces other cells (macrophages) to participate in the immune system reaction, which involves T-cells.

The humoral antibody response refers to antibodies that circulate in the bloodstream and bond to antigens. This bonding renders the antigens easier for phagocytes to ingest and destroy. The humoral antibody response involves B-cells, and activates complement to kill the antigen.

When many antibodies are bound to antigens in the bloodstream, they form a large lattice network called an "immune complex." When the immune complex builds within small blood vessels that nourish tissues, and inflammation initiates there, the effect is harmful. Immune complexes, immune cells, and inflammatory molecules can also block blood flow and ultimately destroy organs such as the kidney. This can occur in people with Lupus. In 2011, autoimmune disease antinuclear antibodies (ANA) were found in 13.8% of the population. A surprising study result was the prevalence of ANA to be lower in overweight and obese individuals than persons of normal weight. Perhaps fat tissues secrete proteins that inhibit antibody production.[36]

Immunoglobulins (Ig)

Antibodies are Y-shaped protein molecules called immunoglobulins (Ig) produced by the B-cells. An antibody does not destroy an invader by itself, but seizes the enemy with one of the branches of its "Y," holding it for destruction by complements C1 through C9.

There are five classes of antibodies: IgA, IgD, IgE, IgG, and IgM. All are functionally distinct from one another, but all are designed to defend against invading bacteria, viruses and microbes in special ways, depending on the location in the body. For example, IgA and IgE are found in our bodily secretions, i.e., in saliva, tears, and in the mucosal membranes of the lungs, genitals, and GI tract.

Characteristics of antibodies are:

- IgA: represents the first line of defense against microbes (especially viruses) invading the body's mucosal barriers. IgA antibody production increases during exercise, lovemaking, and laughter. This explains the phrase "laughter is the best medicine;"

- IgD: antigen receptor on B-cells;

- IgE: primary defense against allergies and parasites. An estimated half million IgE molecules can bind to a single mast cell and trigger the release of histamines that increase immune response and blood flow. IgE is the antibody responsible for allergic (anaphylactic) reactions;

- IgG: the main antibody in blood and tissue fluid; crosses the placenta to give the newborn humoral immunity where circulating antibodies predominate;

- IgM: present on B-cell surface; the secreted form is the main antibody in early response against antigen; good at activating complement; reaches 75% of full potential at 1 year.

Sulfur-containing amino acids are necessary in the diet for antibody formation. These are cysteine, methionine, taurine, and homocysteine. Cysteine is found in poultry, yogurt, egg yolks, red peppers, garlic, onions, broccoli, Brussels sprouts, oats, and wheat germ. Taurine is found in eggs, fish, meat, milk, clams, squid, octopus, and oysters. Methionine is found in animal products, and is important to control fat levels in the liver and the arteries. Plant foods that contain methionine are beans, seeds, onions, peanuts, lentils, and some grains.

Cytokines

Released primarily by activated T-cells, but also by other immune and non-immune cells. Cytokines are small, short-range, multifunctional, short-acting mediators of cellular immune system activities. They have a variety of roles including chemotaxis, cellular growth, and cytotoxicity. Owing to their ability to control immune activity, they have been described as the "hormones" of the immune system. There are four classes of cytokines: Interleukins, interferons, colony-stimulating factors (CSFs), and Tumor Necrosis Factors (TNF-α and TNF-β).

Interleukins

Interleukins are hormones that coordinate the battle conducted by immune system cells against invaders. One type of interleukin attracts T-cells to their targets and tells them when to create interferons, to escalate the immune system response by calling upon NK cells, and to stimulate B-cells to produce antibodies. The body creates interleukins naturally when one is exercising, happy, and generally enjoying life. Both interferons and interleukins are lymphokines, the type of hormone that both infected cells and antigen-activated T-cells create to mobilize the other cells in the immune system. The U.S. Food and Drug Administration (FDA) approved synthetic interleukin therapy against cancer in 1992.[37]

Interferons

When a cell is attacked by a virus, it can create an interferon that will warn other cells of an impending infection. The uninfected cells can then arm themselves with antiviral substances for protection. The name "interferon" derives from its function: the ability to interfere with viral infections. Studies have shown that natural interferons and interleukins are extremely effective and have no side effects. Synthetic interferon has been found to help patients with chronic Hepatitis C.[38]

Colony-Stimulating Factor (CSF)

CSFs are secreted glycoproteins (integral membrane proteins) that bind to receptor proteins on the surfaces of stem cells. The binding process activates intracellular signaling pathways that can cause the cells to proliferate and differentiate into a certain kind of (usually white) blood cell.

Tumor Necrosis Factor (TNF)

TNF is a chemical that macrophages produce to destroy tumors. This has some benefit for cancer patients, but studies have shown that over a long period of time, high TNF levels can lead to tissue (rather than tumor) destruction and eventually to death. This accounts for the wasting syndrome in AIDS patients. TNF has been synthesized with the hope that it can be a controlled treatment for cancer.[39]

Autoimmunity

The ability to react against self-antigens is known as autoimmunity. The causes of autoimmune diseases are multifactorial, a result of breakdown of one of the immuno-regulatory mechanisms. The main predisposing factors are age, gender, infection, and genetics.

MHC molecules and their cell surface proteins are the essential elements of T-cell induced immunity. There is a strong correlation between these proteins called human leucocytic antigen (HLA) and certain systemic, chronic illnesses.[40] One of the most important areas of research today is the association between HLA and autoimmune disease, as exemplified by the relative risk of suffering from Ankylosing Spondylitis (AS) where the prevalence of HLA-B27 is 90%. HLA-B27 is discussed in Chapter 6.

THE ENDOCRINE SYSTEM: HORMONES

Scientists in the 1950s were convinced that hormonal deficiency was the cause of RA. Hormone therapy may provide some relief for RA sufferers; however, the benefit derives from the regulation of the immune system. Since every cell in the body participates in the immune system, a discussion of the endocrine system and hormones is in order.

A wide variety of physiological processes are carried out by the endocrine system through chemical messengers called "hormones." The endocrine system is a collection of glands that produces hormones necessary for normal bodily functions, e.g., coping with stress, fighting infection, dealing with trauma, and adapting to changes in temperature. Hormones control sexual reproduction, growth, and the development of essential bodily fluids. The brain contains at least 45 different kinds of neurotransmitters, many of which act as hormones elsewhere in the body.

Endocrine system glands include the hypothalamus, thymus, pituitary, thyroid, parathyroid, adrenal medulla and cortex, pancreas, testicles, ovaries, and, during pregnancy, placenta. The gut makes several hormones that regulate digestion. The kidneys generate a hormone that stimulates red blood cell production. The endocrine system's ductless glands and the hormones they secrete on demand enable changes in the metabolic actions of the body's tissues.

The adrenals produce steroid hormones, including cortisone, which reduce inflammation by strengthening the membrane of lysosomes, the cell structures that release inflammatory substances. Inflammation of local tissues is designed to stop the spread of infection to other parts of the body. When excess cortisone (natural or synthetic) is present, the lymph glands wither, and this in turn depresses immunity. The natural hormones usually have no harmful side effects, unlike their synthetic counterparts. When the body produces too little of a particular hormone or enzyme, physicians can usually treat the condition successfully by augmenting or replacing the substance. In cases of hormone excess, surgery or radiation is the usual treatment.

The hormone estrogen exerts partial control of the gene that stimulates the production of corticotropin-releasing hormone. The process starts with cholesterol being synthesized through a series of adrenal gland modifications to become various steroid hormones. One end product of this process is cortisol, which may explain why women tend to have slightly elevated cortisol levels. These higher levels, in combination with other factors, such as falling estrogen levels associated with menopause, may be the reason why women are more vulnerable than men to autoimmune diseases like Lupus and RA.[41] Cortisone is the inactive precursor molecule of cortisol (discussed in Chapter 3).

Since the 1970s, it has been known that certain cellular elements of the immune system are intimately involved in the inflammatory reaction characterizing Rheumatoid Arthritis.[42] Specialized T-cells ($\gamma\delta$T and CD4+ T_{reg} cells) gather at inflammatory sites in autoimmune disorders such as RA, Lyme Disease, celiac disease, and Sarcoidosis. Evidence suggests that these T-cells may have a regulatory role in suppressing inflammation, representing an important link between the innate and adaptive immune responses through stimulation of dendritic cells. This activation occurs through a substance called Fas ligand (a surface protein in the TNF family).[43] A 2010 experiment successfully demonstrated a sustained therapeutic reduction in RA disease activity by increasing the numbers of CD4+ and CD8+ T_{reg} cells to ameliorate inflammation.[44]

EMOTIONS AFFECT THE IMMUNE SYSTEM

There is a comparatively new science in Western medicine called psychoneuroimmunology: determining the effect of emotions on the immune system.[45] Studies show that human immune cells have receptors for chemicals produced by the brain, and thus by our thoughts. Even more recently, it was found that the immune cells actually generate some of the chemicals that were for some time assumed to be created only by the brain. A positive mental attitude has been recommended for years as a strategy to deal with a chronic or fatal disease.[46] The Noetic Institute in Petaluma, CA[47] has collected case histories of over 3,000 patients who experienced spontaneous remission of cancer. Common to all cases was their ability not only to transcend their cancer, but also to overcome their <u>fear</u> of cancer.

Hate and fear are negative emotions that are like a deadly toxin to the immune system. This is where meditation, counseling, and love can play a role in healing. Learning to meditate—to still the mind—can be as powerful as the best medicine ever prescribed. It is free and available at any time. Self-hypnosis and other methods are discussed in Chapter 7.

Endnotes and continuing research on topics in Chapter 2 can be found at www.RA-Infection-Connection.com

3. HOW INFECTION WORKS

Inflammation is the way the body generally responds to infection or other form of trauma, such as impact or muscle damage. We are all familiar with the signs of pain, swelling, warmth, and redness associated with this kind of trauma. These symptoms are beneficial because cells of the immune system are attracted to the injured area where they fight the infection, then clear away the debris in preparation for tissue regrowth and repair.

CAUSES OF INFLAMMATION

Chemicals known as cytokines and prostaglandins control the infection process, and are released in an orderly and self-limiting manner. When the immune system is functioning properly, inflammation is beneficial. It is the body's way of ridding itself of potentially harmful agents such as bacteria and viruses.

A significant problem arises when the process does not end at the appropriate time. That is, trauma or infection may trigger inflammation, but the immune system continues to fight in an unabated active state. This explains the autoimmune label that the medical community assigns to Rheumatoid Arthritis. During this complex process, the body responds by moving calcium to the site, forming nodules of dry, gritty, calcium hydroxyapatite crystals that clump around the invading microbes. These may be mistaken for the uric acid crystals of gout. These nodules can be seen as "hot spots" on a radioisotope scan or MRI.

Many of the natural chemicals generated by the immune system's inflammatory response are those that cause the pain of RA and, over time, can damage cartilage. The drugs prescribed to relieve RA pain and associated chronic fatigue are aimed at inhibiting this natural chemical overproduction but the drugs do not remove the root cause.

In RA, inflammation is directed toward the synovium, or joint lining. Nearby blood vessels enlarge, new blood vessels form, and joint fluid increases, creating tenderness and pain in and around the joint, usually with stiffness, visible swelling, and redness. A low-grade fever, along with swollen lymph nodes—glands of the immune system that produce lymphocytes—may indicate systemic or regional inflammation. Calcium nodules of accumulated inflammatory tissue may appear in the lungs and/or just beneath the skin. The more prominent and painful these nodules, the more serious the RA condition. Many patients with chronic infections exhibit RA signs and symptoms although they are not formally diagnosed with RA.

All forms of RA have an inflammatory component, show evidence of connective/synovial tissue damage, and are under the aegis of a process *resembling* an autoimmune reaction. This is perhaps because the invaders bind to or stealthily invade normal cells and can still occasionally be detected as foreign. In a genuine autoimmune reaction, the body attacks its own cells, but in RA, the reaction is actually the body's natural defense against an infection in the connective tissues. This struggle is the cause of the inflammation, pain, and disfiguring effects of RA since the disease agent is connected to the cell. When the disease agent is removed, the fight ceases.

However, the autoimmune theory has become so entrenched in U.S. medical school teaching that other options or considerations, e.g., the role of pathogenic microbes or genetics, were not considered until the mid-1990s when Human Genome Project findings were published. Before those breakthrough insights were known, autoimmunity needed to satisfy four postulates first formulated by Ernst Witebsky's and his colleagues in 1957:

1. identification of circulating or cell-bound
   antibodies in patients with the disease;

2. demonstration of the specific antigen against
   which the immune response is directed;
3. induction of antibody against this antigen in
   experimental animals; and
4. development of pathological changes similar to
   the disease in question in the appropriate
   tissues of the experimental animal.

These outdated rules were modified in 1993[1] and the revisions were not incorporated into medical textbooks until after 1995.[2] We can thus assume that physicians who graduated before 1997 are probably reluctant to accept the notion of an infectious polymicrobial infection as the underlying cause of chronic illness, since they were taught to rely on Witebsky's postulates from the 1950s and Koch's from the 1800s. These are discussed in Chapter 9.

One example of a misnamed "autoimmune disorder" where the linkage to mycobacterial infestation is usually undetected is the development of acute rheumatic fever following a streptococcal infection. Individuals who show evidence of nodules at the joints—a classic and disfiguring symptom of RA—are frequently those who have a history of streptococcal infections, usually from childhood.[3] Streptococcus is discussed in Chapter 4.

Dr. Brown found that diagnostic tests could detect streptococcal antibodies still present, along with the residual strep bacterial cell wall-deficient (CWD) L-forms. He recommended that anti-streptococcal treatment using penicillin (or one of its derivatives) first be used to lower the streptococcal level before attempting to eradicate these L-forms. Mycobacteria and other bacteria have the ability to lose part or all of their cell walls when attacked by antibiotics. Transformation to a CWD form allows these microbes to elude antibiotic attack and regrow cell walls later. The problem with using penicillin derivatives is that drug allergies may occur over time, and this limits their usefulness. Also, penicillin *induces* the bacteria-to-CWD transformation but is ineffective in combating the L-forms.

Now, however, with Polymerase Chain Reaction (PCR) analysis of synovial fluid it is possible to detect the genetic material of mycoplasmal microorganisms, L-forms, and other agents of RA and reactive arthritis. A detailed discussion of PCR testing appears in Chapter 6. Much of the research is originating outside the U.S., but American scientists are gradually beginning to explore the possibility of bacterial infection in RA, confirming the findings of Dr. Brown.[4] Patients with other diagnoses such as Lyme Disease or Fibromyalgia and who test positive for Mycoplasma or Chlamydia also exhibit RA signs and symptoms.

Studies have isolated antigens to several gastro-intestinal pathogens from the synovial fluid in patients with reactive arthritis. The most common pathogens the scientists found were Salmonella, Shigella, Yersinia, Borrelia, and Campylobacter.[5, 6, 7] *Proteus mirabilis* and *E. coli* antibodies have been found in RA patients.[8] Urease-positive Proteus bacteria account for 15% of upper urinary tract infections (UTIs). Urease-negative *E. coli* bacteria account for an estimated 75% of UTIs in the bladder. *Staphylococcus saprophyticus* accounts for about 5 to 15% of UTIs, mostly in younger women.[9]

The Pathogen-Cortisol Loop

The stress hormones produced by the hypothalamic-pituitary-adrenal (HPA) glands exert an important effect on the autonomic nervous system, which controls vital functions of heart rate, blood pressure, and digestion. In response to stress, the brain region known as the hypothalamus releases corticotropin-releasing hormone (CRH). In turn, CRH acts on the pituitary gland to trigger the release of another hormone, adrenocorticotropin (ACTH) into the bloodstream. There, ACTH signals the adrenal glands to release a number of hormonal compounds, including norepinephrine (formerly known as noradrenaline), epinephrine (formerly known as adrenaline), and cortisol. All three hormones enable the body to respond to a threat caused by stress or infection.[10] The hormone cortisol, called the "stress hormone," is an essential part of the "fight-or-flight" response. Small amounts of cortisol offer a burst of energy enabling us to survive a stressful situation, lowering sensitivity to pain temporarily, and providing a short–term increase in memory capability and immune system function. Stress triggers a wide-ranging set of bodily changes designed to prepare the body to meet a threat. Continuous stress to the point of misery causes mental despair, depression, and lack of motivation to make positive adjustments to avert a downward emotional spiral. Stress control is discussed in Chapter 7.

Cortisol is key to regulating the inflammatory response of the immune system in so-called autoimmune disorders like RA. In response to an infection, the immune system produces three substances that start the process: Interleukin-1 (IL-1), IL-6, and TNF. These substances, working either alone or in combination, cause the release of cortisol, which in turn takes glucose from the body's reserves to fuel the muscles and brain. Normally, cortisol initiates the gradual reduction of the inflammation process once the threat situation has passed. But in some cases, infectious pathogens find the generated cortisol to be useful since it gradually suppresses the inflammation process before it (the pathogen) can be killed, as shown in the notional pathogen-cortisol loop in Figure 4.

Problems arise when chronic stress puts a constant demand on the immune system to produce higher amounts of cortisol than needed, tipping the healthy cortisol balance. One example of excess stress is disrupted sleep. A little-recognized result of cortisol over-production is known as the Metabolic Syndrome.[11, 12] Also called Insulin Resistance Syndrome, this is a set of risk factors occurring together that can lead to serious conditions such as: impaired cognitive function, blood sugar imbalance (e.g., Type 2 diabetes, hyperglycemia), decreased bone density, decrease in muscle tissue, high blood pressure, persistent inflammation, chronic fatigue, decreased ability to fight infection, greater risk of heart disease, cholesterol imbalance, and stroke. All risks are related to obesity. This syndrome is becoming increasingly common in the U.S. and other industrialized nations.[13]

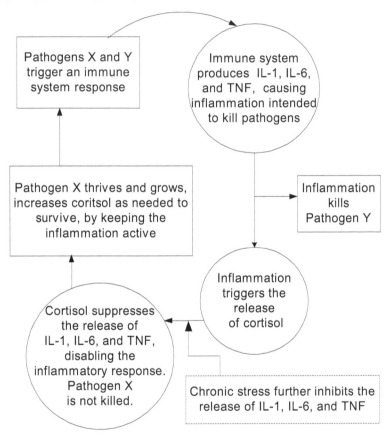

Figure 4. The Pathogen-Cortisol Loop

Research[14] shows that chronic infection plays a role, specifically cytomegalovirus, herpes simplex virus type 1 (HSV-1), *H. pylori*, and *Chlamydophila pneumoniae* (Cpn).[15]

People with insulin resistance feel compelled eat more food to obtain the glucose their bodies have been accustomed to crave. The so-called "hunger hormone" ghrelin may be overactive.[16] The problem is not knowing when to stop eating, and surplus glucose is converted to abdominal fat. When this cycle happens consistently, the result is a potbelly.[17] Vitamin C modulates cortisol production, as shown in Appendix V.

Inflammatory gut conditions such as celiac disease are on the rise in the developed world. The stimulating antigen is dietary gluten, which breaks down into the glycoprotein gliadin. The gliadin attaches to the opiate receptors in the brain, stimulating an appetite for more bread, leading to higher carb intake and eventual obesity. The 2011 book *Wheat Belly* explores this premise, pointing out that modern, genetically modified wheat contains gliadin. Natural wheat pre-1960 did not contain gliadin.

Lack of Sleep Influences Cortisol Production

Chronically disrupted, non-restorative sleep leads the overactive adrenals to produce more cortisol until a relative state of immunosuppression is reached. According to Dr. Franco, Mycoplasmas are commensal "innocent bystanders" that become more aggressive and reproduce when the immune system becomes dysfunctional.

Obstructive sleep apnea is stressful, and has been associated with numerous ailments, including major depression and hopelessness, which are strongly linked to elevated levels of cortisol. One study[18] found that subjects who slept with continuous positive airway pressure (CPAP) machines had measurable reductions in their cortisol levels.

Other consequences of less than 6-9 hours per night of restorative sleep are: lack of focus, memory loss, irritability, constipation, tendency to gain weight (through increased cortisol production), stomach ulcers, and hastening of age-related conditions such as Type 2 diabetes and high blood pressure.[19]

Dental Infections [20]

Sucrose and tobacco are both very harmful to health, and lead to periodontal disease. A 2009 study showed that a low carbohydrate, sugar-free diet prevents almost completely the initiation of periodontal lesions. Incidence of gum disease decreased when study subjects from the city were put in a primitive environment. They were not allowed to brush or floss, but ate a simple, natural food diet compared to their former processed food diet. One conclusion is that perhaps oral hygiene is helpful but not essential to dental health; that proper diet is enough to maintain healthy mucosal balance.[21,22] Inflamed and bleeding gums, symptoms of periodontal disease, are also signs of a severe ascorbic acid (vitamin C) deficiency, indicating scurvy. [23]

An ongoing landmark study (begun in 1986) of autopsied brains of deceased nuns revealed that bacteria and inflammatory mediators originating in the mouth may lead to increased risk of dementia in older adults. The research has shown that folic acid may help stave off Alzheimer's disease; that small, barely perceptible strokes may trigger some dementia; and that early language ability may be linked to lower risk of Alzheimer's.[24] Periodontal disease and cognitive impairment have a number of common risk factors that can influence immune system function and enhance chronic inflammation, including depression, smoking, and diabetes.[25] The *Porphyromonas gingivalis* bacterium plays a key role in Rheumatoid Arthritis.[26, 27]

Plaque deposited under the gum or gingival sulcus is a known gingival irritant leading to inflammation, gingivitis, and periodontal disease. Note that two individuals can have plaque under their gums but one might exhibit a severe inflammatory response and other none. The former may have inflammation in the gums <u>and</u> in the coronary arteries.[28]

Infections occur when bacteria invade the bones of the jaw and the area around the tooth root. Undetected dental infections can cause or exacerbate lymphoma, chronic pain, chronic fatigue, and RA.[29] Failing root canals can often be a source of undetected dental infections, and can be the trigger for other chronic illnesses, especially cardiovascular disease.[30, 31] Root canal failures are difficult to diagnose from traditional 2-D x-rays and may not exhibit any symptoms. A dramatic improvement in diagnoses is the use of digital 3-D cone beam volume tomography, now a dental standard. This type of improved imaging is especially useful for detecting bone disease in the jaw. Oxygen/ozone therapy may be an effective treatment option to tooth extraction or dental surgery.[32]

A research team of 60 leading physicians, dentists, and scientists sponsored by the American Dental Association in the 1990s sought to identify the numerous disease-causing organisms that mutate from aerobic to anaerobic forms after tooth extraction or root canal surgery.[33] The team, headed by Dr. Weston Price, found that microorganisms such as *Entamoeba gingivalis* locked in the root canal produce deadly toxins daily affecting other bodily tissues and resulting in a range of chronic illnesses, including rheumatic diseases.[34, 35, 36]

The toxic effects of amalgams and other metals can cause serious health problems, as discussed in Chapter 7.[37]

Slow-Growing Infections Over a Lifetime

As scientists learn more about the complexities of the immune system and are able to use new research tools and improved testing methods, it may be possible to detect certain destructive pathogens that may not manifest symptoms for decades. Two examples are described in the next sections.

Chlamydial infections [38]

Chlamydia species are ubiquitous, unique micro-organisms, characterized by three distinct life forms: extracellular infectious, intracellular replicating, and intra-cellular cryptic. Hosts that are known to be susceptible to Chlamydial infections are frogs, fish, clams, birds, mammals (cattle, opossums), and humans. Chlamydia is responsible for a variety of mammalian illnesses including: intestinal infection, pneumonia, diarrhea, encephalomyelitis, mastitis, polyarthritis, urogenital tract infection, spontaneous abortion, hepatitis, and inflammation of upper abdomen membranes.

The Chlamydiaceae family consists of two genera and three species, all causing bacterial infections. *Chlamydophila pneumoniae* (Cpn)[39] is discussed here because it is more widely communicable than *C. trachomatis* (the most common of the sexually transmitted diseases in the U.S.) or *C. psittaci* ("parrot fever," carried by any species of birds).[40] Cpn is also a much more stealthy pathogen.

Cpn is an airborne pathogen that infects epithelial cells in the respiratory tract, causing an infection that can be carried to other parts of the body including nerve tissue, the brain, muscles, blood vessel linings, and immune system cells. The standard 1-2 week antibiotic treatment only kills Cpn in one of its three life phases, leaving live forms of Cpn bacteria that are in other stages to renew the infection as they evolve.

The Cpn bacterium has a rugged cell wall and disseminates via the blood stream. It attaches to host cells via heparin molecules, is internalized and becomes a reticulate body. This is an intracellular form having a fragile cell wall with "spikes." Cpn requires host cell energy for replication, and is able to condense back to its elementary body form. The cryptic body form of *C. pneumoniae* is the least understood form of Chlamydia. It does not replicate and form inclusions, but may shift to an elementary body or reticulate body form, and is relatively resistant to antichlamydial agents. Treatment requires a combined antibiotic protocol.[41]

Cpn contains at least two endotoxins that cause tissue damage and inflammation. It can survive lethal attack by macrophages. Cpn is commonly found in mononuclear white blood cells (monocytes), and can also infect epithelial and endothelial cells, smooth muscle cells, lymphocytes (B- and

T-cells), macrophages, astrocytes in the central nervous system, glial and microglial cells, causing chronic infections. Cpn infection has a devastating effect on host cells: replication is followed by cell death; it causes impaired host cell function and signaling; it negatively influences host cell production of nitric oxide, growth factors, cytokines, and chemokines; it inhibits host cell apoptosis by activation of the COX-2 enzyme. All diseases caused by *C. pneumoniae* are characterized by intense and chronic inflammation that is initiated and maintained by re-infection or persistent infection. Diseases where Cpn plays a role are: atherosclerosis, stroke, Alzheimer's dementia, COPD, asthma, Multiple Sclerosis, Pyoderma gangrenosum, heart disease, and interstitial cystitis.

Chronic *C. pneumoniae* is an especially difficult intracellular infection to test for and to eradicate. A wide variety of tests are available, but there is much controversy about which are useful. The clinician must take a detailed patient history and track symptoms, as with Lyme Disease. Important clues can be found by measuring visual contrast sensitivity,[42] discussed in Chapter 6. This test is especially useful when treating patients with mold-related illnesses.[43]

An antimalarial quinine derivative, quinolone AM-1155, investigated in Japan in the 1990s, was shown to be a useful antimicrobial agent for *Mycoplasma pneumoniae* infections and strains of *Chlamydia pneumoniae*.[44]

HSV1 and Alzheimer's [45]

There is strong evidence that Herpes Simplex Virus Type 1 (HSV1) along with Cpn are both major factors in Alzheimer's Disease (AD). Long-term survivors of acute HSV1 brain infection exhibit severe memory loss. The same brain regions are involved in AD. HSV1 infects 90% of adults, and explains the high prevalence of AD in the elderly. HSV1 antibodies were found in the cerebral spinal fluid of elderly patients (with or without AD) but not in younger patients, showing that HSV1 can remain latent throughout life after early infection. PCR tests find HSV1 DNA in a high proportion of elderly patients. This immune response inside the spinal canal confirms that HSV1 is present in the aging brain and that the virus has replicated there, causing an acute, perhaps recurrent, infection persisting for years.[46]

Research results show that 72% of viral DNA is plaque-associated, and that HSV1 is a major cause of plaque formation. Knowing this connection between HSV1 and AD can lead to appropriate, timely antiviral treatment and possibly prevention of AD.[47] Recent studies have shown that while the adaptive immune system has limited access to the brain, the central nervous system (CNS) can still mount a robust response to invading pathogens via antimicrobial peptides (AMPs) and the innate immune system. AMPs are broad-spectrum natural antibiotics our bodies produce to target bacteria, mycobacteria, enveloped viruses, fungi, and in some cases, cancer cells. AMPs are potent immune system modulators that mediate cytokine release. AMPs function in the brain's innate immune system.

A large body of data supports a central role for neuroinflammation in Alzheimer's Disease. Amyloid beta (Aβ) is a peptide of 36–43 amino acids that appears to be the main constituent of amyloid plaques (deposits found in the brains of patients with AD). The inflammatory response in the CNS is mediated by the innate immune system.

A 2010 independent genome wide association study[48] of thousands of European AD patients found the presence of a genetic signature suggesting a viral risk factor in AD. The Aβ peptide showed antimicrobial activity and acted as a defense molecule of innate immunity. The accumulation of plaque deposits may derive from an over-production of Aβ peptides directed against a virus attacking the brain. Therefore, we can surmise that if the normal function of Aβ is to act as a defensive AMP, then an absence of this peptide could mean increased vulnerability to HSV1 infection. Knowing this with certainty can help scientists develop preventive measures for AD.[49]

HSV1 requires arginine to replicate. Foods high in arginine are chocolate, nuts, peanut butter, protein shakes and drinks that contain arginine, oats, porridge, and muscle-building formulas. Lysine inhibits HSV1 replication by competing with arginine. Therapies that use antioxidants and lysine supplements, and adopting a Mediterranean diet high in fresh fruits and vegetables can neutralize the oxidative component of progressive AD and maintain the healthy lysine/arginine ratio.[50]

L-lysine (the L-form of lysine) is one of nine essential amino acids that our bodies cannot make. L-lysine and L-proline are the precursors of hydroxy-lysine (HL), and hydroxy-proline (HP), two constituents of collagen. Collagen is an essential component of arterial linings and joint cartilage. Vitamin C, a strong antioxidant, is also essential for the production of collagen.[51] Linus Pauling found that supplementing the diet with two amino acids, L-lysine and L-proline, can reduce the sticky plaque that clogs the arteries and reduce "bad" cholesterol, especially when combined with vitamin C and CoQ_{10}.[52, 53] Add green tea extract and this therapeutic approach to heart disease could also be an excellent anti-cancer regimen.

THE ROLE OF MYCOPLASMAS

Mycoplasmas were discovered in 1898 and given different names starting in 1910. In 1941 the first classification and nomenclature system was established, but did not catch on because of the ambiguity between Mycoplasmas with bacterial L-forms. In 1956, the current classification system was adopted consisting of a single order, *Mycoplasmatales*, containing a single family, *Mycoplasmataceae*, with a single genus, *Mycoplasma*, and at least seventeen species. Today there are over 100 documented species, although more recent PCR analysis indicates that some previously named species may be identical. Not all Mycoplasmas are harmful. Some are benign (in the tissues, blood, and gut) but others can be pathogenic (in the joints and synovial tissue.)[54]

Mycoplasmal organisms commonly contaminate tissue cultures in lab tests, in which they act as intracellular parasites that alter both cellular and viral molecular events. Since these organisms are difficult to eliminate, questions arise regarding the validity of molecular biology results from tissue culture experiments.[55]

Mycoplasmas are but one type of hundreds of micro-organisms residing in our bodies, part of the indigenous microbial flora primarily in mucosal surfaces, the respiratory and urogenital tracts, but they can invade the bloodstream and travel to organs and tissues throughout the body.[56] Most of the time, these cell wall-deficient microbes are benign, but when they increase in abnormal numbers, a new strain is detected, or they are invaded and colonized by pathogens, the body's immune system reacts to suppress the condition, just as it does when an externally caused infection occurs.[57]

Dr. Brown found that mycobacteria, Mycoplasmas, and their L-forms could cause Rheumatoid Arthritis as well as Lupus and Scleroderma, since they seem to bind to host cell membranes and make those cells a target for a defensive immune system response. Certain dietary fats, e.g. lauric acid (found in coconut oil) and palmitic acid (found in palm oil, palm kernel oil, and coconut oil), form surfactant molecules that can block this binding, interfere with cell signaling pathways (ligands), and even dissolve the microbe/virus's cell membrane.[58] The Western diet, except in tropical countries, includes very little of the unmodified natural forms of coconut, palm, and olive oils.[59]

Mycoplasmas seem to have an affinity for certain parts of the body and attach themselves there, often in biofilm colonies,[60] waiting for the right time to emerge. Experimental animal research has shown that some strains of Mycoplasmas, once isolated, migrate without exception to the joints.[61] Doctors Joel Baseman and Joseph Tully point out that, "It has been suggested that [*M. arthritidis*]-related superantigen-like molecules may exist in Mycoplasmas of human origin triggering autoimmune and other inflammatory pathologies."[62] When this assertion is credibly tested, it will show that mycoplasmal infections are the trigger for autoimmune disorders and will perhaps lead researchers to look beyond the traditionally held belief that such disorders occur because the immune system is malfunctioning. Microorganisms stimulate an autoimmune reaction in the following ways:

- Incorporating host antigen structures into their cell membranes. I.e., when Mycoplasmas are released from cells they bud from the cell membrane like viruses but in contrast to viruses, they do not exclude all host glycoproteins (antigens) from their membranes when they are released. These hybrid (host/microbe) antigens can stimulate an immune response when the host responds against the parts from the microorganism;

- Certain microorganisms, such as Mycoplasmas and some bacteria, use molecular mimicry to "hide" from the host's immune system. This can set off an autoimmune response to the normal antigen being mimicked;

- Some bacteria carry "super antigens" that strongly stimulate the host's immune response; and

- Some bacteria and viruses kill normal host cells, releasing large quantities of normal antigens that may trigger an autoimmune cleanup response.

Problems arise when vaccines are introduced. Vaccines have adjuvant molecules that have been selected to enhance immune system learning and to encourage persistent antigen memory. However, vaccines in the presence of chronic infections teach the immune system to respond more aggressively to the infection-related antigens, as well as to the antigens in the vaccine.

The current medical theory regarding autoimmune disorders is based on the notion of the immune system attacking a single invading/infecting organism in the *in vitro* form, as observed in a lab test culture, not *in vivo*, i.e., within the body. Infections such as malaria, protozoas, and streptococcus have been studied *in vitro* at prestigious medical centers such as the Lister Institute in France. However, Mycoplasmas and L-forms are resident, *in vivo* parasitic "invaders" that become active from time to time to obtain nutrients, expel wastes, breed, and migrate out of the body to form new colonies. These actions precipitate an allergic reaction that only appears to be an autoimmune disorder since no external cause for the reaction is detected by current lab testing methods.

Shape-Changing Organisms

We know from the study of many forms of life that metamorphic changes during the lifespan of an organism run from initial seed through several shape and structure changes, with interim stable forms that adapt to the particular life phase and to the environment, and then change back to seed form again. This ability to alter shape and structure is called pleomorphism. It is probably the combined result of evolution and the many climatic and environmental changes the evolving organism has faced and to which it has had to adapt over hundreds of millions of years and perhaps trillions of trillions of generations. Thus, the vulnerability of one shape or form to an attack or environment change can be circumvented by a defensive adaptation the organism evolves to ensure its resistance to a future attack. Along with this adaptation comes an alteration of the active set of genes in its microbial DNA.

At one time all Mycoplasmas were referred to as L-form bacteria because both lack cell walls. According to Dr.

Brown, Mycoplasmas and bacterial L-forms are vulnerable to various attacks by tetracycline antibiotics in a different way than penicillins, which attack the normal streptococcus cell/cell chain forms, causing Mycoplasmas to transition to the L-form (with reduced or absent cell wall) as an act of survival. Erythromycin and the tetracyclines have broad-spectrum effects on Mycoplasmas and other forms of infection when used in a low-dose, long-term manner. Sometimes to kill both forms of an organism it is necessary to use both a penicillin and a tetracycline, but not at the same time. A tetracycline drug like minocycline will not just negate the effect of penicillin; used together, the combination could exacerbate a Mycoplasma infection.

Penicillin antibiotics temporarily decrease the phagoctyic (germ eating) capacity of leukocytes. The tetracycline family of antibiotics is different from other antibiotics in that it affects the interior of the cell and not the membrane. Specifically, tetracycline inhibits 30-40% of the bacteria's normal folic acid synthesis, which eventually kills the invading pathogen, but the antibiotic also interferes with folic acid synthesis by helpful gut bacteria. NSAIDs like aspirin, ibuprofen, and naproxen—used conventionally in high doses to treat RA—also deplete folic acid.[63]

The question is: should folic acid supplements be used to offset the loss caused by tetracycline or NSAIDs, or will restoring folic acid to the normal level help the infectious microorganism survive? The answer is: bacteria cannot use pre-formed folic acid and must synthesize their own. In contrast, mammalian cells use folic acid obtained from food or from supplements. Therefore, it is worthwhile to take folic acid along with medications for RA.[64]

Chronic pneumonia is a good prototype for what happens when a Mycoplasma infection becomes active around a certain area.[65] Nodules of granulation material—inflamed tissues that surround the infectious organism for months—produce the characteristic cough of the disease. A similar phenomenon happens around the RA sufferer's joints.[66] The body must be trained to defend itself with minimal help from external agents such as antibiotics. This is the reason for very low tetracycline dosage over a period of weeks or months. However, there are certainly circumstances where the only means to cure a chronic cough or other persistent polymicrobial infection like COPD (Chronic obstructive pulmonary disease) are antibiotics of a specific type, prescribed for short duration.[67, 68] Since COPD has other contributing factors, e.g. the Epstein-Barr virus, antiviral medications and vitamin D supplements are also needed.[69]

Souvenirs of Childhood Illnesses

We carry Mycoplasmas and L-forms with us as remnants of childhood infections such as pneumonia, strep throat, bronchitis, rheumatic fever, or other early illnesses. Mycoplasmas are not viruses, since they do not require living cells in which to grow. Mycoplasmas are included within a separate class (Mollicutes) of bacteria because they have lost the ability to develop a cell wall. This makes them harder to see and much harder to culture *in vitro*.[70] They are specifically adapted to certain cellular environments by their genetic nature, which is quite robust in its complexity, having adapted and evolved over millions of years.

Fastidious microorganisms such as Mycoplasmas often lie dormant in the joints or in the organs, waiting for conditions to be favorable for replication as intracellular invaders. This opportunistic latency explains conditions such as RA, CFS, or Gulf War Illness, which only <u>seem</u> to strike suddenly. It also reveals the error of the traditionally held autoimmune disease theory that the apparently healthy, infection-free body mysteriously decides to attack itself.

It is not necessary for the whole Mycoplasma microorganism to be present for a reaction in a joint or tissue to be provoked. Mere fragments are sufficient to create a powerful antigenic reaction that causes the body to produce antibodies to counter it. These antigens are constructed by the host's cells from bits of pathogenic protein and cellular proteins called major histocompatibility complex (MHC) molecules. The processing and assembly of antigens are the keys to understanding the flexibility, specificity, and thoroughness of all immune responses.[71] The antibody reaction may be mainly against a "host antigen" carried on the mycoplasmal membrane.

The affinity of Mycoplasmas or L-forms of cellular bacteria for the tissue and fluid of the joints has been recognized since the 1890s. Experiments by Dr. Brown and Jack Nunemaker in the 1930s demonstrated that the L-form they studied was a variant of the streptobacillus organism. The cellular bacteria was able to lose its capsule and cell wall and enter a state in which it could become invisible, pass through a filter, and return to the parent form, re-growing its cell walls. Chlamydia is another example of a bacterial organism capable of both walled and wall-less states.[72] L-forms can reproduce but the rates are slower than that of the cellular form.

This cloaking capability explains how L-forms are able to "go underground," transmutate, and re-emerge after the immune system attack on the bacterial form has subsided, returning to assault injured cells again, aggressively. An immune system weakened by addictive drugs, anti-depressants, or improper diet is unable to produce the quantity and quality of natural antibodies to stave off this new attack.

Viruses are also able to manufacture proteins that switch off or dampen cellular immune responses. This explains why the common cold can cause a Streptococcus flare. A virus's DNA is capable of infecting or destroying a cell, eluding the immune system by mutating and gene swapping.[73]

Studies in the mid-1990s on ear infections in children concluded that L-forms as atypical forms of bacteria may play an important role in the bacteriologic aspect of secretory *Otitis media*. Both Turkish[74] and New Zealand[75] research groups pointed out the failure of conventional culture methods to identify the responsible pathogen(s).

Further, the researchers showed that some agents are capable of changing bacterial behavior and consequently the clinical course of action. A Russian study identified persistent bacterial forms that performed antigenic mimicry or otherwise protected themselves against the host's immune system response.[76]

Mycoplasmas and Autoimmune Diseases

There are several reasons why mycoplasmal infection can play a role in autoimmune diseases:

- **Cell shape modification.** As Mycoplasmas replicate within invaded host cells and are released from host cells, they seize antigens from the surface of the host cell and incorporate these within their outer surface membranes.

- **Mimicry of normal cells.** Mycoplasmal antigens seem to be able to mimic host antigens or to attach to familiar blood lipoprotein molecules. The body's immune responses become confused, and cross-reactivity results.

- **Infiltrated T-cells.** Standard microbiology textbooks state that the host's cells carry MHC molecules on their surfaces. In infected cells, these MHC molecules bind to and display small peptides from the parasite. It is this combination of MHC molecules and peptides that forms antigens recognizable by T-cells and what makes them candidates for destruction. Infiltrated and compromised T-cells may not function in recognizing or successfully attacking fellow/ different cells that carry parasitic organisms.

- **Apoptosis simulation.** Another possibility is that Mycoplasmas can cause apoptosis or "programmed death" of host cells, after which normal host antigens are released and the body reacts with an autoimmune response.[77] A defective apoptosis gene has been found to be a factor in prostate cancer, possibly contributing to the continued viability of Mycoplasma-invaded prostate cells.[78] Mycoplasmas have been found in seminal fluid.[79] Ascorbic acid in high concentration (at least three grams every four hours for several days) can enhance apoptosis of invaded cells.

SUPPRESSING MYCOPLASMAS AND CELL WALL-DEFICIENT (CWD) MICROBES

Dr. Brown and his colleagues accumulated significant evidence that Mycoplasmas and their CWD L-forms were at the root of RA, as seen in the impressive list of published laboratory results included in *The Road Back*. They discovered that tetracyclines were a group of antibiotics that could kill or radically suppress Mycoplasma and L-form growth in the laboratory. They also found that tetracyclines, together with antihistamines, could relieve RA patients' symptoms when given in a low, controlled dose over a long period (months to years). Dosage and duration depended on the severity of the condition.

In the most serious RA cases, Dr. Brown began with intravenous tetracycline, then transitioned to lower levels after the patient's symptoms had subsided. Where there were other bacterial complications adding to the sensitizing process, Dr. Brown advised using other antibiotics specific to those organisms. Dr. Trevor Marshall's patented but controversial 2007 multi-antibiotic protocol successfully treats CWD bacteria responsible for Sarcoidosis and many other chronic diseases such as cancer and AIDS.[80]

CWD forms of bacteria often have latent and intracellular forms that antibiotics do not reach. Intravenous ascorbic acid (vitamin C) can be used to kill intracellular-infected host cells and tumor cells. Unfortunately, few doctors understand the pharmaco-kinetics of ascorbic acid and its short half-life.[81]

Dr. Brown's research findings explain why arthritis remedies such as quinine, bee venom, gold salts, and copper have been used over many centuries: it is because these substances have also been found to be effective in suppressing the growth of Mycoplasmas *in vivo*.

Quinine

The colonial British stationed in Africa learned of the benefits of quinine in the 1800s as a cure for malaria, a mosquito-borne Plasmodium intracellular parasite. Quinine is derived from the bark of several species of *Cinchona* and during the 17th century was brought to Europe from South America, where it was used to allay fever and pain, dilate the larger blood vessels, and generally relax muscle tissue. Quinine contains alkaloids, which are active organic compounds containing at least one nitrogen atom. Traditional usage is a very small dose, which is more toxic to the parasite than to the host. Alkaloids are potentially toxic in large amounts (e.g., morphine).

Until very recently, quinine sulfate was available inexpensively over the counter (OTC). This drug has been shown to be active against a variety of parasites and also to reduce bursitis, tendonitis, synovitis, and arthritis pain and inflammation. Sadly, it has been removed from the commercial market in the U.S., Europe, and South America for two reasons: (1) malaria is not considered the global scourge it once was, and (2) in rare cases, a severe and possibly fatal Herxheimer reaction can occur.

Other antimalarial drugs are effective against arthritis pain, but they are costly and require a prescription. Quinine sulfate in high doses can be harmful. OTC low dose homeopathic remedies made with trace amounts of quinine are benign but very effective, e.g., for Restless Leg Syndrome. Look for *Cinchona officinalis* on the label.

Bee Venom

Analysis of bee venom shows that it contains some 18 active substances, including mellitin, one of the most potent anti-inflammatory agents known. Bee venom treatments (apitherapy) have been used since ancient times to relieve the inflammation and swelling associated with both RA and Osteoarthritis.[82] Because apitherapy runs the risk of fatal anaphylaxis in some individuals, it is usually avoided by the medical profession for insurance reasons. A skilled clinician, partnering with a beekeeper, can use apitherapy safely. Other documented applications are glaucoma, MS, Alzheimer's, cancer, and leprosy.[83] Ascorbic acid can control the severity of bee venom Herxheimer reactions. See Appendix V.

DR. BROWN'S ANTIBIOTIC PROTOCOL

Since 1949, Dr. Brown's persistence in claiming that RA should be viewed as a bacterial allergy, treatable with anti-Mycoplasma tetracyclines, has run counter to the prevailing view of how antibiotics should be administered. Antibiotics such as penicillin have always been seen as a short-term, high-dosage response used to treat pneumonia, strep throat, bronchitis, and other cell-walled bacterial disorders. They are not usually prescribed over an extended period because physicians believe, correctly, that germs will become more resistant to the antibiotic.

This reasoning applies to the typical course for a prescribed antibiotic treatment, which is 10-14 days. If the patient shows no signs of significant improvement, another class of antibiotic is usually given. Also, if the tetracycline antibiotic *is* effective so that the Mycoplasmas die and the patient experiences an uncomfortable Herxheimer reaction, s/he may opt to discontinue the treatment and not resume. The form and dosage of tetracycline are very important, but pills are more convenient than injections or sometimes painful intravenous drip infusions. However, the latter methods are the best since concentration is higher and more controlled. Also, infusion or injection avoids the GI tract and thus minimally changes the environment of the hundreds of useful microorganisms residing in the gut.

Tetracyclines

Dr. Brown emphasized that a low dose of tetracycline over a long period of time will not have the usual effect of a sudden influx of strong antibiotics, which can interfere with the ability of the immune system to limit fungal infections like *Candida albicans.* Since the mid-1980s, streptomycin-resistant forms of bacteria have developed because of the use of antibiotic pills, which were not 100% effective, and their short-term assaults left behind a cadre of evolved, resilient pathogenic organisms.

The most commonly used types of antibiotics are: tetracyclines, aminoglycosides, macrolides, penicillins, fluoroquinolones, and cephalosporins. The tetracyclines include doxycycline, minocycline, and oxytetracycline.

Dr. Brown's research showed that when tetracycline is used to suppress the defensive lipid envelope the micro-organism builds around itself, the body's own disease-fighting capability can combat it effectively and the RA is eventually driven into remission. Tetracycline antibiotics are among the few that are effective against virtually all species of Mycoplasmas, with relatively low toxicity and few side effects.[84] For decades, physicians have used oxytetracycline to treat adolescent acne with minimal adverse effects.

Doctors Baseman and Tully further vindicated Dr. Brown and his antibiotic approach, saying in 1997, "The occurrence of various Mycoplasma and Ureaplasma species in joint tissues of patients with Rheumatoid Arthritis, sexually transmitted reactive arthritis, and other human arthritides can no longer be ignored. A clinical trial of long-term (6 to 12 months) antibiotic (doxycycline) therapy before cartilage destruction might prove beneficial in managing such frequent and often debilitating infections." This assertion was proved true in a 2005 thirty-month study.[85]

Dr. Brown also found that those individuals who use oxytetracycline over a period of months or years tend to avoid colds, pneumonia, and other respiratory diseases. Other benefits include elimination of the chronic cough associated with COPD[86, 87, 88] and reduction of Irritable Bowel Syndrome (IBS). Tetracyclines are effective against a wide range of bacteria and CWD L-forms.[89] The cautions and guidelines for using tetracycline are: [90]

- not advised for pregnant women or children younger than 8 years;

- depletion of, or interference with, potassium, folic acid, vitamins B_2, B_6, B_{12}, C, and K;

- increased sensitivity to sunburn;

- supportive interaction with probiotics, vitamin B_3 (niacin or niacinamide);

- adverse herbal interaction with goldenseal, Oregon grape, barberry;[91]

- avoid dairy products two hours before and after, as calcium inactivates tetracycline;

- some prescription drug interactions (use the Internet to search[92] or ask your doctor);

- reduced drug absorption/bioavailability of certain minerals (aluminum, calcium, zinc, magnesium, iron).

Dr. Garth Nicolson recommends taking probiotics at least 3 hours after ingesting antibiotics for maximum benefit, otherwise the effects cancel each other. Probiotics are discussed later in this chapter.

Minocycline

According to Dr. Mercola, who has prescribed Dr. Brown's protocol with proven success, minocycline (trade name Minocin) has a distinct and clear advantage over tetracycline and doxycycline in three important areas:

1. Extended spectrum of activity
2. Greater tissue penetrability
3. Higher and more sustained serum levels

Dr. Mercola stresses that Minocin not be given with iron, else over 85% of the dose will bind to the iron and pass through the colon unabsorbed. Dr. Nicolson further advises that *all* metals and mineral supplements be avoided while taking Minocin. Full details of Dr. Brown's antibiotic protocol, modified and improved by Dr. Mercola and written for physicians, are shown in Appendix II. The November 2008 Townsend Letter published a summary of history, use, and efficacy of minocycline for RA.[93]

Test results from individuals suffering from arthritis who participate in double-blind trials with tetracyclines are not typically interpreted correctly because these tests are designed to look for a rapid linear response within a six-month period. Some chronic disease conditions like Lyme Disease may require years to treat. They do not respond to a long-term, low-dose antibiotic regimen for such a short duration, so when the treatment is stopped, a relapse occurs.

The landmark 1995 year-long MIRA study[94] showed that RA may be caused by, exacerbated by, or have relapses triggered by a persistent infection of Mycoplasma or Chlamydia. Another minocycline study showed as much as 50% improvement for 65% of the test subjects.[95] Dr. Gabe Mirkin notes that five significant controlled studies show that minocycline drops the rheumatoid factor towards zero and helps both to alleviate pain and to retard cartilage destruction in RA patients.[96, 97] Dr. Mirkin cites a 1999 study[98] showing that more than half of RA sufferers are infected with Mycoplasma. He has treated hundreds of patients successfully with minocycline and doxycycline.

Dr. Mirkin deplores the fact that despite countless scientific papers showing that many different polymicrobial infections either cause or can contribute to arthritis, most rheumatologists continue to treat RA only with immuno-suppressing drugs because they consider RA to be a so-called "autoimmune" disease.[99, 100] These drugs are extremely expensive, merely dull pain rather than target the pathogens, and predispose the patient to other infections by inhibiting normal immune system functions.[101]

Dr. A. Robert Franco, head of the Arthritis Center of Riverside, CA, has treated thousands of grateful RA patients with Dr. Brown's antibiotic regimen since 1988.[102]

THE PUZZLE OF RA FLARE-UPS

One of the enduring puzzles of so-called autoimmune disorders is that they all go through cycles of exacerbation and remission. Researchers and physicians must integrate the insights from their specialized fields with the knowledge gained about nutrition.

Recognizing that bacteria and their L-forms trigger allergies, which can be suppressed, and that remissions can be maintained by low-dose (or pulsed dose), long-term anti-Mycoplasma antibiotic therapy is an important beginning for treating Rheumatoid Arthritis. Hundreds of experiments on animals have proved that Mycoplasmas are important co-factors in RA and other chronic rheumatic disorders and that the tetracycline family of antibiotics suppresses these mycoplasmal infections. Periodic hyperbaric oxygen therapy (HBOT) works well but cost may be prohibitive.

Mycoplasmas are capable of long-term intercellular *in vivo* survival and slow replication, so they may be resident and waiting for some trauma or barometric pressure changes to activate them when the host's immune system has moderated its operation. Thus, the progression of the infection is cyclical, with waves of re-emergence followed by withdrawal to less detectable forms.

Therefore, when Mycoplasmas act as antigenic substances, triggering internal allergic responses, they release toxins intermittently to a sensitized area, subsiding and then reappearing. Antibodies move through the body via white blood cells and platelets, and it is through this means that RA migrates from shoulder to hand to knee as the antibodies launch counterattacks against local colonies releasing toxins. The antibodies move on to new battlefields whenever migrating antigens like Mycoplasmas flare up. Dr. Brown compares the antibodies' movement and fight against antigens to smoke jumpers carried by airplane from one brush fire to the next. Wherever some "fires" are temporarily quenched, the body enjoys some brief respite.[103]

Clinical evidence shows that two environmental factors can cause flare-ups: (1) a sudden drop in barometric pressure and (2) the presence of high humidity in conjunction with this drop.

Dr. Joseph Hollander, head of rheumatology at the University of Pennsylvania in the 1930s, performed studies of the effects of barometric pressure on rheumatoid disease along with such other factors as temperature, humidity, and oxygen. Volunteers were confined to sealed, climatically controlled rooms, recording their impressions of how they felt each hour while subtle changes in their environment were made. The barometric effects were approximately those of atmospheric conditions prior to a storm. The aches and pains reported by volunteers corresponded to a sudden release of antigens to a sensitized area, confirming Dr. Brown's assertion that shape-changing or migrating Mycoplasmas could be antigenic triggers.

The mechanism of migration of the infectious forms from host to host has not been determined. It might be related to this barometric pressure change. Prior to storms and wet weather periods, there are increases in colds. As the microorganisms stimulate respiratory distress, they seek ways to migrate out of the body to escape the discomfort of the pressure change, spreading their "seeds" via effluvia (e.g., sneezing, coughing) to other mammalian hosts.

RA patients also experience a higher incidence of flare-ups in the late spring and early fall. Some physicians[104] see an allergy connection, but attribute these reactions to specific environmental substances that are assimilated into the body and reach reactive sites throughout the body via the bloodstream. However, such externally caused allergic reactions do not explain sensitivity to barometric pressure. The closer one gets to sea level, the higher the concentration of oxygen. Arthritics do not fare as well at higher altitudes as they do nearer sea level, because in the thinner air their cells are starved for oxygen. This explains the pain and swelling in the joints arthritis sufferers experience after a long airplane journey. It also accounts for the success of HBOT.

Trauma to joints and tendons may cause structural changes, further reducing oxygen transport and limiting removal of fluids and wastes in the region of the injury. The lack of oxygen in the traumatized area increases pressure and swelling. Several of the herbal remedies described in Appendix I improve blood oxygenation, as does CoQ_{10}.

The Jarisch-Herxheimer Effect

If an antibiotic is working against the microorganism effectively, a phenomenon called the Jarisch-Herxheimer (also called a "Herxheimer" or "Herx") effect sometimes occurs. The symptoms are those of a severe allergic reaction[105] that may occur when a physician treats, for instance, a streptococcal infection with a penicillin-group antibiotic. One explanation is that streptococcus is not found at the site of the irritation, nor is it protected by inflamed or scarred tissue, as Mycoplasma would be.

The Herxheimer effect may at first appear to be an allergic reaction to the drug itself, and the physician (or the patient) may discontinue antibiotic treatment for that reason. However, these two responses can be distinguished. Allergic reactions to drugs are typically immediate and rapid, involving different actions of cytokines, and may manifest as stomach upset, rash, or headache. On the other hand, a Herxheimer reaction is an exacerbation of existing symptoms. It is caused by the rapid death of a colony of parasitic microorganisms releasing their internal toxic contents *in situ*.

According to Dr. Brown, with a bacterial allergy the Mycoplasma creates a barrier around itself that keeps the immune system's natural disease-fighting antibodies at bay. Bacteria develop resistance by shielding themselves with one type of protein and creating another to eject the antibiotic from the cell.[106, 107]

Mycoplasmas' membranes are unique among bacteria in having lipids called sterols that they require for growth and that help protect them from lysis (rupture) by β-lactam antibiotics like penicillin.[108] However, antibiotics acting at the level of protein synthesis or DNA modification molecules are highly effective against this membrane. The tetracyclines, fluoroquinolones, and macrolides eliminate Mycoplasma efficiently both *in vivo* and *in vitro*.[109] They do this by binding to specific ribosomes inside the membrane.

Mycoplasma organisms cause infection primarily as extracellular parasites, attaching to the surface of epithelial cells of the respiratory, GI, and urogenital tracts. A unique group of membrane proteins allow this adherence, after which, the organism may damage the epithelial cells by generating hydrogen peroxide. This chemical causes cell dissolution when the usual immune system's antigen-antibody reactions lead to an inflammatory response.[110]

The fact that tetracycline causes the Jarisch-Herxheimer reaction demonstrates the presence of an infection,[111] but there may be more to it than that. With precise testing for Mycoplasmas and L-forms, perhaps by PCR or biochip methods, it may be possible to trace the infection's origin and to see the relationship, for instance, between folic acid and fat-molecule destruction.

Dr. Joseph Mercola, D.O. has found that those patients who follow his strictly prescribed nutritional guidelines in parallel with his improved Dr. Brown protocol rarely experience a Jarisch-Herxheimer reaction.[112] This is probably because, as a result of improved nutrition, an increased amount of vitamin C present in tissues is available to suppress the histamine reaction.

Natural antibiotic or antibacterial substances such as immune system-enhancing herbs and supplements may also produce a Herxheimer effect. As soon as this "allergic reaction" is experienced, the individual should stop intake of the substance because the body's immune system needs time to train itself to deal with the infection and become stronger. Supplements of vitamins C and B_6 are helpful in countering the body's excessive histamine production during the course of the reaction.

A treatment that actively seeks an allergic reaction may seem counterintuitive, but it follows standard allergen immunization principles. The Jarisch-Herxheimer effect to some extent indicates success, but it cannot be endured for long without considerable discomfort, so treatment should be temporarily suspended or dosage reduced. Periodic resumption should be tried until the person gradually becomes immunized to the allergy trigger. The allergic reaction diminishes as the population of the invading organism is minimized.

As Dr. Brown suggested, cortisone or other corticosteroids or antihistamines may be used together with tetracyclines to permit higher doses of the antibiotic with acceptable levels of allergic reaction. Two of the best OTC antihistamines with non-drowsiness effects are loratadine and chlorpheniramine maleate.

Specific and detailed physician-to-physician advice for administering the antibiotic protocol, written by Dr. Mercola, is given in Appendix II. Dr. Charles Malis also provides treatment advice to other doctors online.[113]

ACHIEVING MUCOSAL BALANCE [114]

Mucosal surfaces are the moist inner linings of the body's internal tissues that provide a mechanical antimicrobial barrier in the respiratory, gastrointestinal, and genitourinary tracts. Because the mucosal surfaces routinely contact the environment outside the body, they are particularly vulnerable to pathogenic infection at the contact points (nose, mouth, anus, genitals, and eyes). Recurrent infections of the sinuses, middle ear, bronchial tract, and lungs occur in individuals who have an impairment of the elements of this barrier.

Mucosal Balance is a general term describing the state in which the immune system is rendered non-reactive towards self or non-self antigens. It is a complex process that involves deletion of reactive T-cells and induction of regulatory (or suppressor) T-cells.[115] Multiple factors must combine to disrupt the sophisticated immune system balance that allows tolerance between "good" and "bad" intestinal flora in order to trigger an inflammatory response. Effector T-cells (NK cells) figure prominently in this adaptation of the immune system to fight disease and inflammation.[116] T-cell types and actions are described in Chapter 2.

Certain bacterial and viral infections target mucosal epithelial cells for invasion. The immune system then tries to kill and remove the infected cells. Mucosal surfaces are thus a perpetual battleground. Epithelial cell invasion at the site of the pathology is common. Microbes are "fastidious" and some pick specific targets. Others, like *Chlamydophila pneumoniae*, are equal opportunity invaders, happy to infect any tissue or organ they can exploit for their own survival.

Bacterial colonization of the esophagus leads to GERD (Gastroesophageal Reflux Disease)[117] and in turn, greatly increased risk of tumors (adenocarcinoma) in the esophagus.[118] According to Dr. Sandra Macfarlane, only one in twenty of these cases are correctly diagnosed. The aim of her research on microbial colonization of the gut mucosa was to see how resident bacteria play a role in a chronic peptic ulcer condition called Barrett's Esophagus. A surprise discovery was that high levels (57%) of three types of Campylobacters were found, but not *Helicobacter pylori*. These organisms cause enteritis, and periodontal and bile duct or gallbladder infections. They convert nitrates to nitrites, toxins that are carcinogenic.[119]

Dr. Macfarlane is at the forefront of research in microbial biofilms in the gut.[120] She asserts that a considerable number of chronic conditions could be traced to mucosal balance dysfunction and the various infections that result.[121]

Long-Term Effects of Antibiotics

Despite its success in fighting infection, long-term use of oral antibiotics runs the risk of upsetting the balance of intestinal microbiota. This imbalanced condition is called dysbiosis (or dysbacteriosis). Rotating the antibiotic every 4-5 years, even within the same antibiotic family, decreases the possibility of developing tolerance to a specific antibiotic or damaging the ecology of the GI tract.[122] The goal is to prevent chronic intestinal Candidiasis, but Clostridium toxins could present an even bigger problem.

Unappreciated until the mid-1970's, the major pathogen *Clostridium difficile* causes a spectrum of antibiotic-associated intestinal diseases from ordinary diarrhea to severe, life-threatening enterocolitis. It is usually contracted in hospitals and nursing homes where proliferated spores are difficult to eradicate in areas adjacent to infected patients (e.g., beds, bathrooms). Botulism, tetanus, and soft tissue infections are linked to other forms of Clostridia. *C. difficile* disease is caused by the overgrowth of the organism in the intestinal tract, primarily in the colon. The pathogen appears unable to compete successfully in the normal intestinal ecosystem except when antibiotics disturb the normal flora balance. *C. difficile* then replicates and secretes two toxins: an enterotoxin that causes fluid accumulation in the bowel, and a potent cytotoxin.[123] These toxins are similar to the Borrelia-produced Lyme Disease toxin as well as other fat-soluble toxins resulting from exposure to substances like pesticides and molds.

Lyme Disease and toxins are discussed in Chapter 5.

Reintroducing Beneficial Bacteria

Medical researchers are recognizing that much of our immune system lies along the gastrointestinal tract. The average human gut contains at least 5,600 different kinds of bacteria.[124] The beneficial bacteria, such as bifidobacteria, stimulate the immune system and control the growth of other bacteria, while harmful bacteria, such as species of the Clostridium family, lead to chronic diseases like arthritis and cancer.

Studies have found that ingesting slow release, natural sugars found in grains, fruits, certain kinds of seaweed, and legumes encourage growth of the desired bacteria, while eating refined sugar, starches, too little fiber, too much meat and other animal-based foods favors the harmful bacteria.[125]

Maintaining a healthy environment for natural, beneficial bacteria can be done by eating certain fermented foods such as yogurt, tempeh, cheese, sourdough bread, red grape juice, and red wine (in moderation). Freeze-dried probiotic supplements are helpful to counter Candida yeast infections.[126] Health food stores carry products such as dairy-free

Lactobacillus acidophilus and caprylic acid products (lauric and palmitic acids) to maintain flora balance.[127]
It is very important that the lactobacillus is properly refrigerated on its way from manufacturer to consumer. Temperatures higher than 80 degrees can kill this beneficial bacterium and render it useless as a treatment. Most health food stores keep lactobacillus in a cold case, but it may be shipped in standard unrefrigerated delivery trucks. If in doubt, contact the supplier directly and ask about shipping methods. Until gut balance is achieved (usually about 7-10 days), avoid or drastically minimize yeasty foods.[128]

If an individual is allergic to yeast, s/he should resolve to avoid yeast and mold-containing foods indefinitely. If there is no allergy, one can reintroduce these items gradually back into one's diet, consuming them in very small amounts. Those individuals with chronic yeast-connected health problems are usually allergic to several, often many, different foods.

Specific laboratory tests can pinpoint these allergens and assist in developing a tailored health diet that avoids them.[129] The Immunodiffusion test is an FDA-approved procedure designed to confirm late stage Candidiasis with significantly high antibody levels. The *Candida albicans* Assay has the advantage of detecting intermediate levels of Candida. The high sensitivity and specificity of the ELISA test detects the earlier stages of Candidiasis. There are several symptoms known to affect both people with gluten intolerances and those with Candida infections. Blood Ig tests are available to confirm leaky gut syndrome, Candida, and gluten allergy.[130]

Antifungal diet supplements sold commercially to kill yeast infections are not fully effective, since they only work in the gut. It is when the Candida bacteria migrates through a tear in the gut wall and moves into the systemic portion of the anatomy that an individual experiences the mental and emotional symptoms of Candidiasis and begins the onset of allergic reactions that are indicative of that disease.[131]

Persistent epithelial intracellular infections have been shown to respond well to treatments with vinegar, enzymes, prebiotics/probiotics, and healthy natural oils.

Detoxing the Colon

The practice of natural colon cleansing dates back to ancient Greece. An improperly functioning colon (the large intestine) affects every system and organ of the body. Up to 40% of what is eliminated from the colon are bacteria, and the rest is indigestible solid matter. When the colon is sluggish or weak, digestion and elimination processes are inefficient. Toxins remain in the body rather than being eliminated. To protect itself, the body stores these toxins in fat cells or in the mucosal lining of the intestines. Start with a gentle colon cleanse to purge the gut of accrued waste.[132]

Next, detoxing the gut with apple cider vinegar can be effective in dissolving the waxy coat of various harmful microbes, making it easier for the immune system to attack, kill, and remove them. Apple cider vinegar is rich in natural enzymes that can regulate the presence of Candida in the gut by balancing the pH level. It helps encourage the growth of healthy bacteria, which in turn minimizes Candida overgrowth.[133] After "rebooting" the system with enzymes and probiotics, the next step is to normalize the gut by including prebiotics as part of the daily diet regimen. Regular garlic intake is a highly effective method for controlling Candida and improving immune system function.[134, 135] Sugar must be assiduously avoided.[136]

Prebiotics and Probiotics

While probiotics are the actual bacteria that help to maintain a healthy digestive tract, prebiotics are the foods that feed and nurture these bacteria so they can grow and thrive. This balanced gut environment helps to boost overall immunity and may play a role in preventing and treating a variety of diseases including inflammatory bowel disease (IBD) , infectious diarrhea, and even certain types of cancer.

Prebiotics figure in pathogen inhibition, reduction in *Clostridium difficile* toxin, and the inflammation response.[137] Food sources include most greens, legumes (e.g., soybeans, lentils, split peas, kidney beans), garlic, corn, berries, sweet potatoes, asparagus, artichokes, peas, nuts, carrots, jicama, green beans, onions, bell peppers, mangoes, apples, lemons, red grapes, watermelon, and tomatoes as well as unrefined grains such as barley, oatmeal, and whole grain wheat.[138]

Probiotics are preventative rather than therapeutic. By inhibiting the growth and attachment of pathogens, they help reduce inflammation. Among the many health benefits are enhanced colonization resistance and immune modulation for conditions such as allergy and eczema, traveler's diarrhea, urogenital tract infections, and IBD. Natural probiotic sources include yogurt, kefir, sauerkraut, dark chocolate (in moderation), microalgae (e.g., chlorella, spirulina), buttermilk, miso soup, pickles, and kimchi.[139]

Supplementing the diet with *Lactobacillus acidophilus* and *L. bifidus* in refrigerated or freeze-dried powdered form helps maintain the ecological balance of normal intestinal flora that may be killed during antibiotic therapy. These probiotics are usually made from concentrated globulin whey protein. Those allergic to milk or dairy products should seek alternatives to these substances.

According to Dr. Joseph Mercola, recent studies show that up to one third of beneficial bacteria products labeled "probiotics" do not contain the amount of live bacteria listed on the bottle. Moreover, they may actually contain some harmful strains. Ask for specifics on product content from the health food store or contact the manufacturer. This information is usually on the label. Get recommendations on a trustworthy brand from Dr. Mercola's website.[140] Dr. Julian Whitaker's Wellness Institute in Newport Beach, CA can also design a tailored detox regimen.[141]

Limiting the presence of antibiotics in the GI tract is important for another important reason. When antibiotics cause bacteria to change to their CWD forms, the pathogens are then more able to share and exchange plasmids—a virus-like form that enables genetic swaps between micro-organisms. The result of plasmid exchange can be a mutated bacterium that has learned how to combat antibiotics.

Enzyme Therapy [142, 143]

Enzymes are bioactive molecules that are the catalysts controlling the speed of molecular transformations in living systems. Catabolic enzymes facilitate digestion by breaking down molecules and structures. Anabolic enzymes build new molecules out of molecular components. Growth and regrowth of tissues, organs, and other body components depend on both anabolic and catabolic enzymes.

Enzymes come to us from different sources. Some are contained in our food (many are made from the plants we eat). Microbes in our gut flora make enzymes and essential vitamins. The two-stranded DNA in our genes makes one-stranded RNA enzymes; these in turn make other enzymes and molecules. We sometimes have more than one gene encoded to make the same enzyme or its variant forms.

The microbes that live inside us have a kit bag of genetic recipes to generate enzymes and molecules that can be helpful or harmful. The harmful products we call toxins, and the strains of microbes that make them are called pathogenic. When these pathogenic microbes invade and colonize us, the result is disease. Dysbiosis and other dysfunctional mitochondrial gut conditions are the result of microbe-caused enzyme direct actions or imbalance, or the result of the toxins that microbes make from enzymes.

There may be more than three enzymes for each molecule that we make and use. Several different enzymes may make variants of a molecule; other enzymes may work with an enzyme as a functional system; others may destroy, control, or disable a molecule that is itself an enzyme. Enzymes also differ by location—in blood, circulatory system tissues, peripheral or heart muscles, liver, lymph nodes, central nervous system, brain, joints, glands, etc.

Three types of enzymes work together to regulate the biochemical reactions in the body: (1) digestive, which break down food into nutrients for absorption into the bloodstream (2) metabolic (or systemic), which deliver nutrients to the cells and tissues for nourishment and regeneration, and (3) those obtained from foods we consume.

Digestive enzymes: Many are named by adding the suffix "–ase," which means "dissolving." Thus, protease is protein-dissolving; cellulase digests cellulose; lipase works on lipids (fats); cholesterol esterase splits cholesterol. Pepsin, trypsin, and chymotrypsin work together to convert proteins to amino acid components. The results of this activity can be building-beads to make other organic molecules by systemic anabolic enzymes where molecular assembly is needed.

The plant enzymes bromelain (pineapple) and papain (papaya) assist in food protein digestion, and attack parasites' protective coatings in the gut. Note that merely eating these fruits does not provide enough enzymes to be medicinally effective. Bromelain can heal soft tissue injuries, has anti-tumor ability, prevents/minimizes angina attacks, can denature the toxin in bee stings, and can debride burn wounds to speed healing. Bromelain can calm inflammation in patients with active, normal immune systems, but is able to stimulate inflammation if immune system functions are suppressed.[144]

Combining bromelain and antibiotic therapy has been shown to be more effective than antibiotics alone in a range of conditions including pneumonia and chronic bronchitis.[145]

Systemic enzymes: (like hormones) are transported via blood and lymph to locations where they can be used to interact with location-specific pathways and cycles to control processes or to be themselves processed. These enzymes can have anti-inflammatory properties and have been used to treat Osteoarthritis, RA, MS, and other chronic disorders.[146]

Systemic enzymes may be catabolic anabolic or metabolic. Metabolic enzymes participate in energy flow and regulation of process rates. Catabolic enzymes are vitally important because they can dissolve arterial plaque, strengthen blood vessels, and prevent blood clots. They force rejuvenation of muscles, cells, nerves, tissues, bones, endothelial tissues, and glands. Regulatory systemic enzymes and hormones balance other hormones, regulate the immune system, and enhance mental clarity.

The liver and pancreas produce essential systemic enzymes. Pancreatic dysfunctions cause digestive and sugar metabolism problems related to the enzyme/hormone insulin. Excess sugar causes widespread pathogenic systemic imbalances. The hormone cortisol controls sugar use, fat storage, and cholesterol production.[147]

In different locations in the body, there are multi-metabolic/anabolic enzyme systems called pathways that perform a specific function, much like a factory assembly line makes a product component that is used elsewhere. Some pathways are loops. The citric acid cycle[148] (aka Krebs cycle)[149] makes adenosine triphosphate (ATP, the energy fuel for our cells) from carbohydrates, fats, or proteins from our food.[150] The Krebs cycle uses Co-enzyme A (CoA) in the cellular mitochondria.[151]

The mevalonate pathway[152] makes cholesterol, hematin (heme iron), ubiquinol (CoQ_{10}) , and other essential molecules from fats in our food. Cortisol is made from cholesterol in the steroid hormone pathway.

Statin drugs are designed to block a key enzyme (HMG-CoA reductase) in the liver as part of the mevalonate pathway in order to decrease cholesterol levels. But cholesterol is essential for making steroid hormones and for brain function.[153] Cholesterol starvation is harmful. There are serious consequences in using these "life-saving" drugs.[154] One statin drug patent describes the need for high levels (at least 300 mg daily) of CoQ_{10} to be co-administered with the drug to avoid harm. However, physicians are not urged to recommend supplemental CoQ_{10} so the patient is unaware of the dangers.

Altering the mevalonate pathway initiates a cascade of metabolic dysfunctions, making cells much more vulnerable to oxidative stress unless enough ascorbic acid is consumed to chemically offset the free radicals produced and the collateral damage they cause. E.g., sharply reducing CoQ_{10} results in lower energy, adverse psychological changes, mitochondrial DNA dysfunction, cholesterol oxidation, T-cell disruption, muscular dystrophies ("statin myopathy"[155]), kidney function impairment, liver dysfunction, onset of Parkinson's and Alzheimer's symptoms, premature aging, and many more.[156]

When there is either an excess or a shortage of key enzymes, essential body systems/processes may be under- or over-controlled. E.g., a lack of amylase, the enzyme that digests starch, leads to blood sugar imbalance that characterizes diabetes. A protease deficiency can affect the immune system adversely.

Fibrinolytic systemic enzymes clean out unneeded tissue and dissolve excess fibrin that forms in various organs and tissues during the normal wound healing process. Excess fibrin can form in the kidneys (leading to high blood pressure), carotid arteries (stroke)[157], muscles (Fibromyalgia, Carpal Tunnel Syndrome[158]), the brain (senility), and the respiratory/pulmonary tracts (sinusitis, fluid retention, COPD, and inflammation).

The strongest fibrin-eating enzyme is serrapeptase,[159] a natural anti-inflammatory that is available commercially as a dietary supplement. A powerful agent by itself, serrapeptase teamed with antibiotics delivers increased concentrations of the antimicrobial agent to the site of the infection. Bacteria hiding in biofilms are usually resistant to antimicrobial agents. In an attempt to prevent this bacterial immunity, researchers have experimented with various means of inhibiting biofilm-embedded bacteria.[160] Caution: too much of a tear-down enzyme can cause the same muscle pain symptoms associated with statin myopathy.

Another COPD-related study[161] found that palmitoyl-oleoyl-phosphatidyl-glycerol (POPG), a lung surfactant, suppresses respiratory syncytial virus (RSV) and Mycoplasmas, while making breathing less work.[162] POPG is derived from palmitic acid, a beneficial fat sorely lacking in our Western diet.

Food enzymes are most abundant in raw fruits and vegetables harvested ripe from the tree or vine. Because our produce is often picked unripe to survive the trip to market, enzyme levels can be deficient in our modern diet. According to the late Dr. Edward Howell, a deficiency in digestive enzymes reduces the availability of metabolic enzymes, and this shortfall is the root cause of most chronic conditions.[163]

Enzyme supplementation and therapy is common in Europe and Asia, but is not considered worthwhile in the U.S. According to Dr. Gabe Mirkin, Dr. Howell's assertion that heating food above 118^0 F destroys food enzymes is a myth. The body makes its own enzymes for digestion. Enzymes in food are treated like any other protein, and heat does not destroy protein.[164] Juicing offers an optimal method to obtain maximum benefit from food enzymes in fresh, organic produce.[165]

Combinations of enzyme deficiencies can lead to IBD, Crohn's disease, and cancer. By taking digestive enzyme supplements with meals and metabolic enzymes between meals, systemic dysregulation conditions could be reversed and healed.[166] Minerals[167] activate metabolic enzymes. Magnesium, copper, zinc, calcium or other mineral supplements may be needed because our croplands are being steadily depleted of vital nutrients.[168] A qualified nutritionist should be consulted to determine any deficiencies and to advise on specific mineral and vitamin requirements.

Natural Antimicrobial Oils

Because there are just a few antiviral prescription medicines available, the antiviral aspects of common and ethnic foods deserve mention.[169] Over 100 scientific articles archived by the U.S. National Library of Medicine and National Institutes of Health can be accessed online through Pub Med by typing *antiviral oils* in the search window. The search term *antimicrobial oils* yields over 5,300 results. France has been at the forefront of aromatherapy practice in general, and the anti-infectious use of essential antimicrobial oils in particular. Pharmacists display the term "Aromatherapie" on their store windows, but this is inconceivable in English-speaking countries, where the term "Aromatherapy" has a rather negative connotation.[170] Healthy dietary fats and oils are discussed in Chapter 7.

TOXIN BUILDUP

When antigens and antibodies clash, the result is destruction of cells and a sudden release of toxins, triggering a cascade of immune system functions and components—proteolytic enzymes, kinins, kallikreins, histamines, ROS/RNS (Reactive Oxygen/Nitrogen Species) and other irritants.[171] The result of the struggle is pain and inflammation. As the CWD microbes spawn a new generation, antigens migrate to a new area. The antibodies follow it to this new combat zone, leaving the former battlefield to rest and heal, but toxins are left behind. Ideally, they are flushed away, but if circulation (blood and lymph), digestion enzymes, and elimination systems are dysfunctional, toxins accrue to cause more inflammation. Gentle massage, serrapeptase, and vitamin C supplements consumed frequently can help neutralize the irritating ROS and relieve the pain.

This pattern illustrates the system-wide nature of RA. Arthritics complain of shoulder pain for a week or so, then pain in the hands or feet. The toxins released by the antigen-antibody conflict are often trapped in pockets of the bursa and are not promptly expelled through the various elimination organs of the body. These trapped toxins can create a mass of fluid or scar tissue that can bring pressure to bear upon the joints when blood vessels expand.

Catch-22: pain inhibits motion, but motion is needed for the body's ability to flush the toxins. Gravity draws toxins to the lower extremity joints of the knees and feet. Excess weight[172] and ill-fitting shoes, especially high heels, will increase pressure and pain on swollen, irritated tissues.

One aspect of RA allergic flare-up appears to be related to certain toxins, for example, salmonella toxin, where studies have found the arthritis-linked protein HLA-B27.[173,] [174] HLA-B27 is discussed in Chapter 6.

Pathogenic bacteria synthesize toxins. For example, Sarcoidosis bacteria invade host cells that then make an active form of vitamin D, which in turn stimulates an excessive immune reaction called "vitamin D intoxication"[175] and sun sensitivity. Dr. Trevor Marshall recognized the infection connection with Sarcoidosis and developed a multi-antibiotic protocol to counter it.[176]

While the immune system is busy battling a chronic inflammatory condition, clearance of bacteria from soft tissues appears to be of low priority importance to the host's defense mechanism during soft tissue infection or injury.[177] This may be the reason Mycoplasmas are able to establish a foothold early and have time to adapt to later assault by antibiotics.

Cloaking microbes like *Mycobacterium tuberculosis, Mycoplasma pneumoniae,* and *Chlamydia pneumoniae* seek out and bind to specific types of molecules, especially fats found in the blood (lipoproteins). Fats are diverse in sizes and shapes. Not all fat cells provide ideal camouflage for these organisms; some are only marginally useful, so the cloaking mechanism is rendered defective for these unsuitable fat cells. If the fat monolaurin is present, cloaking fails; this fat dissolves the pathogens' lipid cell membranes.

Coconut oil contains beneficial monolaurin. The relative concentration of useful versus harmful fats[178] is well described by the papers written by Dr. Mary Enig, world-renowned expert on fats and oils.[179, 180, 181]

The characteristics of CoQ_{10}, ascorbic acid, monolaurin, monopalmitin and folic acid, including their membrane-dissolving properties should be studied in relation to the activities of shape-changing, cloaking microorganisms, such as those mentioned above. It would be worthwhile to test all monoglycerides of saturated long chain fats like monolaurin.

Other natural methods to eliminate toxins from a variety of sources are found in Chapter 7.

Neutralizing Toxins and Harmful Enzymes with Antibiotics

Dr. Brown realistically asserted that harmful microbes could not be completely eliminated. The aim of his antibiotic protocol is to keep the pathogenic Mycoplasmas within manageable bounds so that the body's own immune system can keep them from becoming uncontrollably virulent and invasive. Considering re-infections, periodic tetracycline doses and other wide spectrum antibiotics can help lower the total microbe load. In those cases where the particular pathogen is unknown or in doubt, it is more effective to target and neutralize the irritants as a first step, without putting a priority on identifying the organism(s) producing them. Clues might be found in the toxin or enzyme made by the microbe, e.g., the correlation between *Mycoplasma pneumoniae* and the COX-2 enzyme.[182]

Certain enzymes generated in turn may reveal the particular strain of pathogen responsible. The Arthritis Trust's findings confirm Dr. Brown's research that *M. pneumoniae* was a prime candidate as a causal factor of Rheumatoid Arthritis.[183] However, today's commonly available tests are not definitive or comprehensive enough to identify all strains of a given pathogenic organism.

Strain-specific antibiotic susceptibilities are needed to permit selection of the most effective antibiotic/*M. pneumoniae* vaccine combination. *M. pneumoniae* vaccine is used to treat pigs but is not yet available for humans because these vaccines are too dangerous.[184] A similar problem exists with the *Streptococcus pneumoniae* (Spn) vaccine, which is supposed to protect against multi-strains of that bacteria.[185] The vaccines stimulate attack by immune cells. We know that Spn invades epithelial and endothelial cells. If a new Spn strain also invades and compromises the attacking immune cells, as Mycoplasma does, the vaccine would be useless in stopping Spn colonization.

Gamma globulin, also known as Immunoglobulin (Ig), a blood extract similar to an anti-toxin, was used in the past as a non-specific anti-infection passive immune booster.[186] The purity of such blood extracts is subject to question today because of the levels of contaminants in the blood supply (see Chapter 5).

ALLERGIC REACTIONS

If, as Dr. Brown asserts, RA is due to a kind of infectious allergy where mycoplasmal microorganisms and CWD L-forms reside in joints and emit irritants to which the body reacts, this would explain why the person afflicted with RA has periods during which s/he feels reasonably well. During these lulls, it could be that bacteria or their L-forms are hidden or dormant and release just a small bit of the toxin. Other explanations may be that the L-form reverts to a cellular form temporarily, or the organism may develop a cholesterol "coat," or performs a sort of cloaking that is somewhat imperfect. We now know that the life cycles of all persistent parasitic microbe forms must replicate in our bodies before leaving to infect a new host. We also know that many (perhaps most or all) forms invade epithelial, endothelial, tissue, and various attacking immune cells to replicate.

When a cell is invaded, its mitochondria must feed the invader and the cell experiences various mitochondrial dysfunctions. E.g., ROS is amplified. Without ascorbic acid intake, scurvy results and we see the scurvy as an allergy flare, as an acute new illness, or as a chronic relapse. The need for daily ascorbic acid intake increases in parallel with the number and variety of microbes in the host.

Mycoplasmas, Lyme organisms, Cpn and many other parasites are cyclic in nature. They even can persist in metabolically inactive states, when only a few inactive forms transform back to active form; or invaded cells mature and many infant L-forms are released as if from an incubator. Over a period of months or years, the body creates fixed-tissue antibodies that are poised and ready to react to the released L-forms and toxins whenever and wherever they appear.

The body thus learns to react to Mycoplasmas in the same way it learns to react to a substance like poison ivy. The first contact causes the body to produce a specific type of antibody tailored to the allergen. The periodic reaction between antibody and antigen causes irritation. Antibody reactions alone cannot suppress mycoplasmal infections. The multiple polymorphic stages may be why efforts to develop vaccines against Mycoplasmas and other complex microbes have not been successful. The vaccine stimulates recognition of only one polymorphic stage.

Control Theory Applied to Allergic Reactions

Keeping the body's systems in balance requires acceptance of the fact that our bodies are constantly changing. Living organic systems are always in a dynamic state. In the branch of mathematics called Control Theory, the optimum state is where "balance" means oscillating within an acceptable range. Figure 5 is a notional view of the oscillation cycle occurring during an allergic reaction.

An allergic response, whether to an internal or external substance, is really a stimulation of the immune system to develop a specific antibody, immunoglobulin E (IgE). The

IgE antibodies attach themselves to mast cells—specialized immune cells found in the skin, nasal passages, and the gastrointestinal and respiratory tracts—to prepare to ward off the invaders. As the offending substance (e.g., ragweed pollen) enters the body, it bumps against these primed mast cells and sets off their histamine chemicals.[187] Hydrogen peroxide (H_2O_2) is also released.

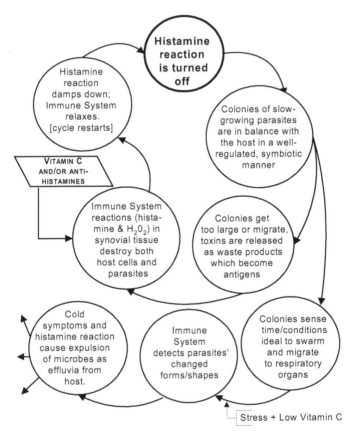

Figure 5. Histamine Reaction Cycle

Vitamin C blocks the initial production and action of histamine, a chemical produced by the immune system. Histamine is usually bound up in granules found inside mast cells. Commercially produced chemical antihistamines work by blocking the action of histamine once it has been released. OTC antihistamines have a long track record of success and are considered safe if used in moderation and according to directions. Loratadine and chlorpheniramine maleate have been shown to reduce the severity of arthritis joint pain.

Do not rush to swallow antihistamines at the first sign of symptoms. Instead, try to find ways to avoid allergens from animals, molds, grasses, detergents, and foods by identifying the circumstances under which allergies strike, then removing the offending agents. The process may be as simple as replacing furnace filters often or installing electrostatic air cleaners in the home or office to minimize dust levels.[188] Low levels of ascorbic acid (vitamin C) allow allergens to trigger a histamine reaction.

Naturopathic remedies

If external remedies are called for, one might try a gentler approach than OTC drugs. No matter what the allergy, German researchers have discovered that eating onions reduces the amount of histamine produced by mast cells.[189] Vitamin C (with bioflavonoids) and pantothenic acid have been shown to be natural antihistamines. Vitamin E and selenium stabilize cell walls, while Vitamin A decreases the permeability of cells in skin and in the mucous membranes. Strong cells walls are important because undesirable pathogens can invade and compromise weakened cells during an allergy attack.

Vitamin B-complex, especially vitamin B_6, has been shown to decrease allergic reactions, especially when taken together with vitamin C in large amounts.[190] This is because the B vitamins enhance the immune system. Those individuals with chronic illness have a low absorption rate so liquid B vitamin supplements in sublingual form (drops administered under the tongue) are the most effective.[191]

Sinusitis and/or allergic rhinitis may be linked to nasal polyps. Symptoms include nasal block, loss of sense of smell, sinus pain/inflammation, and secondary infection leading to severe headache. Applying tea tree oil to the nasal passages with a Q-tip should dissolve polyps.[192]

Homeopathic Remedies [193, 194]

Homeopathic relief for allergy and sinusitis usually consists of:
- *Belladonna* 3X;
- *Sanguinaria canadensis* 3X; and/or
- *Spigelia* 3X.

Endnotes and continuing research on topics in Chapter 3 can be found at www.RA-Infection-Connection.com

4. OPPORTUNISTIC PATHOGENS

Antibiotic-resistant bacteria were practically unknown 60 years ago. Today they are a worldwide health problem. Illnesses such as strep throat, pneumonia, meningitis, and tuberculosis are becoming increasingly harder to treat. Reducing deadly methicillin-resistant *Staphylococcus aureus* (MRSA) in both healthcare and community settings continues to be a high priority for the CDC. New prevention procedures resulted in a 17% drop in MRSA infections from 2005-2008. However, healthcare-associated infections still present a major public health problem in the U.S., affecting 5 to 10 percent of hospitalized patients annually, resulting in 2 million infections, 90,000 deaths and adding $4.5 to $5.7 billion in healthcare costs.[1] Vancomycin is the first choice for antibiotic treatment for MRSA.[2]

Until 2000, *Streptococcus pneumoniae* infections caused 60,000 cases of invasive disease each year. Up to 40% of these were caused by Pneumococci resistant to at least one antibiotic. These statistics have improved substantially following the introduction of multivalent pneumococcal conjugate vaccines. However, some major challenges remain: (1) by including antimicrobial agents in household cleansers, cosmetics, and lotions, industry is exacerbating the problem and making it easier for pathogenic microbes to develop resistance; (2) some clinical laboratories have not adopted recommended methods for identifying and defining drug-resistant *S. pneumoniae* (DRSP); and (3) underuse of the 23-valent pneumococcal polysaccharide vaccine recommended for older adults and high-risk children. However, no vaccine protects against all strains of Pneumococcus.[3, 4]

As of 2011, over 30% of all Enterococcus infections in U.S. hospitals' intensive care units and in nursing homes are now resistant to vancomycin, until recently considered the most effective antibiotic.[5] Researchers are hunting for new antimicrobial agents, and pharmaceutical companies are developing synthetics like Zyvox and Cidecin to combat microorganisms that have become resistant to traditional drugs thought to be "magic bullets" since the discovery of penicillin in 1944. By the 1950s, most Staphylococcus infections had become highly resistant to penicillin. Part of the problem was that doctors prescribed penicillin indiscriminately for all sorts of complaints, often in response to patients' demands for antibiotics. Research shows that 87% of children aged 0-5 years have had at least one ear infection. We know now that ear infections and some sinus infections may not only be caused by bacteria, but also by viral and/or fungal infections.[6]

THE WIDESPREAD USE OF PRESCRIPTION DRUGS

Overuse of prescription drugs, like the overuse of insecticides, is a Pyrrhic victory. In time, as a drug is used more and more frequently, the susceptible germs die off but the resistant, pernicious ones reproduce as mutated strains. The more people use antibiotics, the more pressure is put on bacterial populations to develop immunity until the pathogenic germs become resistant to multiple drugs. Physicians may eventually be forced to return to less effective treatments abandoned many years ago, before antibiotics were introduced, as the number and type of omni-resistant germs continue to grow.

Much of the fault of this untargeted and widespread drug use in the United States lies with the American patients, who have come to expect a prescription for a quick fix for their discomfort.

Antibiotics

Antibiotics work in one of five ways:

- Interfering with cell wall synthesis, preventing the microbes from repairing their cell walls, which weaken and eventually burst, leading to cell death;
- Disrupting cellular processes, preventing cells from making proteins or other essential components they need to grow and multiply, thus making it easier for the immune system to destroy them;
- Competing with nutrients, by attracting the germs to a substance that they need to survive, such as para-aminobenzoic acid (PABA). Sulfa antibiotics are chemically very close in structure to PABA. The germs that require PABA take in the sulfa instead. This inhibits cell growth, making it easier for the body's immune system to kill the colony;
- Blocking DNA synthesis, interfering with their ability to make the DNA they need to multiply;
- Blocking of metabolism, preventing germs from taking in nutrients and expelling their metabolic waste products. This process both starves the germ and makes it store internal toxins that kill it.

Bacteria can generate overt enzyme counterattacks to break down antibiotics. They also can adapt to the new chemical environment by building a tougher membrane wall or changing slightly whatever biochemical process the antibiotic was supposed to affect.[7] They accomplish this by generating new enzymes that are not blocked by the antibiotic.

Hospitals try rotating the use of antibiotics they routinely administer to avoid resistance. E.g., alternating penicillin, streptomycin, tetracyclines, macrolides, and sulfonamides with chloramphenicol in 3- to 4-year cycles. Antibiotics like vancomycin, ristocetin, neomycin, colistin, and polymyxin are reserved for special, severe cases. However, this rotation strategy is not practical because strains are constantly reacting to attacks and evolving.[8]

Microbes' adaptations can occur at a rapid rate if recipe swapping is facilitated by the use of cell wall-dissolving antibiotics that do not kill all forms of the bacteria. Humans could thus be viewed as the result of four billion years of gene swapping.

Studies of various pathogenic *E. coli* strains showed that there was a tradeoff between genes for virulence and those for antibiotic resistance. Discoveries of new CWD strains that demonstrate stronger resistance to tetracycline and erythromycin antibiotics sustain the disturbing assertion that Mycoplasmas may become undefeated in the long term.

In June 2005, the FDA approved tigecycline, an intravenous antibiotic designed to fight complicated skin infections and intra-abdominal infections caused by *E. coli*, MRSA, *Klebsiella pneumoniae*, several Streptococcus strains, and other microorganisms. Tigecycline, a derivative of minocycline, is active against many anaerobic bacteria,[9] but with an increased risk of death compared to other antibiotics prescribed for similar severe infections.[10]

Agricultural antimicrobial additives

Animal arthritis traced to *Bovis pleuropneumoniae* was first documented at the Pasteur Institute in 1898. These viral-like microbes are a particular strain of a pleuro-pneumonia-like organism (PPLO), which we now know as is highly transmissible *Mycoplasma mycoides*. PPLOs can cause a variety of arthritic, respiratory, reproductive, and neurologic disorders in different animal species.[11] Since the early 1950s, farm animals have been routinely dosed with antimicrobial compounds and hormones to keep them healthy so they will grow faster to be ready for market. Production of medicated feed additives is big business.[12] Nearly 29 million pounds of antibiotics for food-animal use was sold in 2009[13] representing about 80% of total antimicrobial drugs manufactured, as shown in Table 3.

Table 3. FDA-Approved Antimicrobials [14]

Food-animal use	Pounds	% of total
Tetracycline	10,167,481	28%
Ionophores	8,246,671	23%
NIR	4,910,501	14%
Macrolides	1,900,352	5%
Penicillins	1,345,953	4%
Sulfas	1,141,715	3%
Aminoglycosides	748,862	2%
Lincosamides	255,377	1%
Cephalosporins	91,113	<1%
Sub-total	28,808,024	**79.8%**
Human medical use	7,275,255	**20.2%**
Total	36,083,279	100%

(Source: FDA)

The original aim was to keep animals disease-free but the unintended consequences are that waters polluted by the waste from pigs, poultry, and cattle increasingly culture antibiotic resistance genes.[15] Whether or not antimicrobials in food production pose a serious human health risk has been hotly debated for the last forty years. Determining how someone becomes infected is easy; determining how the microorganism acquired the genetic profile giving it antibiotic resistance is very difficult.

Genes for drug resistance are carried not only on the bacterium's chromosomes but also on extrachromosomal elements called plasmids, which control their own replication. The plasmids of bacteria found in the small intestine are called "R-factors." These plasmids may carry several resistance genes—to sulfonamides, streptomycin, erythromycin, tetracycline, and penicillin. As a result of plasmid transfer, resistant R-factors were found in pathogenic *Staphylococcus aureus* soon after penicillin was introduced in the 1940s. The plasmids from livestock make their way into our food chain.[16]

The U.S. government tracks antibiotic resistance through the National Antimicrobial Resistance Monitoring System (NARMS), a cooperative program including the FDA, CDC, the USDA agricultural research service, and various independent research groups. In 2004, the FDA warned feed manufacturers that adding subtherapeutic doses of antibiotics to feed was "high risk." The amended Animal Drug User Fee Act (ADUFA) of 2008 directed the FDA to collect data beginning in 2010 on antibiotic use from animal drug sponsors. In 2010, Dr. Thomas Frieden testified to Congress on the CDC's ongoing efforts to control antibiotic resistance as a threat to public health.[17] That year, the FDA issued draft *voluntary* guidance on limiting subtherapeutic dosing.[18] The compliance matter is highly controversial and outside the scope of this book.[19]

Regrettably, one cannot tell whether the meat and animal products, including eggs, dairy products, and fish, carry drug-resistant microorganisms such as *S. aureus*, Campylobacter strains, *E. coli,* or salmonella.[20] The consumer must resolve either to eat fewer animal products, seek out organically grown farm products, or accept the risk of absorbing strains of resistant bacteria. Part of the problem is improperly prepared food (notably chicken, sausage, and hamburger), e.g., prepared under unsanitary conditions or being undercooked.[21] Ideally, the FDA should post regular online updates on food safety (domestic and imported) for easy public access.[22]

SURVIVAL STRATEGIES OF MICROBES

Antibiotics were first commercially available in the 1940s.[23] By 1965, there were over 25,000 antibiotic formulations on the market.[24] Many of these drugs were only marginally effective for various reasons: pleomorphic organisms shifted to a resistant form; the concentration was too low; microbial resistance was too high; the target organism was not a bacterium but a virus, fungus, or parasite; or the antibiotic did not match the strain of the pathogen.

Bacteria are determined to survive. This may mean changing shape, modifying cell walls, transforming into L-forms, mutating, encysting, conjugating, adopting camouflage, going dormant until a suitable opportunity to emerge again presents itself, hitchhiking on another organism, migrating to another host, or developing a protective (cholesterol) coating to deflect attack. Not all microorganisms use all of these techniques, but such actions and capabilities are encoded in the DNA of many microbes, to be used when the need arises.

Author Mark Lappe's book *Germs That Won't Die*, published in 1982, decried the improper use of antibiotics and predicted wholesale production of pathogenic new organisms. His critics charged that he grossly exaggerated the problem's scope. Ten years later, he was vindicated, but the problems remained. By then, a number of organisms, including strains of cholera, *E. coli*, Legionnaires' Disease bacteria, and Cryptosporidium had developed a tolerance to chlorine. Microbes were able to survive in doses of chlorine that in the past had nearly killed their species. To ensure safe drinking water, higher and higher doses of chlorine are being used. Evidence of chlorine failure can be seen in the surge of Legionnaires' Disease, cryptosporidiosis infections, and Giardia infections among users of chlorinated hot tubs, swimming pools, and public spas.[25] All icemakers should have a filter to block microbial spores.

By 1993, nearly every common pathogenic bacterial species had developed some degree of clinically significant drug resistance, and over two dozen of these strains posed life-threatening crises to humanity by having learned to tolerate the most commonly available antibiotic treatments.

Resident bacteria that we all carry in our bodies at any given time can outwit antibiotics as they evolve chemical weapons to overcome competitors for survival. Killing all but a few percent of a colony of bacteria still leaves the equivalent of "weed seeds" to spawn the next resistant generation.

Streptococcus pyogenes [26]

There are several bacteria capable of inducing RA. E.g., Streptococcus experiments using lab animals have shown that systemic injections of Group A *Streptococcus pyogenes* (GASp) lead to acute RA that peaks in a few days, then subsides, only to manifest as inflamed joints several weeks later, eventually causing joint destruction.[27] GASp and HHV-1, -2, or -4 make a deadly combination as their flesh-eating genes lyse protein cells and tissue. If we humans all contract and harbor some form of Human Herpes Virus (HHV) during our lifetimes, we are more vulnerable to pathogenic GASp.

According to the CDC, another form of the virus (HHV-6) replicates in the salivary glands and saliva is the usual transmission medium. The virus remains latent in lymphocytes and monocytes and persists at low levels in cells and tissues. HHV-6 infection is a major cause of opportunistic viral infections in the immunosuppressed, typically AIDS patients and transplant recipients, but HHV-6 can induce Autoimmune Hepatitis and may also be linked to Multiple Sclerosis.[28, 29]

There are several enigmas in the streptococcal arthritis model that parallel those of reactive arthritis, one of which is that arthritis and other chronic disorders such as Chronic Fatigue Syndrome and Fibromyalgia can be triggered by an assortment of completely different overlapping co-infections. This type of ebb and flow explains the types of flare-ups that RA sufferers describe. It also explains the apparent causal relationship between changes in the weather and RA pain, as seen in Chapter 3.

The cause of strep throat, scarlet fever, impetigo, and rheumatic fever, *S. pyogenes* bacteria colonize connective tissue, causing arthritis-like pain in the joints and potentially lethal infections of the heart. This bacterium was believed to have been wiped out by the 1970s in industrialized nations, yet a rheumatic fever outbreak in 1987 occurred in Salt Lake City, Utah (150 cases) and another in 1997-98 (72 cases).[30] The Merck Manual cited the U.S. national average as 3,000 cases per year in 2006.[31]

A cluster of seven deaths in 1994 attributed to Group A *Streptococcus pyogenes* (GASp), dubbed "flesh-eating bacteria," attracted attention to this virulent strain.[32] In 2008, the CDC reported about 9,000-11,500 cases of invasive GASp disease occurring each year in the United States, resulting in 1,000-1,800 deaths annually.[33]

Streptococcus pneumoniae

As of 2009, *S. pneumoniae* is a leading cause worldwide of illness and death for young children under five, persons with underlying medical conditions, and those over sixty-five. It is the most commonly identified cause of bacterial pneumonia. Since the widespread successful use of the flu vaccine against *Haemophilus influenzae* Type B, *S. pneumoniae* has become the most common cause of bacterial meningitis in the United States.

Streptococcus pneumoniae is also linked to *Otitis media,* bacterial pneumonia, sepsis, bacteremia, peritonitis, sinusitis, and reactive arthritis. Pneumococci are in the upper respiratory tract of 15% of well adults; in childcare settings, up to 65% of children are colonized.[34] The World Health Organization (WHO) estimated in 2009 that nearly 1 million of the annual deaths among children worldwide were caused by *Streptococcus pneumoniae.* Pneumococcus strains have shown increasing resistance to penicillin, the preferred drug for treating this type of infection.[35]

Pneumococcal vaccination since 2001 has led to markedly decreased rates of infection in the U.S.[36] Unfortunately, general respiratory infections caused by Streptococcus have not decreased much at all in the world's poor countries. In developing nations where antibiotics are available, village paramedics, lacking training and laboratory support to correctly distinguish viral from bacterial infections and mild from acute disease, may overuse or mis-apply antibiotics. The result is a set of antibiotic-resistant pneumococcal strains thriving globally, some able to defeat the actions of several antibiotics administered simultaneously.[37]

T-Cell Infiltration and Molecular Mimicry

The notion of individual susceptibility has been studied only recently as a part of the research effort to investigate human genetics. It is logical to assume that chronic arthritis develops because genetically susceptible individuals handle infection differently depending on the robustness of their immune systems. If a dysfunctional immune system is faced with an invader skilled in molecular mimicry, the contest is over before it has begun. A powerful antigenic agent with cloaking capability is able to activate a massive T-cell response to a nonspecific target, leading to the development of inflammatory chronic arthritis and the appearance of an autoimmune disorder.

Shortly after retroviruses were discovered in the early 1970s, research scientists theorized that if a retrovirus inserted itself near certain host genes, those cellular segments of DNA where transposons rarely go would be activated and cause wild cell growth. Animal experiments demonstrated that cancer could be caused by retroviruses by virtue of their ability to invade and modify activation of cellular DNA.

In 1979, researchers found evidence of a virus *inside* the immune system's T-cells (disease-fighting white blood cells discussed in Chapter 2) in human patients.[38] Despite this (and other) evidence of microbes infiltrating T-cells, the body's front line of defense, a 1995 study at the Mayo Clinic admitted surprise at finding that sets of T-cells are "different" for patients who have RA and those who don't.[39]

The disease process initiated by mycoplasmal micro-organisms is usually very slow, characterized by periods of dormancy. Because many are able to hide themselves in various ways inside animal or human tissue and even, as viruses sometimes do, within the T-cells, they are very difficult to detect. Different types of T-cells have various proteins protruding from their surfaces that serve to identify their function and form to other parts of the body. These sugar/protein markers allow cells to recognize each other in a "friend or foe" fashion. It was only in the 1980s that scientists achieved the ability to distinguish one population of T-cells from another. Much more is known about the actions of T-cells today, as seen in the discussion of New Immunology Models in Chapter 8 of this book.

HOW MICROBES SPREAD

Disruptive influences over the course of history have forced microbes to adapt to a much wider range of ecological conditions. Examples are the opening of new trade routes, increasing urbanization, the Industrial Revolution, the development of irrigation farming, air travel, and the systematic use of antibiotics in the treatment of a potpourri of ailments. It is little wonder that infection, spread so easily, can account for a wide variety of chronic health problems. Pathogenic microbes seek stability in their relationship with their human hosts. Virulence decreases as parasite and host mutually adapt to one another.

The more people infected, the greater the chance of mutation by microorganisms. As populations increase and people become more mobile, better opportunities exist for bacterial and viral spread and mutation. Person-to-person sharing of strep throat, pneumonia, and other respiratory diseases lead to the development of organisms that later show up as elements of RA.

Opportunistic infections such as pneumocystis, meningitis, and candidiasis attack immunodeficient humans. Even a healthy immune system overloads if exposed to too many microbes, many of which have pleomorphic forms that invade immune cells, reducing immune system efficiency. As we age, we accumulate a variety of parasites in the form of viruses, bacteria, and fungi. Keeping vitamin C levels high can ward off infections.[40] See Appendix V.

Pneumocystis carinii is an organism that often causes pneumonia. It is resident in nearly every human being and kept in check by the immune system until that system fails to perform optimally for a variety of reasons such as: poor diet, stress, fatigue, drug use, negative environmental factors, vitamin deficiencies, and so forth. E.g., when the time is ripe, the opportunistic *P. carinii*, which is associated with AIDS, will assert itself, grow, and spread to another human host. Similar etiology operates for *Mycoplasma pneumoniae* and *Streptococcus pneumoniae*. Researchers estimate that more than 2 million cases of *M. pneumoniae* infections occur annually. In a 2011 study, *M. pneumoniae* infection was linked to a higher risk of ischemic stroke.[41]

Adaptation Strategies of Microbes

Recent research in cellular biology and virology has identified shape-shifting organisms, but much more remains to be done. Plasmids and transposons[42] move among microbes trying to gain entry to cells. L-forms, viruses, and CWD Mycoplasmas can readily interact with plasmids.

Plasmids play a role in the evolution not only of bacteria but also possibly of all species on earth. Many contain genes called "integrons" that facilitate the integration of their DNA into any of the host organism's genomes. DNA thus moves not only between assorted bacterial species but interacts with entire families of organisms, e.g., between:

- bacteria and yeasts;
- plants and bacteria; and
- complex parasites and host cells, including T-cells and macrophages.[43]

Streptococcus pneumoniae bacteria are not very efficient at absorbing plasmids, compared to other bacteria, but they compensate for that failing by being voracious DNA scavengers.[44] *S. pneumoniae* L-forms minus the cell wall can easily interact with foreign plasmids.

Staphylococcus also uses plasmids, genes, mobile DNA, mutations, and conjugative sharing of resistance factors to overcome whatever drugs are set against it.

Staphylococcus is everywhere—in human bodies as well as in mammalian pets, on object surfaces, and in garden soil. Many varieties of Staphylococcus are not pathogenic. We interchange Staphylococci on a daily basis, through handshakes and by handling common objects, but most of the time, our immune systems render it harmless. If the bacterium enters a cut or wound, it finds an environment favorable to growth and stimulates an immune system response. While the cut or wound takes the full attention of the immune system, the bacteria find a home.

Pneumonia Epidemics

During the Spanish Flu pandemic of 1918-19, the human immune system could make antibodies against only two of the over 700 proteins that were observed to protrude from the outer envelope of the virus. Those who were able to generate these antibodies survived. The Flu sickened one billion people worldwide, and killed over twenty million.[45] Analyses of the complete genome of the 1918 influenza virus suggest that the source was an avian virus that adapted to humans.[46]

Virologists in the mid-1970s discovered that as flu viruses invade a cell and multiply in great quantities, their packaged chromosomes migrate to the outer wall of that cell and push through the cell membrane just hard enough to pull a glob of the membrane around themselves to create an outer protective coating. This process is called "budding." The newly created virus buds protrude from the host cell, attached by a strand of cell membrane until the time is right to detach and migrate to the lungs, nasal passages, or tear ducts of their human host. The new shape causes reactive immune system responses that promote the expulsion of the virus from the body of the host, allowing it to spread.

This process explains high transmissibility and virulence, such as that evidenced by the 1968 Hong Kong flu pandemic[47] and the 2003 worldwide outbreak of severe acute respiratory syndrome (SARS). The WHO proclaimed a novel coronavirus, never before seen in human or animals, as the cause SARS.[48]

Each year a new flu virus is cultured based on a guess as to which mutations will be troublesome so that a vaccine can be developed. The guess is almost always wrong.

Pneumonia Mutations

According to Doctors Baseman and Tully, "Today *M. pneumoniae* remains an important cause of pneumonia and other airway disorders, such as tracheobronchitis and pharyngitis, and is associated with extrapulmonary manifestations such as hematopoietic, exanthematic, joint, central nervous system, liver, pancreas, and cardiovascular syndromes."[49] *Chlamydophila pneumoniae* (Cpn) is also associated with these extrapulmonary symptoms. Cpn is discussed in Chapter 3.

Using multiple pathways of interaction with target cells is how Mycoplasma species and other CWD forms operate. Associations of Mycoplasmas to human diseases remains controversial because of the difficulty in identifying each CWD form in a polymicrobial soup of many chronic parasitic co-infections. We can determine that the host has a list of infections but identifying which specific microbes are at the root cause is very hard to do.

Application of PCR techniques to samples from a wide range of arthritic and other potential infection sites has shown multiple strains of cooperating organisms including assorted intracellular, CWD forms, viruses, L-forms, and Mycoplasmas.[50] This leads to the conclusion that multiple antibiotics, carefully combined and precisely directed to specific organisms, are needed to effect a rollback of multiple co-infections. The Marshall Protocol utilizes several antibiotics in staged treatments for RA, Fibromyalgia, and Sarcoidosis.[51]

Persister cells

In 1944, researcher Joseph Bigger added penicillin to a culture of Staphylococcus resulting in cell decomposition (lysis). After cells lysed, the transparent liquid was placed in a new Petri dish, and surviving colonies were noted. When recultured, and again lysed by penicillin, a new subpopulation of "persisters" was noted; these cells were not resistant mutants. Bigger concluded that penicillin did not have the ability to completely sterilize an infection. We now know that all antibiotics have this deficiency due to persister cell hardiness.

Persister bacteria cells may be the main reason for stubborn resistance of chronic infectious disease to antibiotics. Biofilms serve as a protective habitat for persisters. Stress responses may generally activate persister formation.[52] In healthy persons, persisters enable pathogens to survive at sites poorly accessible to the immune system (especially the central nervous system and the GI tract) and in places where antibiotics fail to penetrate. In persons with compromised immune systems, persisters enable pathogens to survive antimicrobial therapy.

POSSIBLE LINKS WITH OTHER DISEASES

The immune system requires hundreds of distinctly different types of cells—from tiny, free-floating lymphocytes to huge, slow-moving macrophages—to recognize a harmful incoming microorganism and then do the appropriate signaling to the immune system to muster its defenses and destroy it. If incoming microbes are small enough to disguise themselves as friendly cells, even to the point of hiding within T-cells, they can take root in the body and modify genes in normal cells. Here they can switch on/off any molecule generating gene recipes, including the cellular detection genes, thus living like reproducing bacteria clumps to form cysts, benign tumors, and/or cancerous masses. The question is: if there is a link to cancer, what other diseases could trace their root cause to shape-shifting, evasive microbes? Mycoplasma infections are commonly found in a wide variety of diseases: neurodegenerative, neurobehavioral, autoimmune, respiratory, gastrointestinal, genitourinary, fatiguing, rheumatic, and immunosuppressive conditions. Mental illnesses such as schizophrenia, Tourette's Syndrome, and psychosis have been found to be associated with Mycoplasma infection.[53, 54, 55] The percentage of patients with chronic illness who test positive for Mycoplasma infection is remarkable, as seen in these examples:[56, 57]

- Chronic Fatigue Syndrome: 50%
- Gulf War Illness: 40%
- Fibromyalgia: 60%
- Multiple Sclerosis: 50-60%
- Autism Spectrum Disorders (ASD): 60-70%
- Rheumatoid Arthritis: 45%
- Lyme Disease: 65%
- ALS (Lou Gherig's Disease): 85-90%

Mycoplasma infection can influence disease outcome. E.g., in breast and ovarian cancers, patients with systemic Mycoplasma infections die more often and sooner than uninfected patients at the same stage of the disease.[58]
Mitochondrial dysfunction also plays an important role in these diseases. The host cell compromised by Mycoplasma becomes a pathogenic "super antigen" that:

- Releases toxins and host antigens;
- Competes for metabolites and energy;
- Alters cellular structures;

- Can make different bioactive molecules (e.g., vitamin D); and
- Stimulates reactive oxygen species (ROS) to oxidize and damage mitochondrial membrane lipids and proteins, and nuclear DNA.

Oxidative stress occurs as a result of cellular aerobic metabolism, whose byproducts (such as ROS) can damage cells, including neurons. Oxidative stress is associated with cancer progression, aging and age-related degenerative diseases. The brain may be especially sensitive to damage from free radicals. It is caused by an excess of ROS and reactive nitrogen species (RNS) over cellular antioxidants, resulting in harmful oxidation of cellular structures.[59] Symptom severity is statistically related to multiple chronic intracellular infections. Antimicrobial treatment can often result in suppression of infection and relief of symptoms.[60]

It could be argued that oxidative stress is related to histamine over-production leading to ROS. The destructive effects might be the result of ascorbic acid depletion. This would explain the Herxheimer reaction to ROS and RNS, linked to hydrogen peroxide and nitrogen oxide byproducts of the inflammation process.[61]

Rheumatoid factors (or R-factors) have been observed in a number of diseases other than arthritis, for example: chronic infectious diseases like leprosy, various parasitic diseases, tuberculosis, and subacute bacterial endocarditis; liver disease (in the form of chronic active hepatitis); lympho-proliferative syndromes, and Sarcoidosis.[62, 63]

Dr. Joseph Tully, in an article[64] for the International Organization for Mycoplasmology, lauds Dr. Brown and his colleagues for their basic research, clinical expertise, and persistence in advocating antibiotic treatments for a variety of chronic illnesses traceable to mycoplasmal infection.

The Arthritis Center of Riverside has tabulated an impressive list of arthritis-causing microorganisms.[65]

Ongoing research is documenting the clearly causal relationship between a wide range of diseases and mycobacteria, Mycoplasmas, bacterial L-forms and the R-factor. A few of these disorders are described more fully below as examples. AIDS and Lyme disease are discussed in Chapter 5.

Gulf War Illness/Gulf War Syndrome

A range of as-yet undiagnosed illnesses continues to be reported by Gulf War veterans and their families long after that 1991 conflict.[66] In 2010, more than 250,000 troops returning from the Gulf suffer from chronic, unexplained symptoms.[67] The sum of the conditions documented is called collectively Gulf War Illness (GWI). However, some conditions are not unique to Gulf War veterans and were reported before 1990 (i.e., before the war began).

A variety of infections are common in the Persian Gulf region—sandfly fever (also called Phlebotomus fever, pappataci fever, or three-day fever), Dengue fever, Sindbis, Rift Valley fever, typhus, brucellosis, spotted fever, schistosomiasis, and echinococcosis—but these have not been diagnosed among the veterans.

Dr. Garth Nicolson's hypothesis is that the combined effects of multiple toxic exposures (including multiple vaccines) may have produced symptoms of GWI in predisposed, susceptible individuals. Gulf War troops were exposed to a wide variety of toxic substances, low level nerve agents, fumes and smoke from burning oil wells, blow-back from bunker demolitions, and inhalation of fine sand.

A 2011 Baylor study[68] suggests that GWI prevalence is based on the residual effect of varying levels of toxic exposures encountered by troops in specific battlefield areas. However, the study does not explain the complex GWI symptoms manifested by family members and associates in the U.S. after the afflicted veteran returned home. Testing of these non-deployed individuals revealed that *M fermentans* infections were being passed to immediate family members who then became sick with CFS or FMS (adults or teens) or Autism Spectrum Disorders (young children).

Troops were also given several vaccinations against possible biological warfare pathogens: acute agents like anthrax (*Bacillus anthracis*), Brucellosis, Clostridium species (*C. botulinum* and *C. perfringens*), *Coxiella burnettii*, Mycoplasma (notably *M. fermentans* and *M. genitalium*), and *Francisella tularensis*.[69]

Dr. Nicolson proposes that these vaccines may have been given too close together, and that 4 of 5 (AVIP) anthrax vaccine lots have failed FDA tests for potency and contamination.[70] He estimates that commercial vaccines are about 6% contaminated with Mycoplasma. This assertion is still hotly debated and outside the scope of this book. A 2003 study showed that adjuvant persistence for months or years can upset immune functions, leading to GWI symptoms.[71, 72]

Dr. Nicolson's multiple-vaccine theory for those afflicted with GWI extends to children with autism, a neurological condition typically striking children between 18 months and 3 years of age. As of 2010, pre-schoolers are routinely inoculated with as many as 26 assorted vaccines[73], compared to just three given in the 1940s.[74, 75] Vaccines are a multi-billion dollar industry. Price lists per dose are on the CDC's website.[76]

Autism was relatively rare (one in ten thousand) until mass vaccination programs were mandated in the 1990s, with the introduction of the Hepatitis B vaccine and the HiB (meningitis) vaccine. Fourteen studies are usually cited to disprove all association of vaccines with autism. However, these vested-interest studies were funded either by the CDC (the agency in charge of the vaccine program) or pharmaceutical company grants or the NIH, and touted in the media by celebrity spokespersons paid by the vaccine manufacturers.[77] The matter is hardly closed, as the government agencies claim.[78, 79]

Studying unvaccinated children may be the best hope for finding the cause of a disorder that now impacts 1 in 110 children. A 9,000% increase in reported cases of autism since 1987 indicates an epidemic in progress.[80] Autism Spectrum Disorder is discussed in Chapter 5.

Most of the signs and symptoms in a large subset of GWI patients can be explained by chronic pathogenic bacterial infections, such as Mycoplasma (all species) and Brucellosis[81] infections. Three types of symptoms were seen to be about three times more prevalent among Gulf War veterans than other test subjects in one 18,075 participant study: chronic fatigue, muscle and joint pain, and neuro-cognitive problems.[82, 83]

In Dr. Nicolson's words, "Once these [infections] are identified, then they can be treated with a regimen of antibiotics, vitamins, and nutritional support.... At least three quarters of the people who start this treatment have recovered. Not everybody recovers and we attribute that to the fact that a lot of people have multiple reasons for their chronic conditions...In some cases people get temporary relief by going on hyperbaric oxygen."[84]

Mycoplasmas are microorganisms that prefer low oxygen tension. That is, when the body's tissues are starved for oxygen, the condition will stimulate the growth of these borderline anaerobes. This explains why symptoms of individuals with Mycoplasma infections are worse after a long airline flight with variations in cabin pressure. GWI is particularly evident in helicopter pilots for this reason.[85] It also explains why deep breathing and aerobic exercise help oxygenate cells and keep anaerobes in check. In 2000, a major study considered childhood autism and adult depression as chronic illnesses linked to mycoplasmal infection for which antibiotics and hyperbaric oxygen treatments could apply.[86, 87] HBOT is discussed in Chapter 1.

At the time of this writing, there are approximately 100 different types of Mycoplasmas; 14 have been found to cause disease in humans and 17 in animals.[88] One species in particular, *M. fermentans (incognitus)*, has been detected in some tested Gulf War veterans and their families.[89] The infected individual will start to exhibit Chronic Fatigue Syndrome (CFS) or Fibromyalgia (FMS) symptoms:[90] a low-grade fever and/or a sense of "coming down with the flu." The condition becomes chronic as more symptoms develop: joint pain, reduced mobility, chronic fatigue, vision problems, cognitive problems, and muscle spasms—all coming on very slowly.[91] Details on FMS symptoms and treatment appear in Appendix II.

Multiple Sclerosis (MS)

MS is a neurological disease in which the blood/brain barrier is damaged. Edema and swelling cause the release of plasma proteins into the central nervous system, triggering an inflammatory response. The disease is intermittent, so initial diagnosis is difficult and is usually made only after several disabling attacks have damaged the nervous system. Abnormal regulation of apoptosis has been implicated in autoimmune disease and in degenerative conditions such as MS. Members of the TNF family of cytokines and receptors are critically involved in the process.[92]

German researchers found in 2011 that gut bacteria might be involved in autoimmune disorders such as MS, juvenile diabetes, and arthritis. They concluded that ordinary commensal gut flora—in the absence of pathogenic agents—are essential to initiate immune processes, leading to a relapsing–remitting autoimmune disease driven by myelin-specific CD4+ T cells.[93] In another study, the stimuli triggering MS have been attributed to Epstein Barr viral infection.[94] Several scientists have found that patients with MS have a high incidence of mycoplasmal infections.[95] Systemic chronic infections (caused by bacteria such as Mycoplasma, Chlamydia, Borrelia, Brucella, etc. or viruses such as cytomegalovirus (CMV), Human Herpes Virus Six (HHV-6), or enterovirus, etc.) can invade virtually every human tissue. These pathogens can not only directly damage and kill nerve cells by apoptosis, resulting in nervous system degeneration, but also can compromise the immune system, permitting opportunistic infections by other bacteria, viruses, fungi and yeast. When Mycoplasmas exit certain cells, such as synovial cells, they can stimulate an autoimmune response in others, e.g., nerve cells.[96]

HHV-6 is a disease contracted in infancy causing a high fever and rash. Although the children recover, the HHV-6 stays dormant in the nerves until an opportune time to emerge. At that time, the virus damages the nerves' myelin sheath, producing the symptoms of MS.[97, 98, 99, 100] HHV-6 DNA is detectable by PCR testing. One could experiment with high levels of ascorbic acid to utilize its antiviral properties against HHV-6.[101]

Cerebrospinal fluid (CSF) is examined using PCR tests to detect the presence of immune system proteins known to be associated with MS. The CSF test can also detect the presence of oligoclonal bands. These bands are evidence of an autoimmune response and are found in over 90% of MS patients.[102] However, since these bands are detected in other individuals with other diseases, their presence does not lead to a conclusive diagnosis for MS.[103] Since the late 1990s, compelling research using CSF tests[104] indicates that MS is either caused by or exacerbated by *Chlamydia pneumoniae* (Cpn) infection.[105, 106, 107, 108]

Dr. Luther Lindner, a physician and pathologist at Texas A&M University, has been researching pathogens and MS for many years. The bacteria in question (unique strains of Methylobacterium) cannot be cleared from the bloodstream with available antibiotics. In fact, antibiotics actually stimulate this bacterium's growth and are <u>not</u> recommended. Milk, fruit juice, and excessive light exposure may make symptoms worse.[109]

Prescription drugs provide some temporary relief, but have not been able to stop the progression of, or reverse, the symptoms of the disease. These drugs also introduce adverse side effects. Persons with MS admit to using a variety of alternative methods and supplements: e.g., high-EPA fish oil, borage oil, and lecithin help to suppress autoimmune reactions and to rebuild the myelin sheath. Coenzyme Q_{10} and vitamin B_{12} (sublingual preferred) are also beneficial for cell rejuvenation.[110] HBOT can help relieve symptoms.[111]

Endnotes and continuing research on topics in Chapter 4 can be found at www.RA-Infection-Connection.com

5. EMERGING EPIDEMICS

Sustained antibiotic treatment has been seen to inhibit mycoplasmal infection long enough for the body's natural immune system to destroy the invaders. Although Dr. Joseph Tully notes that physicians who treat chronic illnesses estimate that more than 25% of their patients benefit from a long-term, low-dose antibiotic regimen, this treatment is not guaranteed to work for all patients diagnosed with arthritis.[1]

Dr. Franco of the Arthritis Center of Riverside conducted a study of 255 of his RA patients. After long-term antibiotic treatment, 78% had a better than 20% improvement, and 53% had a better than 50% improvement; 22% of the patients did not improve. However, those patients whose antineutrophilic cytoplasmic antibodies (ANCA)[2] test results are positive seem to have an increased likelihood of worsening with minocycline treatment. In these cases, Dr. Franco prefers to use the macrolide antibiotics (erithromycin, azithromycin, or clarithromycin) since minocycline can lead to drug-induced Lupus.[3]

A 1997 study from the University of Nebraska focused on patients who had RA for less than one year. After three years on the antibiotic drug, 44% of the patients had improved by 75% or more. Improvement criteria included joint tenderness, stiffness and swelling.[4]

The point has been made repeatedly in this book that there is no single solution to healing RA. Despite thousands of documented success stories, there are still many individuals who do not respond to Dr. Brown's protocol. This could be because they have additional serious medical conditions or co-infections, or perhaps their bodies harbor antibiotic-resistant microbes, or possibly because their symptoms have been misdiagnosed. As we have seen in Chapter 3, food allergies can aggravate arthritis symptoms.

Chronic illness individuals, especially those with gut disorders or bulimia, often have nutritional and vitamin deficiencies that must be corrected in parallel with any treatment against infection(s).

Physicians may be treating mycoplasmal, chlamydial, and other chronic infections but they are often not taking into account the intracellular, persistent phases of these infections. During treatment, the microorganisms may be assuming a dormant phase within healthy tissues until they sense a more opportune time to colonize. The treatment may not address polymicrobial co-infections attributable to insect bites, viruses, mycotoxins, and/or bacteria.

Lyme Disease is one of a growing number of diseases exhibiting a full range of arthritis-like symptoms. This group includes other multi-strain, tick-borne (and sometimes mosquito-borne) illnesses such as Babesiosis, Ehrlichiosis, and Rickettsial disease.[5] Perhaps the best-known example of disease caused by *Rickettsia rickettsii* in the U.S. is Rocky Mountain spotted fever (RMSF). Nine strains found worldwide cause a variety of illnesses, including typhus.[6] Reports of RMSF cases have increased from less than two cases per million persons in 2000 to over eight cases per million in 2008.[7, 8]

Babesiosis is caused by tick-borne *Babesia mircoti*, which are malarial–like piroplasms. Ticks are also carriers of *Ehrlichia phagocytophila*, which causes Ehrlichiosis, a Lyme co-infection that can be fatal in about 10% of cases. At present, it responds to doxycycline but only in the early stages.[9] Sometimes multiple antibiotics must be used; anti-protozoal and antimalarial drugs are needed to treat Babesiosis.

Bacterial infections involving the brain and central nervous system often do not respond to certain antibiotics because the biochemical structure of the drugs makes the molecules too large to cross the blood/brain barrier (BBB). Minocycline can cross the barrier, but tetracycline cannot.[10]

This barrier acts protectively to limit the penetration of harmful substances to the brain. By blocking the transport of curing substances as well, this filtering mechanism acts as a limiting factor for brain treatments with drugs. These neurological conditions require high doses of antibiotics to raise serum concentrations to levels able to penetrate the BBB but at the risk of damaging other organs. Intensive international research efforts are underway to discover a selective penetration method that would guarantee the transport of drugs through the intact barrier. Ascorbic acid passes through the BBB and can act as an antibiotic via intravenous protocols.

LYME DISEASE (LD)

In 1975, fifty-one residents of Old Lyme, Connecticut were afflicted with a mysterious illness that resembled RA. By 1990, what has come to be called "Lyme Disease" was reported in all 50 States and parts of Western Europe. This is not because LD appeared as a new or localized disease spreading from the U.S. east coast; rather, it is because its bacterial origin had finally been recognized and a name given to the condition. LD is as ancient as the insects that carry it. Nantucket, CT now has the dubious distinction of being called the Lyme capitol of the world.[11]

Although formally recognized for over 25 years, Lyme Disease is still one of the most under-, over-, and mis-diagnosed diseases today. Some LD symptoms are common to other chronic illnesses like Fibromyalgia (FMS) or Chronic Fatigue Syndrome (CFS) : fatigue, muscle aches, joint pain and swelling. Neurological complications of LD may include meningitis, chronic Neuroborreliosis, or Bell's palsy.[12] Some patients diagnosed with CFS or autism are later found to have Lyme Disease.[13, 14]

Through diligent pest control measures, improved sanitation, and antibiotics, we have been lucky to prevent serious outbreaks of insect-borne diseases in the United States. Lyme Disease remains a significant problem.[15] Other insects (e.g., lice, bedbugs, flies) are also microbe carriers, but they are not yet associated with huge human or animal infection pools in the U.S. However, invading mosquito strains and the West Nile Virus has recently become endemic in most States, with reservoirs of that virus now in the bird population. Horses are vulnerable if unvaccinated,[16] but human cases are infrequent and can be fatal if not treated with high levels of vitamin C.[17]

Mycoplasma co-infections are common. According to Dr. Nicolson at the Institute for Molecular Medicine, 60% of LD patients with Borrelia, 70% of those diagnosed with Ehrlichia, 40% of those with Bartonella, and 20% of those with Babesiosis also test positive for Mycoplasma.[18] The most common LD co-infection is *Mycoplasma fermentans.*[19]

Lyme Disease Carriers

The disease was traced to a little-studied spirochete bacterium, *Borrelia burgdorferi*, which is transmitted to humans by a tick *(Ixodes scapularis)*. During their two-year life cycle, shown in Figure 6,[20] ticks use a variety of carriers—mostly large mammals such as deer and humans, but also migrating birds[21]—who can be counted upon to disperse them over a wide geographic area as they mature. It is as though gangs of microbial terrorists are using ticks as their own FedEx method to deliver their deadly cargo.

Deer are considered prime carriers of adult ticks, which feed on the deer's blood, then drop from their host to lay their eggs.[22] Known disease carriers like rodents thrive in a fragmented forest environment where their natural predators (coyotes, weasels, and foxes) have migrated away to larger areas or have been killed as pests in urban areas.

Limiting the population of animal hosts as LD carriers is essential to controlling the spread of the disease.

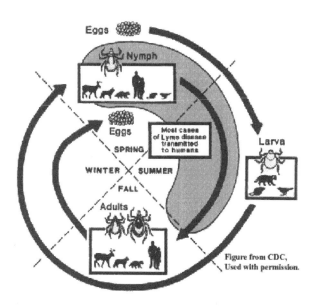

Figure 6. Life Cycle of Lyme Disease Ticks

Entomologists tracking the spread of mosquitoes over 17 years on a coastal Maine island noted a concurrent epidemic spread of ticks carrying *B. burgdorferi* (Bb).[23] The species variants changed, with new Bb strains found, likely imported by birds and then spread to the ticks from animals infected by the mosquitoes from the bird reservoir. Lyme was not detected in the mosquitoes until year ten. After 10 years, Bb in ticks was 4%; at year 17, it was 43%. The scientists concluded that there was a corresponding increased risk of exposure to LD on the mainland of New England and Canada near the island.

As of 2008, there were 5 identified subspecies of Bb with over 100 strains in the United States and 300 strains worldwide.[24] Bb exists in at least 3 different forms: bacterial (spirochete), spheroplast, and cyst form. Only the spirochete can be killed by beta lactam antibiotics. Tetracyclines and erythromycins can kill the spheroplasts, but only the antibiotic metronidazole is effective against cysts.[25]

The disease-bearing tick punctures the skin, introducing the *B. burgdorferi* spirochete. As the tick feeds, it transmits the disease. About 70-90% of those who contract LD are bitten by nymphs. The resulting circular red rash may expand to 12 inches or more in diameter over the next several weeks. By then the bacteria has pervaded muscle, tendons, organs, heart, and even the brain.[26]

LD-infected humans can experience a wide range of neurological, cognitive, and psychiatric symptoms. In the later stage of the disease, patients exhibit memory deficits, loss of fluency of speech, and difficulty recalling motor skills. Dr. Robert Bransfield has developed a psychiatric diagnostic and tracking system.[27] This technique goes far beyond the standard medical approach, combining lab test results with a detailed patient history, physical, and mental status exam to obtain a more accurate diagnosis.

Dr. Bransfield points out that co-infections with other agents leading to interactive infections pose a significant issue. He has also found that effective treatment consists of intramuscular and intravenous antibiotics, sometimes for an extended period of weeks or months. However, Dr. Allen C. Steere, who discovered and named Lyme Disease, cautions against long-term antibiotic treatment for unsubstantiated LD.[28]

In the opinion of some researchers, LD may rival Mycoplasma infection as the causative agent for Rheumatoid Arthritis. One important but subtle difference between classical RA (Mycoplasma infection) and LD (vector-borne infection) is that LD affects the large weight-bearing joints, especially the knees, where RA prefers the small joints of the peripheral extremities, notably in the hand. This contrast may be because Mycoplasmas migrate to the cooler areas of the body while spirochetes prefer warmer areas where the body temperature is relatively constant. Lyme Disease can be as painful, degenerative, and crippling as classical RA.

Tests for Lyme Disease

In 2008, the CDC reported that Lyme disease was the sixth most commonly reported illness in the U.S. and the most common vector-borne disease, with 95% coming from endemic regions. A conservative estimate is that only one in ten cases of Lyme Disease is actually reported to the CDC. Estimates are about four million cases of LD since 1980.[29] The CDC requires a positive test for surveillance purposes in reporting cases of LD, and requires a diagnosis based on a doctor's evaluation of symptoms plus supporting tests.

Criteria for LD epidemiology tests are selected to reduce the number of false positive tests and to increase the false negatives. A problem arises in treatment if the doctor uses these criteria to diagnose LD infection because of the high number of false negative results. Patients who have Lyme infection should seek out a Lyme-literate MD (LLMD) who is skilled at evaluating test results and who knows how difficult and long-term a treatment must be to effect a cure.

All testing methods currently available for LD have serious limitations. Some tests (e.g., *in vitro* culture) may be inadequate for clinical purposes, while others provide results needing skilled interpretation. Bb can be detected by culture in BSK II (modified Barbour-Stoenner-Kelly) but lab culture is not reliable for routine testing.

Several labs have developed research protocols to identify the causative agents of Lyme Disease, Ehrlichia, and Babesia.[30] The Lyme Urine Antigen Test (LUAT) once held promise but was found to return a high rate of false-positive results and now is not recommended.[31] Western blot may become the gold standard for LD testing, although a real problem is that many labs do not perform this test as accurately as IgeneX.[32]

Dr. Joseph Burrascano,[33] an internationally renowned LLMD, notes a paradox with chronic Lyme testing: the more ill the patient the weaker the blood serum test result and the less likely it is to get a positive indicator. He asserts that ELISA tests are of little value; PCR testing requires multiple samples from multiple sources (whole blood, urine, bone marrow, saliva, spinal fluid, etc). Time of day for the test makes a difference in results. Western blot is best, however, it is very difficult to produce and interpret: bands do not easily line up; the sample may be affected by subtle changes in temperature and the chemistry of the test system; and the technician's proficiency is a factor.

According to Dr. Lida Mattman, prominent infectious disease expert, blood samples to culture should be taken from the ears, as LD bacteria tend to cluster there waiting for a mosquito to bite and carry them to a new host.[34]

The specific strain of Borrelia (of hundreds of known strains) being tested for may not match the strain infecting the patient. Standard LD tests look for just one strain. The three or four strains found in the USA are region-specific, so these tests are not likely to be available to all doctors trying to diagnose and treat LD.

Treatment for Lyme Disease

Tick-borne diseases are very complex infections.[35] Diagnoses are often unclear or inaccurate. Treatment is expensive, may be difficult to tolerate, and may not help. Patients may have severe and confusing symptoms, often to the point of disability. LD can be treated with the usual short course of antibiotics but *only* if caught in the very early stages. Antibiotic protocols for late stage LD must be much more intensive and complex than the relatively simpler treatment proposed by Dr. Brown for Mycoplasma infection. Most LLMDs agree that steroids can be very harmful.[36] Controversy still surrounds LD diagnosis and treatment.[37]

Frustrated LD patients often seek out complementary and alternative medicine (CAM) doctors to treat their chronic, painful, debilitating symptoms. According to Dr. Burrascano, antibiotics alone or CAM alone are unable to solve the LD problem. Too gentle dosage may lead to resistance; too strong can cause a setback. Aggressive CAM therapies may not kill the pathogen and just mask the underlying infection, setting the patient up for later damage that could have been prevented. Antibiotics must have both extra- and intra-cellular sites of action since Bb can survive in both places. Antibiotics must act in body fluids (mucosal surfaces) as well as in the tissues, because Bb lives in both sites. Specific antibiotics are needed to target the various forms of Bb as shown in Table 4:[38, 39]

Dr. Burrascano advises a comprehensive assessment of the patient's diet, lifestyle habits, addictions (alcohol, smoking, drugs), exercise regimen, sleep cycle, environment (toxins, stress, work schedule, etc), and so forth. He would begin yeast cleanout/detox, test for and treat other known parasites, initiate a nutrition regimen, encourage keeping a daily diary and temperature record. He would screen for complicating factors such as co-infections and opportunistic infections, the toxic burden, genetic influences, endocrine irregularities, presence of heavy metals, and low cellular energy production (using a cardiac echo screen).[40]

In the absence of diagnostic tools required to identify LD, doctors have little data to form a diagnosis. Insurance companies are understandably reluctant to authorize coverage for treatments based on guesswork. However, they are also inexcusably reluctant to invest in the extensive tests, tools, and procedures required for accurate diagnoses.

CDC criteria[41] miss 90% of LD cases; commercial blood tests miss about half. Co-infections are nearly universal in chronic LD, which renders standard diagnostic tests and evaluation unreliable. Lyme Disease treatments do not treat Bartonella, viruses, or Babesia (a protozoa).[42] Opportunistic co-infections include Candida, Mycoplasma, Staphylococcus, Chlamydophila, and various intestinal parasites. Contracting Lyme Disease can reactivate latent viruses: HSV, CMV, Epstein-Barr, XMRV, parvovirus, and Human Herpes HHV-6, -7, and –8.[43]

Table 4. Bb Forms and Corresponding Antibiotics

Bb form	Characteristics of each *B. burgdorferi* form	Antibiotics
Spiral form (spirochete)	Cell wall; very mobile; spiral/drill shape allows penetration into dense tissue and bone	Penicillins, cephalosporins, Primaxin, vancomycin
L-form	Cell wall-deficient; makes dense colonies	Tetracyclines, erythromycins
Intracellular	Penetrates and remains viable within cells	Extracellular antibiotic, e.g. penicillin, plus an intracellular agent, e.g., telithromycin
Cyst	Dormant form, converts back to spirochete when conditions are favorable	Metronidazole, tinidazole, tigecycline, rifampin

Patients must be proactive in researching their condition, tapping the formidable resources available to them through LD-related foundations and their websites.[44] Because LD's forty-odd symptoms fit a number of medical conditions, it is important to find definitive tests and physicians who have the expertise to evaluate them.[45]

An Anti-toxin Treatment for LD

An effective therapy developed by LLMD Dr. Ritchie Shoemaker[46] has received attention from physicians who treat Lyme Disease patients. The LD spirochete has been found to produce a toxin (a 37 kD protein) that has similar properties to botulinum C2 and other cytoskeletal toxins.

Dr. Shoemaker's therapy[47] uses cholestyramine to bind the fat-soluble toxins into molecules that are too large for the colon to reabsorb, and thus they are preferentially excreted. Cholestyramine is a cholesterol-lowering drug but it is much safer than others usually prescribed because the molecules produced do not find their way back into the gastrointestinal (GI) tract or into the bloodstream. Thus, some of the harmful side effects associated with the newer statin drugs are avoided.[48]

Ascorbic acid is inherently anti-toxin, so any anti-Lyme protocol should include high and frequent (pulsed) vitamin C dosages to disable toxins. Since toxins do not replicate, persistence of their presence implies the existence of an internal generative process or continued intake of new toxin molecules. Toxins can also be created by the ROS/NOS created by our immune system's allergic reactions. Oxidized lipids are rancid fats; cholesterol oxides are neurotoxins.

TUBERCULOSIS (TB)

Drug-resistant TB and malaria are re-emerging as serious health problems in developing countries. TB causes infectious septic arthritis.[49]

In the time frame 1953-2009, the CDC reported that case rates in the U.S. had steadily decreased from 84,304 to 11,545. In 2009, Hispanics and Asians accounted for 80% of TB cases among foreign-born persons, representing 48% of the national case total. The top five countries of origin of immigrants with TB were Mexico, Philippines, Vietnam, India, and China.

Although TB case reports in 2009 and the annual TB rate reached all-time lows in the United States, disproportionately high rates of TB persist among foreign-born persons and racial/ethnic minorities, particularly among U.S.-born blacks.[50] The WHO 2009 Global TB Control Report revealed that one out of four TB deaths was HIV-related, twice as many as previously recognized.

By 2010 the number of reported cases in the U.S. were dramatically down, but challenges remain: (1) increasing high incidence of global TB; (2) more infected patients in immigrant communities where the rate is 76% higher than the U.S.-born population; (3) no TB testing for foreign arrivals; (4) waning collective knowledge/expertise; (5) complacency in reporting TB; (6) reduced TB funding.[51]

FIBROMYALGIA SYNDROME (FMS) [52]

Fibromyalgia has now reached the status of an epidemic. Nearly 6 million Americans (mostly Caucasian women) suffer daily from this puzzling condition, which leaves many barely able to function, even though their symptoms often seem vague and difficult to describe.

For a very long time, doctors insisted that FMS was "all in the head" of the patient. One of these is Dr. Jerome Groopman, who proposed in the *New Yorker* magazine that FMS is caused by the stress endured by middle-class white women unable to cope with modern life.[53] Sadly, these patients are routinely given drugs like Prozac or Xanax for depression and "brain fog." Psychotherapy is often suggested.

According to LLMD Dr. Ritchie Shoemaker, so-called "Fibromyalgia" belongs to a much larger disease scenario in which an entire new constellation of undiagnosed environmental illnesses has been attacking millions of Americans in recent years. He asserts that Fibromyalgia and other chronic conditions are actually caused by a new group of biotoxin-mediated diseases. FMS patients don't need help for depression; their debilitating "brain-fog" is caused by neurotoxins.[54]

In the words of Dr. Shoemaker, "These little-understood diseases make people sick by producing low molecular-weight toxins (aka 'ionophores') that hide out in the body's fat-containing tissues, where they remain impervious to the germ-fighting antibodies that endlessly patrol the human bloodstream."

Advances in biomarking tools, notably the Visual Contrast Sensitivity test (described in Chapter 6) now allows physicians to diagnose toxin-based illnesses such as FMS, Sick Building Syndrome, Lyme Disease, and CFS accurately and to precisely measure the effects of therapy. Additional information and details on the Shoemaker Protocol can be found at www.chronicneurotoxins.com.

Approximately 50% of CFS and FMS patients show Mycoplasma infection and most appear to recover after long-term antibiotic therapy with doxycycline.[55, 56]

Some species of Mycoplasma might have the ability to cause a dysregulation of the neuroendocrine system. In the late 1980's to early 1990's, some diagnoses of Fibromyalgia and rheumatic diseases were subsequently changed to a hypothyroidism diagnosis after thyroid testing was performed. In clinical practice is has been demonstrated that a significant percentage of FMS patients are tested with secondary hypothyroidism.[57] This is missed by many health practitioners who routinely test thyroid function by measuring common thyroid hormones T3, T4, and TSH (thyroid stimulating hormone). The majority of FMS patients will test in normal ranges. However, thyroid dysfunction is often revealed in FMS patients when a TRH stimulus test (thyrotropin-releasing hormone) is given.[58]

Low blood pressure (hypotension) is common in many Fibromyalgia and CFS patients. A tilt-table test can confirm this diagnosis.[59, 60] Treatment can be as simple as increasing water intake or balancing salt in one's diet.[61]

Find a discussion of FMS in Appendix II.

AUTISM SPECTRUM DISORDER (ASD)

Autism has become more common in our children than cancer, diabetes, and AIDS combined.[62] ASD refers to a set of pervasive brain developmental disorders causing severe impairment in thinking, feeling, communication, vision, and eye contact. Hallmarks are repetitive behavior and the inability to relate to others. Variations include autism, Asperger's, and other conditions seen first in early childhood.

Statistics reveal one in 10,000 pre-1990, with increasing numbers of ASD cases each year. The CDC reported that in 2006 one in 110 children in the USA exhibited some ASD symptoms, with total numbers of afflicted children growing 10-17% annually.[63] A 2008 CDC study revised this estimate to one in 88.[64] Note: this number does not include PDD, Asperger's, and other spectrum disorders.[65]

There are countless theories about the causes of ASD, ranging from vitamin deficiencies to genetic susceptibility. Intensive research is underway to solve this complex problem.[66, 67] A few of these efforts and hypotheses are presented here.

ASD treatments include diet, behavior modification, psychoactive drugs, antioxidants, and chelators. Hyperbaric oxygen therapy (HBOT, discussed in Chapter 1) has been shown to be successful in several cerebral hypoperfusion syndromes including cerebral palsy, fetal alcohol syndrome, closed head injury, stroke, and autism.[68] HBOT can reduce oxidative stress and inflammation, two characteristics of neurodegenerative disease.[69] By increasing blood flow to the brain, HBOT normalizes oxygen levels in ischemic tissue.[70]

Dr. Nicolson's extensive research has shown that Mycoplasmas invade immune cells and suppress normal immune system function. He suspects the role of pathogenic Mycoplasmas in ASD because he has observed some children manifest autistic symptoms after an acute childhood infection, multiple childhood vaccinations, heavy metal exposures, and/or chemical exposures.

Professor Nicolson concludes that most autism patients have chronic polymicrobial infections (bacterial, viral, fungal) that cause disease. Such infections could be causative, co-factors, or opportunistic, and should be considered as one of the multiple approaches in the clinical management of ASD.[71]

Assorted Mycoplasma species were found in ASD patients[72] with single infections:

> *M. pneumoniae:* 50%
> *M. fermentans:* 30%
> *M. hominus:* 27%

Overlapping co-infections also detected in ASD patients:

> Mycoplasma species: 40-65%
> HHV-6: 15-30%
> Borrelia species (Lyme): 10-30%
> Fungal infections: 5-20%

Many symptoms of ASD children are the same as that of vitamin A deficiency.[73] In case of proven measles–related chronic infections, there are reports of a few doctors who have used a very high vitamin A dosage of retinol palmitate (100,000 to 200,000 IU) for two days followed by lower but still relatively high dosages. The protocol requires appropriate monitoring of antibody levels and careful control of the vitamin A dosage to avoid toxic effects. The results were far from uniform or repeatable.

However, use of various combinations of antivirals such as cod liver oil (high vitamin A and D content), coconut oil, ascorbic acid (vitamin C), and olive leaf extract (together or in alternation) have resulted in elimination of the measles virus. The association of the ASD symptoms with visual disabilities/symptoms and their reduction or elimination by vitamin A (or other antiviral) intake allows a measure of the effectiveness of different dosage levels.

Dr. John Cannell has written extensively on ASD, suggesting that the primary trigger in autism is gestational and early childhood vitamin D deficiency, based on a 2008 review detailing the devastating effect of this deficiency on developing mammalian brains.[74] Vitamin D[75] deficiency has also been implicated in Parkinson's disease, another neurological disorder.[76, 77] A vitamin B_{12} deficiency has also been suggested as a possible trigger for ASD.[78] A simple blood test can determine vitamin levels in an at-risk child.

A body of research published in 2005-11 concerning the possible role of gut bacterial metabolites in ASD has been listed among the top 50 scientific discoveries in Canada.[79] In 2005, a researcher found that children with autism have higher-than-normal concentrations of Clostridium bacteria.[80] Protozoal parasites were found in high numbers (69% of patients) versus control subjects (30%) in a study of 106 autistic children.[81]

Research shows that 70% of children with ASD suffer from gastrointestinal problems, compared with only 28% of typically developing children.[82, 83] A 2011 study suggests that gut microbes may influence brain development, thus ultimately shaping behavior.[84] Dysbiosis often plays a role.[85] An intestinal barrier defect (i.e., leaky gut) is liked to many systemic disorders, including ASD.[86]

Dr. Aristo Vojdani's excellent illustrated research paper details the role of environmental triggers (e.g., viral infection, dietary proteins and peptides) that lead to gut inflammation/dysfunction, and in turn to immune system dysregulation. Dr. Vojdani's research posted online at glutensensitivity.net shows that toxins, stress, and infections can damage the gut so badly that food cannot be digested properly. This chaos manifests itself in the nervous system where neuroinflammation correlates with a genetic susceptibility to ASD.[87]

The impact of food allergies on autism has also been reported.[88] Many children with autism have allergic reactions to yeast, gluten, casein (dairy), or environmental allergens. Some of these substances are used in vaccine production. Experts advise that if the child is intolerant of yeast, avoid the Hepatitis B shot; for eggs, avoid the measles, mumps and rubella (MMR) vaccine; for Neomycin, avoid MMR or Varisella shots; for a gelatin intolerance, avoid the Varivax vaccine.[89]

Associated with vaccination are tens of thousands of adverse events subject to claims presented to the Office of Special Masters of the U.S. Court of Federal Claims (called the "Vaccine Court"), which administers a no-fault system for litigating vaccine injury claims. The Court hears cases of ASD disability that have chronic viral gut and systemic infections with strains from one or more of the MMR live viruses in the vaccines.[90] By denying all autism claims, new claim filings have stopped. This method alters the statistics but incidents still occur.

Autism/ASD incidence statistics differ widely between vaccinated (U.S., Canada, Australia) and unvaccinated (Cuba) regions.[91] High vaccination rates go with high MMR claims, indicating that something related to our high-rate, high-frequency vaccination program is going wrong. The HHS director now says that reevaluation of the vaccination schedules, rates, and rules is needed, but immediate action is required,[92] as well as more complete disclosure to the public. Vaccines are discussed later in this chapter.

Ultrasound and ASD

Ultrasound has been used in obstetrics since the 1950s. At that time, studies indicated it was safe for both mother and child, but recent research implicates it in neurodevelopmental disorders. The major risk to the fetus come from high acoustic output required for high-definition images, which may take some time as technicians hunt for suitable images. However, an almost equal risk is ultrasound in the hands of operators who may have no medical background or appropriate training.

These variables, along with factors such as cavitation (a bubbling effect caused by ultrasound that can damage cells) and on-screen safety indicators that may be inaccurate by a factor ranging from 2–6, make the impact of ultrasound uncertain even in expert hands.[93]

Other risks to fetal tissue include conduction of heat produced at the contact point with the transducer surface, and also radiation forces leading to streaming in fluids and stress at tissue interfaces.[94] The FDA provides guidance for ultrasound devices, but there is some concern that the upper limit may be set too high.[95]

Prenatal ultrasound warnings were mentioned in a 1982 WHO report which stated, "...animal studies suggest that neurological, behavioral, developmental, immuno-logical, haematological changes, and reduced fetal weight can result from exposure to ultrasound."[96] A 1995 study confirmed dangers of blood vessel spasm and hemorrhage.[97] There have been concerns that epidemiological studies do not always reflect the higher output capabilities of modern scanners.[98]

In 2004 and again in 2011, the FDA warned that "ultrasound is a form of energy, and even at low levels, laboratory studies have shown it can produce physical effect in tissue, such as jarring vibrations and a rise in temperature."[99] Parents requesting nonessential "keepsake" photos using ultrasound are making a serious mistake.[100]

In countries with nationalized healthcare, where nearly all pregnant women are exposed to ultrasound, ASD rates are even higher than in the USA. E.g., in the UK, teachers surveyed in 2002 said that one in 86 primary school children exhibited symptoms of autism, dyslexia, epilepsy, mental retardation, and schizophrenia. One in 152 had a formal diagnosis of ASD, far higher than official prevalence estimates. 67% of teachers noticed more children with ASD symptoms than the previous 5 years. This was consistent across all age groups and in all types schools (special and mainstream).[101]

Autistic children become dysfunctional and often unemployable adults who require lifetime care. One in 100 adults in England has autism, according to official NHS sources (per a 2009 study), but this estimate is closer to one in 64 in the view of autism experts who assert that the study was flawed.[102]

France has made autism awareness the national focus for the year 2012. Their Health Ministry now estimates the rate of autism in France to be 1 out 150 children.[103]

The conclusion is that clinicians must seriously consider the consequences of unnecessary use of fetal ultrasound and electronic fetal heart monitors, which could be dangerously invasive and unsafe if not professionally applied.[104]

Many support groups connect families with autistic children to share treatment information and coping skills.[105]

FUNGAL INFECTIONS

Some researchers theorize that autoimmune diseases such as Rheumatoid Arthritis and Lupus are not explained by the body is not attacking itself primarily; possibly the main target is not the body but a fungus like Candida.

Candida

An estimated fifty percent of RA patients suffer from Candidiasis, an overgrowth of the yeast *Candida albicans*. Many of the symptoms associated with RA are the same as those from Candidiasis or food allergies. Candida species are the most common fungi associated with opportunistic infections, including septic arthritis.[106]

Yeast overgrowth is usually found in the lower bowel, vagina, and on the skin. *Candida albicans*, among other similar opportunistic microorganisms, will spread throughout favorable body sites when the immune system has been compromised.

Candida has seven known survival forms including one CWD form that cannot be recognized by the immune system as a foreign invader because it is in the blood. Candida's most damaging form is the fungal (mycelial) state, which occurs throughout the intestinal tract whenever the resident "good" intestinal bacteria have been killed by the use of various drugs, notably antibiotics.

As Candidiasis (yeast overgrowth) can mimic so many other diseases due to its ability to affect various body targets, such as organs and digestive system elements, the disease frequently goes unrecognized, undiagnosed, and untreated by traditional medical practitioners.[107]

Candidiasis in the digestive tract will prompt cravings for sugary, starchy foods the yeasts thrive on, causing overeating and in turn, weight gain. The hormones in birth control pills promote yeast growth. A yeast infection can also cause chronic irritation of the intestinal lining, and the resulting swelling appears to be excess weight. Self-testing kits are available,[108] or ask for a detailed stool analysis from your physician. A positive result could mean a leaky gut problem or another fungal infection. Tests for food allergies as well as Candida are done by Better Health USA.[109]

Mold and Mycotoxins

An estimated 37 million Americans suffer from chronic sinus infections each year.[110] A 1999 Mayo Clinic study cited mycotoxins from molds as the cause of allergic fungal sinusitis.[111] Yet, tens of thousands of unnecessary sinus operations are still performed when the problem might actually be a mold allergy that can be neutralized without surgery.[112]

Some physicians are beginning to recognize that molds are responsible for allergies, asthma attacks, and negative impact on the immune system, leading to increased susceptibility to colds and flu. The prior prevailing medical view held that mold accounted for less than 10% of chronic sinusitis. The Mayo Clinic study found that number to be closer to 93%. This translates to over 34 million people seeking medical treatment, drugs, and/or surgery for a condition that is easily prevented.

Molds are a subset of the fungi which are found everywhere on the earth. There are more than 400,000 species of molds.[113, 114] Some, like mushrooms and yeasts, are beneficial; others, like mildew and rust, are not. The majority of molds are not pathogenic. Molds are essential for the natural breakdown and recycling of organic matter. However, when molds lose moisture, they release spores because they sense impending death and in turn, the need to reproduce. The process also releases mycotoxins.

Outdoor spores are not usually a source of toxicity but indoor molds have a greater potential to cause illness. Molds and spores themselves can cause allergy and/or infections but much more harmful are the mycotoxins released when the mold's food source (moisture) is removed. Since moisture plays such an important part in mycotoxin production, indoor humidity must be carefully controlled to prevent mildew, mold, and spores.

There are over 400 recognized mycotoxins, with new ones still being identified.[115] Dr. Ritchie Shoemaker is an expert in biotoxins and their neurotoxic effects: a variety of short-term responses such as dermatitis, cold and flu symptoms, headache, fatigue, diarrhea, and impaired immune system function, which may lead to more serious opportunistic infections and conditions like Fibromyalgia and CFS. The long-term effects are potentially carcinogenic and teratogenic (affecting fetal development). Treatment with antibiotics is not advised. Dr. Shoemaker's effective protocol should be considered.[116] One can try preventative measures, plus diet and lifestyle adjustments.[117]

Zygomycosis (or mucormycosis) is a rare, very invasive fungal infection that spreads rapidly among survivors of a natural disaster, with a fatality rate of 50% or higher. It usually afflicts people with weak or compromised immune systems or untreated diabetes, but can affect healthy people who suffer traumatic wounds embedded with contaminated soil or vegetation. Dr. Uwe Schmidt, an infectious disease specialist in Joplin, MO, treated tornado victims in 2011. His zygomycosis patients developed cellulitis followed by an aggressive necrotizing soft tissue infection.[118]

Stachybotrys chartarum mold produces at least 170 known mycotoxins.[119] When this mold dries, mycotoxin production increases up to 40,000 times.[120] The inhaled Stachybotrys mycotoxins accumulate in the body and are receiving increased attention as a phenomenon called "sick building syndrome."[121] When spores enter the body through the nasal passages, the immune system sends eosinophils to attack the fungi. The eosinophils irritate nasal membranes.

Antibiotics and OTC decongestants are widely used to treat chronic sinusitis, but antibiotics are not effective because they target bacteria, not fungi. These drugs may temporarily relieve symptoms, but they have no effect on the inflammation. One recent study indicated that as much as

30% of U.S. buildings have indoor mold. Ingestion of mold toxins will make Lyme Disease symptoms worse and increase the need for ascorbate (vitamin C). Dr. Shoemaker offers an effective treatment.[122]

Stachybotrys atra toxic mold is the designated culprit in illnesses contracted at schools, homes, and office buildings and the focus of multimillion-dollar lawsuits. However, contamination by strains of aspergillus, chaetomium, and penicillium can be just as harmful. Mold has become big business since it has been shown to be associated with serious health problems. Antipollution activists, lawyers, and support groups are suing construction companies, landlords, and insurance companies for damages to property and health. According to Farmers Insurance, there was a 1,000% increase in mold-related claims from 1994-2004. In 2000, there were no mold removal companies; today there are an estimated 20,000 such firms.[123]

Mold and the Mummy's Curse

The legend of the "Mummy's Curse" has some basis in fact. Many archaeology workers and tomb robbers have died soon after opening and entering tombs or handling their contents. Two famous historical cases document the clusters of archeological team deaths associated with opening ancient burial tombs and handling their contents.

King Tut's tomb in Egypt was opened in 1922. Since royal persons were buried with fruits, vegetables, and meats for the afterlife, molds would naturally form in the enclosed tomb as these items decayed. Spores and surface toxins could last thousands of years. The first people to enter these tombs would be exposed to a huge dose of mold toxins. Within five years, eleven people who had entered Tut's tomb were dead. Researchers who examined the mummy of Ramses II in 1976 prudently wore special protective masks. They found over 89 different species of molds in or on the mummy.

In 1973, King Casimir's tomb in Poland was opened. The 15th century ruler's wooden coffin was rotted inside the tomb. Within a few days, ten of the twelve archaeologists died. One of the two survivors suffered with neurological imbalance for five years. Studies of the tomb artifacts found aspergillis and penicillin species that make dangerous mycotoxins (aflatoxins).

AMOEBIC INFECTIONS

Parasitic infestations are part of the missing diagnosis in the etiology of many chronic health problems, including arthritis.[124, 125] Professor Roger Wyburn-Mason, M.D., PhD was the author of several important medical textbooks, a renowned specialist in nerve diseases, and honored by having two nerve diseases named after him during his lifetime. He claimed in 1970s that the cause of RA and other degenerative chronic diseases was a microorganism called "limax amoebae." He theorized that this microorganism could infect any system in the human body, causing collagen tissue diseases.

Dr. Wyburn-Mason stressed that these pervasive, pathogenic microorganisms had the power of independent existence for an extended period. This observation seems to confirm Dr. Brown's theory of CWD, shape-shifting Mycoplasmas. Later research sponsored by the Arthritis Trust showed that while the amoebic cause was probably wrong, the protocol that was developed on the basis of Wyburn-Mason's hypothesis was very effective in treating RA and other related diseases.

Table 5 shows examples of some 100 rheumatic illnesses he found linked to microbial infection, and their locations in various tissues of the body.

Dr. Wyburn-Mason documented his work over 26 years in numerous British medical journal articles and in his book *The Causation of Rheumatoid Disease and Many Human Cancers.*[126]

Table 5. Area Infected vs. Resulting Condition (per Dr. Wyburn-Mason)

Adrenal gland	Addison's disease
Small intestine	Crohn's Disease
Muscles	Dermatomyositis
Thyroid	Graves' Disease, Hashimoto's Thyroiditis
Red blood cell membrane proteins	Hemolytic anemia
Blood	Hemolytic Disease
Platelets	Idiopathic thrombocytopenic purpura
Pancreatic beta cells	Insulin-dependent Diabetes
Nerves, brain, spinal cord	Multiple Sclerosis (MS)*
Nerve/muscle synapses	Myasthenia gravis
Arteries	Periarteritis nodosum
Gastric parietal cells	Pernicious anemia
Skin	Psoriasis
Joints, connective tissue	Rheumatoid Arthritis
Heart, lungs, gut, kidney	Scleroderma
Salivary glands, liver, kidney, brain, thyroid	Sjögrens Syndrome
DNA, skin, platelets, organs, connective tissue	Systemic Lupus Erythematosus
Colon	Ulcerative Colitis

*Caution: the Wyburn-Mason protocol must not be given to anyone with MS or *Helicobacter pylori* infection.

Dr. Paul Pybus continued Wyburn-Mason's work and developed a successful treatment procedure that he called "Intraneural Injections." The aim was to provide relief from joint pain without using harmful cortisone. The late Dr.

Gus J. Prosch, Jr., M.D., refined the technique and trained 600 other physicians in its use. Dr. Prosch claimed a 75% to 80% cure rate with his patients from 1982 to 2005.[127]

The treatment consists of assorted applications of clotrimazole, tinidazole, ornidizole, allopurinol, rifampicin, potassium para-amino benzoate, and furazolidone. While these are prescription medications, they do not have the serious side effects associated with standard RA drugs.

Dr. Prosch asserted that many factors operate in concert to create conditions favorable to the development of rheumatic disease, such as genetics, stress, poor nutrition, injuries, Candidiasis, chemical sensitivities, polymicrobial infections, vitamin deficiencies, allergies, food sensitivities, and so on. These factors must be addressed in parallel with the protocol for complete and permanent relief.[128]

Dr. Jack M. Blount, Jr. of the Philadelphia Medical School was nearly totally disabled by RA in 1974. He discovered Dr. Wyburn-Mason's work after trying all known conventional treatments in an effort to relieve his pain and retard the progression of the disease. Dr. Blount increased the recommended dosage of clotrimazole and within two weeks noticed dramatic improvement. He gave his patients the U.S. equivalent of clotrimazole, Flagyl (known generically as metronidazole).[129]

Since his recovery, Dr. Blount has treated over 16,000 patients with this protocol with significant success. This method could be considered as an alternative for those who do not respond to Dr. Brown's antibiotic regimen.

Because metronidazole is also effective against the cyst form of the Lyme Disease spirochete, it seems to support the theory that as shape-shifting organisms take on different forms during their life cycle, they are vulnerable to specific medications at various times.

Dr. Blount was so impressed with his own personal remission from RA and that of his patients that he founded the Rheumatoid Disease Foundation, now called the Arthritis Trust of America. Dr. Blount conferred with other physicians, including Dr. Robert Bingham of Desert Hot Springs, CA and Dr. Paul Pybus, colleague of Dr. Wyburn-Mason, who also achieved impressive results with their own RA and OA patients. Sadly, their enthusiasm for the treatment was met with hostility from rheumatologists who ignored the many publications and scientific tests performed by Dr. Wyburn-Mason and others.

A detailed history and description of the treatment, with associated essential diet and vitamin/supplement information, is available from the Arthritis Trust.[130] This nonprofit foundation provides the names of over 200 physicians in 16 different countries (but mainly in the U.S.) who apply the protocol with success. The Arthritis Trust provides many publications documenting case histories and scientific studies.

The treatment takes about 6-7 weeks under close supervision by one's doctor. The patient is also given methods to improve the immune system and lifestyle modifications similar to those described in this book. The treatment does not correct the damage already done to the tissues, but the progress of the disease is usually halted and the painful symptoms decrease and in many cases disappear. Some patients may become reinfected and must repeat the treatment, depending on the severity of the infection.

Dr. Blount advises taking measures to limit infection by use of filtration and by making sure home water pipes are made of copper. Waterborne protozoan microorganisms such as *Cryptosporidium parvum* and *Giardia lamblia* colonize in biofilms, growing quickly in swimming pools and spas. Chlorine does not effectively kill them. Copper algaecide is recommended at 4 ounces per 5,000 gallons of water. Copper plates can be placed in the pool.

BLOOD-BORNE VIRUSES AND BACTERIA

The blood is a conduit for a wide variety of microorganisms to travel throughout the body, wreaking havoc along the way to their ultimate targets in tissues and/or organs. New research suggests that arterial inflammation producing an immune system response contributes to heart attacks. Older patients (> 65) who had antibodies to the herpes simplex virus (HSV) had an increased risk of heart attack and cardiac death.[131] HSV is discussed in Chapter 3.

Three well-known blood-borne illnesses described in the next sections are Sepsis, AIDS/HIV, and Hepatitis.[132]

Sepsis (Bacteremia)

This illness is an overwhelming and life-threatening infection of the blood and body organs caused by bacteria that has entered body tissue. Entry is most often through a major trauma site (burns, severe wound), but can happen after organ failure (e.g., pancreatitis, appendicitis). The ensuing infection leads to pus formation and/or to the spread of the sepsis (bacteremia) organisms throughout the body.

Multiple organ dysfunction syndrome (MODS) has reached epidemic proportions, and is now the most common cause of death in most intensive care surgical units (ICUs). Dr. Edwin Deitch notes that MODS is responsible for 50-80% of all ICU deaths because of ignorance of the true origin of this syndrome.

Based on the notion that the gut is the largest immune organ in the body, Dr. Deitch asserts that many gut-derived factors, including bacteria, exit the intestine via the lymph system rather than the portal blood vein in the stomach and intestines. He proposed that the mesenteric lymphatics and the pro-inflammatory properties of the gut are the missing links in the gut hypothesis of MODS. That is, gut-barrier failure allows bacteria to reach distant organs, causing injury in which bacteria, gut ischemia or both invoke an intestinal (and immune system) response that contributes to MODS.[133] Mucosal (gut) balance is discussed in Chapter 3.

Sepsis organisms are resistant to most standard antibiotics, but the disease been shown to respond well to UV treatment, described later in this chapter. The number of deaths from sepsis has almost doubled in the last 20 years in regional clusters in the Southeastern to mid-Atlantic states.[134]

The Arthritis Center of Riverside found *Proteus mirabilis and E. coli* to be associated with septic arthritis.[135] Although bacteria are most commonly the cause, viruses and fungi can also cause sepsis. People with weakened immune systems are more susceptible than others: the very young, the elderly, those with other infections such as pneumonia, meningitis, cellulitis, or AIDS, and those taking steroids or immunosuppressive drugs. Commonly affected areas are the genitourinary and GI tract, the liver, surgical wounds or drains, lungs, and skin eruptions such as bedsores or burns.

HIV and AIDS

Human Immunodeficiency Virus (HIV) and Acquired Immune Deficiency Syndrome (AIDS) are characterized by a reduction to 20% or less of the normal amount of CD4 helper T-cells, rendering the individual's immune system highly vulnerable to serious illnesses such as pneumonia. HIV has been found in blood, semen, saliva, tears, nervous system tissue, breast milk, and female genital tract secretions. HIV is usually transmitted via infected blood and bodily fluids, commonly during illicit intravenous drug use and/or sexual intercourse.

The HIV microbe may also reside inside the infected person's lymph nodes, often for years, before producing detectable symptoms. The documented synergy between

HIV and other microbial epidemics such as malaria, Epstein-Barr virus, tuberculosis, and others is a clear indication that immune system suppression gives rise to a wide variety of chronic diseases.[136] This calls into question all treatments that rely on immunosuppressing drugs and the widespread use of OTC medications such as cold medicines and antihistamines that can cause long-term harm.

Mycoplasmal infections have been found as co-factors in the progression of AIDS, leading to kidney lesions and respiratory complications.[137] Detection of infections in clinical specimens is frequently dismissed as "only Mycoplasmas" even when they appear to be the primary pathogens.[138]

Another reason for the lack of scientific interest in Mycoplasmas may be that they were initially linked to the detection of infections in AIDS patients. Until the mid-1990s, the moral judgment of those who fund medical research politicized and stalled the investigation of this autoimmune disorder.[139] Sadly, this prejudiced stance led to delayed recognition of a latent deadly disease requiring testing, detection, and quarantine that in turn caused the global spread of the virus; the number of cases of infection increased exponentially.[140]

Today, more funds are allocated to AIDS research[141] but at the expense of investigating other infectious diseases. Fortunately, the results of AIDS research have disclosed behavior mechanisms generally applicable to other microorganisms, including mycoplasmal forms. Some 2.5 million deaths have been averted since 1995 when anti-retroviral therapy was introduced.

Sodium lauryl sulfate (SLS) has been shown to be a natural, potent, nontoxic, topical microbicide against several pathogens: Herpes simplex viruses, HIV-1, Semliki Forest virus, papillomaviruses, reoviruses (including rotavirus), and poliovirus by dissolving the microbe's protective waxy viral coating. If SLS use were adopted, the public health impact on STD prevention would be significant.[142]

It is not well known that vinegar and monolaurin also dissolve the waxy coating of the HIV virus in the gut. If these substances are consumed long enough (e.g., 2-3 times per day) the HIV colony in the gut can be eliminated. The detectable HIV in the blood and lymph drops to zero and AIDS remission could result.[143]

Autoimmune Hepatitis [144]

Normal liver function is critical to good health. At least five inflammatory liver viruses (Hepatitis A through E: HAV through HEV) are now recognized:

- HAV is contracted from infected food and water. It causes jaundice and a brief illness. Complete recovery is typical and vaccine is available;

- HBV is transmitted by blood and can cause serious liver damage. Like Hepatitis A, its effects appear in the short term. Vaccine is available, but a 2005 control study found serious autoimmune adverse reactions after immunization;[145]

- HCV was only identified in 1989. It is transmitted by direct blood contact (e.g., transfusions), through sexual intercourse, or via infected needles, and can remain dormant for decades while the liver is slowly damaged;

- HDV is most commonly spread through contact with infected blood or other bodily fluids, such as semen, vaginal fluids, or saliva. One cannot get HDV unless s/he already has HBV. There are two types: acute (recently

acquired) and chronic (life-long). No consensus
on treatment. No vaccine is available;

• HEV spread by fecally-contaminated water
within endemic areas, usually running its course
without treatment.

Together, Hepatitis B and C represent one of the
biggest threats to global health, causing 78% of all cases of
liver cancer and 57% of all cases of cirrhosis, and killing
about one million people per year. In 2010 the WHO
estimated that 500 million people worldwide are chronically
infected with HBV or HCV, and one in three have been
exposed to either or both viruses.[146] Studies continue to find
a prevalence of thyroid cancer in patients with chronic HCV
infection.[147]

Ignorance of hepatitis infection is a barrier to
diagnosis and treatment. The CDC estimates that only about
25% of those infected with HCV are aware of it.[148] The 75%
of the unaware have not been screened, because either they
do not access the healthcare system or because they do not
appear to have risk factors, so they are not screened.

Among the common causes of chronic liver disease is
a fatty liver, which is linked to HCV, but can be found in
non-alcoholics as well as in heavy drinkers. In the U.S., one
in ten Asian-Americans is HBV positive. When the doctor
orders a HBV test, if the result is positive, HCV and HIV
tests should also be run. Lifestyle risk factors for HBV and
cirrhosis are: habitual alcohol consumption, co-infection
with HCV, HDV, HIV, and smoking.

The HCV epidemic in Egypt (to a 20% level) started
in 2007 with shared needles to vaccinate against Schistosomiasis. HCV infections are on the rise in that country
because of poor healthcare and erratic hygiene.[149] In the
U.S., HCV accounts for 40-60% of all chronic liver disease
and is the leading cause of liver transplants. The rate of

HCV progression indicates that this disease alone could bankrupt the U.S. health care system by 2020.[150] Approximately 15%–25% of persons clear the virus from their bodies without treatment and do not develop chronic infection, but the reasons for this are unknown.[151]

Risk factors for HCV infection[152] are:

- Received blood, blood products, or organ transplant(s) prior to 1992;
- Ever—even once—shared drug paraphernalia or used injection drugs;
- Ever been stuck by a used blood needle;
- Are now or have been on kidney dialysis;
- Had a tattoo or body piercing in an unsterile setting;
- Had multiple sex partners or sexual activity involving blood contact;
- Were a combat veteran (dried blood on the battlefield can be aerosolized);
- Have shared personal care items (toothbrush, razor) with someone with known history of chronic hepatitis;
- Previous incarceration;
- Test results show unexplained elevated ALT (normal liver enzyme);
- Tested HIV+.

Hospitals and blood banks are now able to screen blood routinely for the various hepatitis virus strains, but individuals who received a transfusion prior to 1992 should request a test for Hepatitis C. A positive test result should prompt the doctor to try antiviral therapy with interferon-alpha and ribavirin. Do everything possible to avoid infecting others. Avoid alcohol, which increases the rate of liver damage, and request Hepatitis A and B vaccinations to prevent additional liver problems. Antiviral therapy can reduce liver inflammation but cannot cure the disease. Clinicians are encouraged to try intravenous and/or oral ascorbic acid as a benign antiviral treatment.[153]

Aflatoxin from mold is also a risk factor in HCV.[154] Crops that are frequently affected include cereals (maize, sorghum, pearl millet, rice, wheat), oilseeds (peanut, soybean, sunflower, cotton), spices (chili peppers, black pepper, coriander, turmeric, ginger), and tree nuts (almond, pistachio, walnut, coconut, Brazil nut). The aflatoxin can also be found in the milk of farm animals given contaminated feed.[155]

The bifidobacterium blocks the toxic effect of aflatoxin *in vitro*; experiments are underway *in vivo*. This probiotic is a dietary supplement that can keep accidentally ingested toxins under control. It is found in yogurt products.[156] Probiotics are discussed in Chapter 3. Daily vitamin C supplements (≥ 3 grams) will eliminate most toxins. See Appendix V for details.

BLOOD SUPPLY CONCERNS

The FDA is responsible for purity of medicines and the nation's blood supply; the CDC's charter is to keep epidemiological statistics.[157] Since 1985 the FDA has issued repeated warnings to the Red Cross of a "potential for harm" to patients based on failure of federal inspections and noncompliance with mandated good manufacturing practice standards.[158]

However, increasingly tough FDA actions and court orders have not succeeded in correcting problems in the collection, processing, and distribution of blood used in medical procedures. More than 200 safety violations and deficiencies were logged in 2002. Dr. Mark McClellan, then FDA commissioner, said that there is "…continuing evidence of a culture that is willing to accept noncompliance, as in many previous inspections." Since 2003, the Red Cross has paid $37 Million in fines.[159]

The Public Citizen's Health Research Group is demanding that the FDA work significantly harder to protect the nation's blood supply from contaminants like Hepatitis B.[160] The FDA should insure strict compliance with U.S. laws and regulations in every agency that handles blood and blood products. The Red Cross collects about 70% of this supply, representing about 11.5 million units of blood.[161]

We now know that some diseases take many years to develop and transfusions are not the most significant way the average person gets the disease, because there are other primary modes of infection. For example, those infected with AIDS typically do not get the disease through transfusion.

Individual blood testing is expensive and there are too many organisms that could be pathogen candidates. Only a limited number of microbes and viruses are tested for in practice. A complete list (as of 2009) of donor screening assay for infectious agents can be found on the FDA's website.[162] Blood has been collected from donors for decades but not tested for pathogenic Mycoplasmas. Because Mycoplasmas in the blood do not immediately affect mortality statistics, data collectors do not view these microorganisms as an important problem in the quality of the blood supply. Nevertheless, the CDC takes the view that blood purity is still an important issue.[163]

Since the advent of the AIDS epidemic, the blood banking industry has been undergoing a revolution of increased sophistication. Various manufacturers have had products in clinical trials since the 1990s but no truly safe and effective artificial blood product is currently on the market.[164] Lab-created artificial blood is now technologically feasible.[165] European researchers made a major breakthrough in 2011, but availability is at least 3 years away.[166]

Transfusions unwittingly pass along blood cell-invading pleomorphic microbes from donor to recipient in an iatrogenic manner. Very slow acting/growing microbes that have a high epidemiological incidence are nearly certain to be transferred. Most likely the recipient has already been infected, but not with all strains. To be certain, auto-donate your own plasma before an operation.

VACCINES

The slowly progressing rheumatic infections—whether viral, mycoplasmal, or bacterial L-forms—are all prime candidates for suppression by vaccines which, even if they do not target the exact microbe, can also stimulate the immune system to re-energize its defenses.[167]

Where the primary reserve host is the human body, the use of vaccines has reduced the incidence and infection rate of a disease to insignificance, e.g., with smallpox and polio. In persistent disease cases, such as rabies, multi-dose vaccine treatments are necessary. In general, multi-doses (i.e., booster shots) of many vaccines such as tetanus are found useful if not essential to preserve levels of immunity over time. This may also apply to vaccines like the pneumococcal vaccines that work against microbes that express enzymes like COX-2, known to be associated with arthritis.

Vaccines, together with use of appropriate antibiotics, antienzymes, anti-toxins, antiviral drugs, and/or apoptosis-inducing drugs in cases where the microorganism invades host cells would seem to provide a more effective multi-pronged attack on the microbe's vulnerabilities in several of its forms/stages.[168]

Some antiviral drugs act to defeat the cell attachment "ligand receptor" link mechanism. *Mycoplasma fermentans* (*incognitus*) is reported to have a cell link structure on its surface that is very similar to HIV. This implies that its ability to invade host cells may be inhibited by an anti-HIV compound working to disable the ligand receptor. Coconut oil and palm oil do the job of vaccines and drugs naturally by blocking immune system triggers and/or cell invasion mechanisms.[169]

Organizations like the Gates Foundation are funding development of vaccines against epidemics that are again becoming global threats—malaria, tuberculosis, rotavirus-caused diarrhea, pneumonia, meningitis, and polio.[170] Many vaccines against various problem microbes like *E. coli* have been developed for domesticated animals.[171] Use of these vaccines can suppress the microbe in the animal population and reduce the chances of food-borne infections in humans. Human vaccines need to be developed against the same or similar colonizing pathogens such as Chlamydia, Shigella, Salmonella, Giardia, and Clostridium.[172]

However, vaccines are not always effective or beneficial. Dr. Russell Blaylock has published extensively on vaccines and their adverse effects. He asserts that microglia are primed at birth by the Hepatitis B vaccine, and activated by subsequent infection or vaccine(s). The results include developmental delays, learning disorders, seizures, and sometimes death from Sudden Infant Death Syndrome (SIDS).[173] Gut inflammation and immune system suppression can occur after administration of specific vaccines like pertussis (DTP)[174] and rubella.[175]

The nonprofit National Vaccine Information Center (NVIC) seeks to prevent vaccine injuries and deaths through public education and to defend the informed consent ethic in medicine. The NVIC is a consumer-led, nonpartisan, independent clearinghouse for data on diseases and vaccines. They do not advocate for or against vaccines, but merely gather data on post-vaccination problems and report their findings.[176] E.g., chronic health statistics such as:

Diabetes	1969: 1/7100	2008: 1/450
Autism	1970: 4/10,000	2009: 1/100
ADHD	1997: 1.6 million	2008: 4 million

Dr. Stephanie Cave, M.D, asks several probing questions: how did the generation of the Great Depression survive into their 80s and 90s without vaccines? Why do doctors think it is safe to give up to ten vaccinations at a time to a child? Have we been able to change Nature's design of immune balance? Are we creating a problem for future generations?[177]

A prophylactic antibiotic regimen in addition to a targeted vaccine might be a fruitful area for further research, leading toward infection identification and more rapid patient cures. However, there are many more vaccine candidates than funds. Development and production is costly and dangerous to technicians who must culture the pathogen, work with its host and avoid being infected themselves. Such lab facilities may also generate significant amounts of bio-hazardous wastes that require meticulous control and destruction. Progress in vaccine research and development seems to be limited mainly by funding.

Endnotes and continuing research on topics in Chapter 5 can be found at www.RA-Infection-Connection.com

6. DIAGNOSTIC TESTS

"The good physician treats the disease, the great
physician treats the patient who has the disease."
---Sir William Osler

In this chapter, several testing methods are described to
help the arthritis sufferer work with his/her physician to
determine the presence and extent of infection. A typical
routine physical examination will involve blood, urine, and/or
tissue samples. A urine test offers particularly valuable data to
identify potentially infectious agents. A doctor analyzes the
test values to see whether they fall between acceptable ranges.
All laboratory test results must of course be interpreted in the
context of the patient's overall health. A skilled physician will
take a holistic view of each patient, asking relevant, probing
questions that will provide context for, and augment findings
from, lab tests. The doctor must evaluate symptoms from the
viewpoint of the patient, taking into consideration his/her
entire health history, including hereditary influences.

Other factors influencing test results may be drugs the
patient is taking, foods ingested before the test, how strictly
the patient followed pretest instructions (e.g., fasting), and
variations in laboratory procedures and techniques. Some
fundamental questions arise concerning the reliability of any
diagnostic test involving organic samples, which may be
collected exactly according to procedure at the doctor's office,
but may suffer damage in transit to the lab. Sensitivity to time,
temperature, humidity, altitude, and other factors may
influence test results by altering the sample before the lab
technician begins to examine it. False positives or out-of-
range values may result. Several tests may be required to
obtain an average. Internet resources can help interpret test
results and augment the information provided by the
physician's assessment.[1]

According to Dr. Sidney Baker[2], when a patient is suffering from an acute infectious disease, the impulse is to rush to conventional treatments (i.e., drugs) before analyzing microbial persistence in order to develop more effective treatment options. The analysis can come from listening to both the patient and the test data, developing a participatory, team player arrangement between doctor and patient.

Jumping to a conclusion based on a checklist of symptoms and putting a name on a disease does a disservice to the patient. For a chronic condition, the name of the illness becomes the patient's identity and can lead to depression: "I have RA. It will only get worse. My life is over." A quick but incorrect diagnosis (e.g., "JRA explains your symptoms") leads to bad policy ("treat JRA").[3]

Information technology (IT) will empower clinicians with valid statistical tools to let the data "talk" and answer questions they did not know how to ask before. To quote Dr. Baker, "IT will provide a compass to help steer us in the 'terrain wreck' (sic) of chronic illness to the most efficient curative strands in nature's web."

Since disease often begins when the immune system is dysfunctional or weakened, a nutritional analysis should be a starting point. Deficiencies of certain micronutrients is an established factor in a multitude of dangerous health conditions and diseases, including resistance to infection, cancer, cardiovascular disease, osteoporosis, and birth defects.[4] For example, diets that include little or no seafood, meat, and poultry will reflect low vitamin B_{12} values. A nutrition-oriented health care professional can assist with determining deficiencies and help tailor a personalized dietary profile. The patient will likely be required to keep a daily journal of not only food and liquid intake, but also environmental factors, such as workplace conditions, and lifestyle factors such as smoking, drug use, hygiene habits, and exercise. Nutrition guidelines are given in Chapter 7.

ALLERGY TESTING

There is a tendency to call any joint pain "arthritis" when in fact the cause may be something else: food allergy, crystalline/calcium deposits, muscle spasm, sports injury, or repetitive injury. Inflammation and stiffness are not reliable determinants. Many chronic diseases (e.g., Candidiasis) and allergic reactions (to food, mold, chemicals, etc.) can mimic arthritis symptoms, so appropriate testing and constant detective work on the part of both patient and physician is absolutely essential. Candidiasis is discussed in Chapter 5. Tests for food allergies as well as Candida are done by labs such as Better Health USA.[5]

A causal relationship between and a currently active state of food allergy and/or chemical sensitivity has often been reported.[6] The presence of multiple allergens heightens the histamine reaction. Sir William Osler first suggested that dietary proteins were an important cause of inflammatory arthritis. A gluten grain (wheat, barley, oats and rye) connection has been studied in RA patients.[7] Gluten is a mixture of individual proteins belonging to two groups: prolamines and glutelins. The prolamine fraction of gluten is usually the culprit when grain intolerance is suspected. The prolamine gliadin seems to be associated with celiac disease.

Rheumatoid Arthritis is often associated with Inflammatory Bowel Disease (IBD). The mechanisms of food allergy link abnormal gastrointestinal tract function with immune system attacks on connective tissue, giving rise to the mistaken autoimmune theory of some internally-generated origin for the inflammation.[8]

Enzyme Linked Immuno-Sorbant Assay (ELISA) Tests [9]

The cause of food sensitivity is undigested protein components that the immune system does not recognize as beneficial. It responds defensively by producing antibodies and starting an allergic reaction that can result in pain and inflammation. While food allergies usually cause an immediate reaction, food sensitivities may take a few hours or even a few days to develop.[10] [11]

Tests show delayed food allergies to be associated with over 65 chronic conditions, including RA and Candidiasis, and over 200 symptoms including headaches, rash, fatigue, gastritis, fluid retention, joint pain, brain fog, muscle ache, sinus pressure, depression, mood swings, constipation.[12]

Standard patch test or skin prick test[13] exposes the skin to 20-30 extracts of common allergens including hair dyes, medications, fragrances, preservatives, detergents, metals, latex, and resins. The test is not done for food allergies because of high false positive/negative results.

Fortunately, there are options available for more accurate testing. Some laboratories in the United States offer ELISA tests in the form of IgG food sensitivity tests and IgE airborne, mold, and food allergy tests.[14]

Food allergy tests are of two types:

1.   The IgG ELISA Delayed Food Allergy Assay is the Immuno 1 Bloodprint. Allergic foods are commonly favorite foods, frequently eaten, and eaten in larger amounts. Virtually any tissue, organ, or system of the body can be affected, including the so-called "classical" allergic areas. Symptoms often disappear following 3-6 months of avoidance coupled with nutritional therapy.

2.   The IgE Immediate Allergy Assay is the Immuno 3 Bloodprint. Small, even trace amounts of food can trigger an intense allergic reaction. In the worst case, anaphylaxis occurs leading to fatal results within minutes. One example is peanut allergy. These allergies affect the esophagus, skin, and digestive tract triggering symptoms of asthma, rhinitis, urticaria, eczema, vomiting, diarrhea, angioedema, and anaphylaxis.

Self-Testing for Allergy Factors

Undiagnosed allergies may be causing a variety of symptoms that contribute to arthritis. In 80-90% of arthritis with an allergic component, such as RA, removing the external allergen, either by avoidance or methods like kinesiology, can provide dramatic relief from the inflammation as well. Polymicrobial infection may still be present, but the immune system will be better able to deal with it.

Some questions to ask that may indicate the presence of arthritis in one of its many allergic forms are:

- Do you have any of the most common symptoms of arthritis:
    - o pain and stiffness in one or more joints, especially on arising?
    - o persistent swelling, tenderness, and limited motion in one or more joints?
    - o pain and stiffness in a joint, tendon, or bursa that was once injured?
- Do these symptoms come and go, apparently with no reason?
- Do these symptoms appear to correlate with changes in the weather or at high altitude?
- Do the symptoms correlate with time of day? After meals? With the seasons?
- Do you have low energy or lack of initiative?
- Do you experience unexplainable night sweats, or a low-grade fever that comes and goes?
- Do any close relatives have a history of allergies?
- Do you/did you have any allergies like eczema, hay fever, asthma, rashes, rosacea, or hives?
- Do you/did you suffer from frequent strep throat, bronchitis, pneumonia, or ear infections?

- Have you ever had mononucleosis?

- Do you have a history of taking prescribed antibiotics?

- Do you have frequent "indigestion," heartburn, gas, bloating, recurring diarrhea, or constipation?

- Are you more than 20 pounds overweight?

- Do you seem to suffer colds or flu more often than other people? Are your symptoms more severe than theirs?

- Do you have a persistent cough and/or post-nasal drip?

- Have you ever had a blood transfusion?

- Do you have other chronic health problems like migraine headaches, sinus/nasal congestion, colitis, unexplained fatigue, or body-wide complaints?

- Do you experience chronic depression, anxiety, "brain fog" or mood swings?

Affirmative answers to five or more of the above questions should prompt a consultation with one's physician about the possibility of allergy and/or chronic infection(s) as the root cause(s) of the condition.

The survey above is a composite of several questionnaires routinely given to allergy patients. But it reflects a simplistic view regarding the cause of sensitivity as being allergens from food or environmental sources, and not from resident pathogens. The insertion of the questions regarding a history of illnesses such as strep throat, bronchitis, and mononucleosis is an attempt to complete the list to include probable infectious causes, e.g., remnants of an earlier infection involving Mycoplasma and other cell-invading persistent forms.[15]

Allergens are found in cosmetics, chemicals, foods, and/or airborne substances (dust, mold spores, pollen). Of course, it is impossible to discover and remove *all* the dietary and environmental triggers to allergic arthritis, but it is feasible to identify enough of them to reduce the total load on the body's systems and relieve painful inflammation.[16] Joints and muscles must be given a chance to rest and repair while allergy-induced stress is decreased by elimination, reduction, or control of offending substances.

Results from the CDC's 2009 Behavioral Risk Factor Surveillance System survey found that obesity prevalence in the United States was 26.7%, up nearly 2% from 2007. Food allergies can also be a factor in weight gain. When one consumes a food that causes mild irritation in the form of headache, bloating, or gas, the body tries to counteract the discomfort by releasing endorphins. The pleasurable sensations these natural opiate-like painkillers produce are an inducement to eat more of the offending food.

This is the counterintuitive reason why people crave and seek out those foods that cause allergic reactions. They unwittingly become somewhat addicted to these pleasurable chemicals, so more of the so-called "comfort food" is consumed than would normally be eaten, and weight gain often results. Appetite can also be driven by powerful mood swings and stress,[17] as discussed in Chapter 3.

A 2010 study[18] found that high levels of the hormone ghrelin seem to increase the attraction to sweet, high-calorie foods. This "hunger hormone" originates in the gut but acts in the brain to stimulate cravings. Its level rises to high before we consume our food, and declines soon after eating.

TESTS FOR MICROBIAL INFECTION

Early detection and treatment of Rheumatoid Arthritis is possible. RA and other chronic diseases are linked in that they can be traced to the activity of pathogenic microbes and lack of cellular immunity. Unfortunately, the tests may show low values even when infection is active. This is also true of a sizable group of diseases that manifest as "fever of unknown origin" or FUO. In this category are Lupus, rheumatic fever, hypersensitivity angiitis, and Still's disease.

Erythrocyte Sedimentation Rate (ESR) Test

The ESR test, often called "sed rate," is a nonspecific screening test for various infectious inflammatory diseases and suspected rheumatologic disorders such as RA and Lupus. The test measures the distance in millimeters that red blood cells settle in unclotted blood toward the bottom of a specially marked test tube in one hour. The more red cells that fall to the bottom, the higher the sed rate, and the greater the immune system's inflammatory response. Test results and interpretations depend on a patient's age and sex. The normal range of values for males is 0-15 mm/hr (under age 50) and 0-20 mm/hr (over age 50). For females, the range is 0-25 mm/hr (under age 50) and 0-30 mm/hr (over age 50). [19]

Although ESR is a screening test, not a diagnostic test, it can help detect and monitor infections, inflammatory or malignant disease, tissue necrosis, rheumatic fever, tuberculosis, connective tissue disease, anemia, and acute myocardial infarction. It is useful in cases where symptoms are vague or physical findings are minimal.

The advantage of this blood test is that readings will frequently be high when the patient is without symptoms. This is an alert to the physician that the disease is still active. The test must be done in the doctor's office, not in a commercial laboratory, since analysis within one hour of drawing the blood is critical to an accurate diagnosis.

Tetracycline as a Probe

Physicians should use one of the tetracycline family of antibiotics (doxycycline, oxytetracycline, minocycline, etc)[20] as a probe to test whether patients could be afflicted with RA, urinary tract/GI/respiratory tract infections, Fibromyalgia, and/or CFS since the test targets Mycoplasmas and other cell wall-deficient forms specifically. A Herxheimer reaction to the killed microbes would be evidence that antigens or toxins are being released.[21] The tetracycline dosage must be tailored to the individual patient. The assumption is that the average patient weighs 70 kg (155 lbs). Dosage must be adjusted for actual weight. Details are found in Appendix II.

Interferons

Interferons constitute a class of natural cell products from the immune system that stimulate antiviral resistance in cell cultures and in the body. These soluble, hormone-like proteins are produced in response to viral infections or to stimulation of immunocompetent as well as other somatic cells by a wide variety of distinct nonviral materials. These materials are for the most part protein- or cell wall-related organic molecules/shapes. Interferons can also have significantly diverse biological activities. Measurement of levels of specific interferons in blood analysis provides quantitative evaluation of immune function in infection-caused diseases such as AIDS, Lupus, and RA.[22]

C-reactive Protein (CRP) Test

In the 1930s, when Dr. Brown was developing his Mycoplasma theory, researchers at the Avery Laboratory of the Rockefeller Institute in New York were convinced that rheumatic fever was associated with streptococcal infection. By 1946, procedures were established to apply the measure-ment of CRP as a test for rheumatic activity. Results indicated that CRP detection could also be clinically useful as an index of polycyclic infection activity in such diseases as rheumatic fever and tuberculosis.[23]

The CRP test detects a specific protein that appears in the blood during inflammatory conditions. Levels of CRP higher than 8 micrograms per milliliter can help diagnose RA. The test can be an indicator of inflamed arteries and postoperative infection. High CRP levels have been linked strongly to a propensity for heart attack or stroke.[24] A CRP test can be done with blood drawn in the doctor's office.

In the 1980s, experiments binding CRP to the surface of Pneumococcus showed that alternative pathway activation could be blocked.[25] Vaccines are now available for the most common strains of Pneumococcus.[26] A CRP affixed to such invader cells serves as a protective mechanism for the host to ward off potential antigen-reactive cells, thus modulating the severity of the autoimmune reaction. However, it was found that CRP cannot bind to the strain of Streptococci that causes acute rheumatic fever and therefore cannot protect the individual from this particular pathogen.

A few patients with immune deficiency who have no immunoglobulin will nevertheless have a normal CRP response to infection. Although a valuable test for RA patients, CRP may be only moderately increased or even absent in spondylarthritis (affecting the spinal column), Scleroderma, and dermatomyositis. [27]

The Rheumatoid Factor (R-factor)

It is important to test for binding indications and levels of CRP to obtain a correct diagnosis for the anti-antibody called the rheumatoid factor, or R-factor. A Bentonite flocculation test and a latex fixation test will also indicate the presence of the R-factor (RF).[28] Testing for the RF is most useful in severe or fairly mature infections. It may take months for it to rise to levels deemed significant. Even after a positive test result, the RF's discovery may lead simply to an acknowledgment by the doctor that the patient has RA, but will yield no definitive course of action about how to cure the condition.

A surprising finding is that aspartame (used in sugar substitutes) depresses the R-factor and can thus relieve arthritis pain.[29] However, some individuals have experienced adverse reactions to aspartame. Many scientists and experts believe that aspartame has very toxic potential and should never have been approved by the FDA. A wide range (and number) of symptoms makes diagnosis very difficult, since severity of allergic reactions vary from person to person, and symptoms do not persist in every case. Most of the controversy surrounds sensitivity to the chemicals that compose aspartame, which include methanol, formaldehyde, formic acid, aspartic acid and phenylalanine. These chemicals are released as part of the digestion process.[30]

Joint Scan

A gamma camera is used to determine how technetium 99, a rapidly degradable radiopharmaceutical, concentrates in areas of arthritic activity.[31] The radioisotope targets the calcium nodules surrounding sites of infectious activity. These nodules show as "hot spots" in the picture.[32] It appears that the calcium may be the body's natural mechanism for walling off the microorganisms to keep them from obtaining nutrients and to stop them from spreading. In recent years, MRI scanning has largely replaced bone scanning for the diagnosis of localized knee pain.

Anti-cyclic Citrullinated Peptide (CCP) Test

In 2006, the anti-CCP test was developed to be more definitive than the R-factor (RF) test for Rheumatoid Arthritis. Citrullination is a chemical reaction that occurs when inflammatory cells release enzymes in local tissues. Patients with RA have been shown to form antibodies to citrullated peptides. Anti-CCP appears to be more specific for RA (approximately 98%) compared to the RF, which is not particularly sensitive. Some patients who have a negative RF test may be anti-CCP positive, so rheumatologists may wish to order both tests.[33]

Neutrophil Testing

Neutrophils constitute over 90% of cells found in synovial fluid of RA individuals. Electron microscopy reveals that neutrophils degranulate when they encounter cartilage with immune complexes entrapped; neutrophils first degrade and then invade the tissue. The connection between stimulus and secretion of enzymes from neutrophils can be measured during a histamine reaction, and the triggers to infectious bacterial allergy can then be identified.[34, 35]

Animal experiments using *Mycoplasma arthritidis* have resulted in the development of chronic arthritis resembling RA in humans. The disease is characterized by swelling, an influx of neutrophils into the region surrounding the joint, and a mild increase in the numbers of synovial tissue cells. The disease settles in the synovial membrane and adjacent tissues. In the later stages, collagen deposition and destruction of cartilage becomes apparent. Experiments with *Mycoplasma pulmonis, M. bovis, M. mycoides, M. capricolum, M. hyorhinis, M. alkalescens, M. meleagridis, M. gallisepticum,* and *M. hynosynoviae* led to arthritis.[36]

PCR Testing

According to Drs Baseman and Tully, "Sufficient evidence has accumulated recently to establish an important and emerging role for *Mycoplasma fermentans* in human respiratory and joint diseases. For example, *M. fermentans* has been detected by specific gene amplification techniques such as PCR in the synovial fluid of patients with inflammatory arthritis, but not in the joints of patients with juvenile or reactive arthritis. In two other studies using PCR, *M. fermentans* was identified in the upper respiratory tract of 20-44% of both healthy and HIV-infected patients and was associated with acute respiratory distress syndrome in non-immunocompromised persons."

Using PCR tests, four pathogenic Mycoplasma species (*M. fermentans, M. pneumoniae, M. hominis,* and *M. penetrans*) have been found in patients with RA.[37]

Many CFS and Fibromyalgia patients have a systemic cytomegalovirus infection. Dr. Nicolson recommends testing for CMV in <u>any</u> type of suspected autoimmune illness.

Appendix III lists several labs. Immunosciences Lab is a reputable testing facility in California, offering a comprehensive menu of tests for autoimmune diseases, viral infections, gluten sensitivity, and Lyme Disease.[38]

The nonprofit Mycoplasma Registry[39] describes several types of Mycoplasma tests and recommended preparations one should take before having the blood sample drawn. This organization provides a list of laboratories in the U.S. that offer tests for Mycoplasma, Lyme Disease, Candidiasis, Chlamydia, HHV-6, and Rickettsia. The group will provide a printed version of the brochure "How to Get an Accurate PCR Blood Test for Mycoplasmal and Other Infections" for a donation.

It is important not to take any antibiotics, colloidal silver, flax seed oil, or fish oils for at least one month prior to the PCR test. These substances will remove most of the infection from the blood, precluding accurate test results. Suspend intake of immune system-enhancing vitamins, herbs, or supplements since these may reduce the Mycoplasma count. The optimum time for testing is when the patient exhibits symptoms and before antibiotic treatment has begun. Re-testing should be done if test results are negative but the symptoms persist.

Genetic Marker Testing

In 1973, researchers found human leucocyte antigen B-27 (HLA-B27) in 96% of Ankylosing Spondylitis (AS) patients, compared to 8% of the general population. Since then, a considerable body of research has developed to understand the cause(s) and treatment of AS.[40] In general, people with either AS or Reiter's Syndrome (one of the more common types of reactive arthritis) test positive for HLA-B27. Of Caucasians who develop AS, 90% have this gene. The percentage is not as high among other races, but is still strong. About 10-20% of individuals who have a close relative with

AS and who inherit the HLA-B27 antigen eventually develop AS.[41]

More than 50% of adults who have RA also have the inherited gene HLA-DR4, which increases one's risk of developing RA and Lyme disease.[42] Furthermore, research indicates that these genetic markers may predispose individuals to contract reactive, infectious arthritis after particular infections in the urinary tract or gastrointestinal tract, or after diarrheal food poisoning.[43]

Some genes may have a stronger influence than others, and this strength is likely to vary from person to person, predisposing one individual's immune system to respond differently than another's by attacking bones or joints when exposed to a virus or some other antigen. Specific genes may cause some people to be more severely stricken, and sooner, than others. E.g., a 2007 study identified the STAT4 gene as an important risk factor for both RA and Lupus.[44]

AS is often called Rheumatoid Arthritis of the spine because of the synovial inflammatory reaction observed in that area. The high level of lymphoctyes and plasma cells in the synovial membrane suggests an important immune system involvement. A substantial body of research details cellular interactions that occur in chronic synovitis, however, the researchers admit that they know little about the influence of genetic factors and the nature of the inciting stimuli. What is known is the highly associated genetic background signified by the frequency of the HLA-B27 marker.

There are two molecules in the bowel microbe Klebsiella showing molecular mimicry, one against HLA-B27 and the other against spinal collagens. Elevated levels of antibodies to *Klebsiella pneumoniae* have been reported in many AS studies.[45] People with AS are more likely to have genital or intestinal symptoms and/or infections with Mycoplasma, Chlamydia, and Ureaplasma.[46]

There are tests that measure the B27-positive lymphoctyes of the RA patient compared with the antigens of gram-negative organisms. Results can be used to see microbial interaction in relation to HLA background and thus develop a course of treatment that avoids the infectious trigger(s) for arthritis. The trigger(s) can be an episode of intestinal disease such as salmonella or dysentery, or an instance of venereal disease.[47]

An estimated 90% of RA patients possess the HLA-DR1 shared epitope but the frequency in the general population is only about 35%. The prevailing theory to explain this is that the HLA-DR1/HLA-DR4 molecules resemble some external bacterial or viral antigen. An example of this theory is the Streptococcus microbe, which has molecules that resemble cardiac and brain antigens, but infects tonsils and causes upper respiratory infection.

The microbe *Proteus mirabilis* contains sequences that resemble HLA-DR1 and HLA-DR4. Researchers have found that AS and RA are linked to *P. mirabilis* infection and that antibiotics, vegetarian diets, high water intake, and cranberry juice are effective treatments.[48, 49, 50]

Antibody Tests

Antibody tests are usually given for yeast infections. *Candida albicans* fungi stay benign in the gut until a dysfunctional immune system permits the yeast to flourish or strong doses of antibiotics kill off normal intestinal bacteria that keep Candida in check. Yeast infections, especially among women (but not limited to women) in Western societies, are common today. The related symptoms of fatigue, muscle ache, and joint pain overlap those of RA, but Candida arthritis is designated a separate form of fungal arthritis that may be mistaken for acute bacterial arthritis. Diagnosis depends on synovial fluid analysis.[51]

A yeast infection is sometimes misdiagnosed as a bladder infection or IBS *Candida albicans* thrives in a sugary environment. Yeast sends tendrils through the gut wall allowing leakage of larger protein food-molecules into the blood where they stimulate the Ig reaction to the food protein.

Anti-Candida antibody tests are extremely comprehensive and can indicate the level to which one's body is producing antibodies to fight off bacteria and food-molecules gone astray. An amino acid chromatography test is another method to test Candida status.

For patients already taking antibiotics whose PCR test results show a false negative for mycoplasmal infection, antibody tests offer an alternative. Although these tests are not as accurate as PCR, they can reveal whether the patient has developed antibodies to Mycoplasmas. The longer the individual has taken antibiotics, the more accurate the test results may be.

Antinuclear Antibody (ANA) test [52, 53]

The ANA is a blood test that is used in the evaluation connective tissue disorders such as RA and Lupus. It measures the presence of abnormal antibodies. A positive ANA indicates an autoimmune disorder, but alone it can't lead to a diagnosis. False positives are common. A negative ANA, however, means that the patient does not have Lupus. This is important because some RA medications can make Lupus symptoms worse.

The ANA profile includes basic ANA plus tests for other related abnormal antibodies. The profile test may find cryoglobulins. These are antibodies that may be high in a variety of different diseases, including Rheumatoid Arthritis, Lupus, Hepatitis B and C, Sjögren's syndrome, Waldenstrom's macroglobulinemia, multiple myeloma, lymphoproliferative disorders, Raynaud's phenomenon, polymyosis, dermato-myositis, and other infections. The doctor may order ESR and CRP tests in conjunction with the ANA profile.

51Chromium Release Assay

Individuals having illnesses characterized by chronic fatigue, autoimmune disease symptoms, cancerous tumors, and viral infections are likely to have low NK cell activity. The 4-hour 51Chromium release assay test can reveal the influence of synovial virus infections such as Epstein-Barr virus (EBV), CMV (a β-herpes virus), and parvovirus B19.[54] These viruses are known to be linked to several types of chronic arthritis, including RA. Anti-tumor necrosis factor (TNF-α) treatments for RA can keep the viruses under control without interfering with normal T-cell activity.[55]

A 2008 study found that 45% of a subgroup of 1027 children with autism suffered from low Natural Killer (NK) cell activity. Researchers concluded that low intracellular levels of glutathione, interleukin-2 (IL-2) and IL-15 may play an important role.[56] A 2009 study showed dysfunction of NK cells may predispose to adverse neuroimmune interactions during critical periods of a child's early development.[57]

Eosinophil Testing

The Absolute Eosinophil Count test measures the number of these active white blood cells to indicate certain allergic conditions, infections, and other chronic illnesses.[58] [59] Test results for persons with infectious mononucleosis include an elevated white blood cell count, an increased percentage of certain atypical white blood cells, and a positive reaction to a "mono spot" or heterophile test.

When infection with EBV occurs during adolescence or young adulthood, it causes infectious mononucleosis 35% to 50% of the time. However, direct detection of EBV in blood or lymphoid tissues is a research tool and is not available for routine diagnosis.

A 2006 CDC article[60] shows the gaps in conventional testing. "Although the symptoms of infectious mono-nucleosis usually resolve in one or two months, the Epstein-Barr virus remains dormant in cells in the throat and blood for the rest of the person's life...[the virus] also establishes a lifelong dormant infection in some cells of the body's immune system." To which one might add: "...as it does for other persistent pathogens like herpes, Varicella-zoster virus (chicken pox and shingles), measles virus, HIV-1, and CMV."

Thyroid Testing

According to the Thyroid Society, twenty million Americans have some form of thyroid dysfunction but many are undiagnosed or misdiagnosed.[61] The thyroid gland controls the body's metabolism by producing hormones that regulate energy, control heart rate and body weight, and determine how the body uses nutrients. Thyroid test results, therefore, can be a valuable indicator of nutritional balance and efficient use of hormones. A significant percentage of FMS patients are tested with secondary hypothyroidism.[62]

Thyroid dysfunction, notably Hashimoto's Thyroiditis and Grave's Disease, has been shown to be linked to mycoplasmal infection.[63] One of two types of antibodies— thyroperoxidase or thyroglobulin—is found in nearly all patients with hypothyroidism (Hashimoto's Thyroiditis) and in approximately 50% of those with hyperthyroidism (Grave's Disease). Mary Shomon has created an excellent Internet resource for those who wish to know about thyroid conditions and to find a qualified practitioner for diagnosis and treatment. This detailed overview is called "Thyroid Disease 101: Basic Information on Hypothyroidism, Hyperthyroidism, Goiter, Nodules, and Cancer."[64]

JUVENILE RHEUMATOID ARTHRITIS (JRA) [65]

Clinicians arrive at a diagnosis of Rheumatoid Arthritis (in particular, JRA) based on particular symptoms such as persistent arthritis pain in one or more joints for at least six weeks that cannot be attributed to another cause. Other signs are an enlarged liver or spleen, swollen lymph nodes, anemia, heart problems, and eye inflammation.

Laboratory tests that can help diagnose JRA and rule out other disorders are:

- Complete blood count (CBC) – to evaluate the child's red and white blood cells and hemoglobin to detect anemia and/or a decreased white blood cell count;

- ESR and/or CRP to detect inflammation;

- Antinuclear antibody (ANA) to detect the presence of auto-antibodies; this is the most common test to be positive in children with JRA. About 80% of those with eye inflammation will test positive for ANA;

- Comprehensive Metabolic Panel (CMP) to help evaluate and monitor the child's kidney and liver function;

- RF may be positive or negative based on the type of JRA;

- Blood culture to rule out infection:
  o HLA-B27 test to detect this gene, which is present in 70-90% of patients with arthritis affecting the spine;
  o Ferritin levels, though not used to diagnose the condition, may be elevated with JRA. Note that test results for patients with inflammatory conditions like RA may have falsely elevated ferritin levels;[66]
  o Synovial fluid analysis is sometimes ordered to detect crystals that may be present in the joint and to look for signs of joint infection;
  o Other laboratory tests, such as a test for Lyme Disease, may be ordered as indicated to rule out other conditions with similar symptoms.[67]

Non-Laboratory Tests helpful in diagnosing JRA:
  - X-rays of the joints to identify the presence of inflammation;

- X-rays of the chest to check for fluid build-up around the heart or lungs;
- Eye exam to detect the extent of inflammation;
- EKG to detect heart inflammation.

UNCONVENTIONAL TESTING METHODS

Because some degree of success has been reported using the following tests, they merit mention, even though they are considered controversial in some medical circles. The tests described in the following sections are endorsed by well-known and credible physicians and scientists.

Darkfield Microscopy [68]

This instrument is used by blood-imaging researchers and specialty diagnostic laboratory scientists to observe living whole blood cells. The microscope projects the dynamic image in high contrast, magnified 1,400X onto a video screen. The object appears bright against a dark background. The skilled physician can detect early signs of illness by looking for microorganisms known to cause disease.[69] The length of time the blood stays alive is also an indicator of the overall health of the patient. Distortions of red blood cells indicate nutritional status, possible bacterial or fungal infection(s), and blood ecology patterns offering clues to illness. Routine blood tests and cultures do not show the rich detail necessary to make these diagnoses.

Dr. Philip Hoekstra, director of ThermaScan, Inc.,[70] has found that the blood samples of virtually all RA patients studied contain significant amounts of *Propionibacterium acnes* in an altered state, i.e., the bacteria are cell wall-deficient.[71] *P. acnes* is a relatively slow-growing, anaerobic gram-positive bacterium linked to the skin condition called "acne." It can also cause chronic blepharitis (inflammation of the eyelash follicles) and endophthalmitis (inflammation of the internal coats of the eye) . *P. acnes* was first identified in

1981.[72] It is passed from mother to fetus through the placenta, perhaps explaining how RA reappears in generations within a single family. It also explains why RA patients respond to the same tetracycline treatment given to those with acne. The late Dr. Lida H. Mattman, professor emeritus of biology at Wayne State University and Dr. Hoekstra's mentor, extracted this bacteria from the synovial fluid of RA patients, injected it into chicken embryos, treated the hatched chicks with antibiotics, and observed the RA disappear.[73]

Dr. Hoekstra has tested blood samples of Multiple Sclerosis patients, finding another stealth pathogen, *Borrelia mylophora*, a bacterium resembling *B. burgdorferi* that is linked to Lyme Disease. *B. mylophora* has a special affinity for the myelin sheath covering nerves. White blood cells and their antibodies attack and destroy the myelin sheath in their efforts to get at the bacterium as it skillfully cloaks itself. Treatment of MS patients over several weeks with doxycycline has met with considerable success in subduing this bacterial infection.[74, 75]

Although useful in some applications, one serious deficiency with darkfield microscopy is that it is unable to find intracellular infectious agents.[76] The FDA has not approved darkfield blood analysis, so this prevents some doctors from even considering the controversial technique.

Phase-Contrast Microscopy [77, 78, 79]

A specialized microscope allows the physician to examine blood cells as a diagnostic test of the performance of the immune system. The following are a few examples of observable indicators:

- Platelet aggregation and adherence to damaged blood vessels causing impaired circulation, high cholesterol, or candidiasis;

- L-forms, indicating a condition of immune system dysfunction, high blood sugar, or bacterial infection;

- Arterial plaque, linked to poor circulation, calcium imbalance, and fatigue;
- Protein linkage, a condition that shows improper digestion of protein;
- Spicules or fibrin, showing toxicity of the liver and/or bowel;
- Eosinophils, elevated count of large white blood cells found under conditions of allergy, parasite infestation, and edema;
- Rouleau, an aggregation of red blood cells caused by physical or mental stress, leading to poor circulation, fatigue, and depleted oxygen; and
- Neutrophilic viability, a measure of poor immunity, infectious state(s), and malabsorption of nutrients.

Phase Contrast Microscopy is considered the easiest and most cost-effective periodontal exam technique to view dental plaque.[80] The sight of the living "bugs" from their own mouths on a high-resolution, big screen monitor is a powerful means to motivate patients to adopt good oral hygiene habits.

The Ergonom microscope, invented in 1991 by Kurt Olbrich, has only recently (in 2010) become commercially available.[81] Exciting improvements by Olbrich, working with Grayfield Optical, Inc., allows observation of detailed structures otherwise invisible with conventional phase contrast microscopes. E.g., one can see the *in vitro* decomposition processes of blood. During this transitional phase new viruses and structures arise, which can give insights about processes involved in cell replication diseases such as cancer.[82]

Applied Kinesiology

Techniques using applied kinesiology (muscle testing) in skilled hands can have significant positive effect in reversing chronic disease by identifying and eliminating allergens. The Total Body Modification (TBM) method and its derivative, the Nambudripad Allergy Elimination Technique (NAET), not only work, they are non-invasive, drug-free, and less expensive than ELISA tests.[83]

TBM and NAET represent an effective but still controversial approach that employs muscle testing to diagnose allergy, followed by acupressure, acupuncture, or chiropractic methods to eliminate the specific irritating allergen.[84] The goal is to retrain the brain and nervous system to deal with the allergen not as a poison to be attacked but as a benign substance temporarily present in the body. Dr. Mercola has three TBM-trained therapists on his staff. The theory behind TBM and NAET is that an allergic response is not only a physical problem but also an indication of dysfunction or blockage of chemical and neural pathways.[85]

A veterinarian may prescribe prednisolone (a type of prednisone) for a pet with allergy symptoms. The nontoxic TBM or NAET reprogramming usually is permanent, and the treatment includes suggested nutritional changes.

Hair Analysis

The Journal of the American Medical Association's 2001 study of this controversial clinical test to determine nutrient (mainly mineral) deficiencies and excesses from hair samples concluded that test results vary so widely that the procedure should be considered worthless.[86] Dr. Joseph Mercola and other physicians took exception to this study,[87] characterizing it as flawed and pointing out that hair analysis can be a useful diagnostic tool if, and only if, the hair sample is not washed prior to laboratory analysis. This important step is essential to preserve the essential mineral ratios, but has minimal effect on toxic metals. Other studies confirm the validity of hair analysis, if done properly.[88, 89] On his website, Dr. Mercola provides data on two recommended laboratories —Trace Elements and

Analytical Research—for accurate, reliable analysis and high standards.[90]

It is advisable to check whether the facility doing the testing is associated with a drug/vitamin supply company. If so, the tests may reveal, not surprisingly, that the test subject has deficiencies in those particular supplements sold by the lab's commercial affiliate and sponsor. This association has probably led to the prevailing prejudice against hair analysis that the medical community still maintains.

Visual Contrast Sensitivity (VCS) Test [91]

Standard medical diagnostic test results are usually normal for patients who have chronic illness caused by exposure to biotoxins/neurotoxins, making the condition difficult to diagnose and treat. Biotoxins are produced by organisms such as Borrelia and Babesia (Lyme spirochetes), water-dwelling dinoflagellates and cyanobacteria, fungi (as airborne mold) and some types of bacteria.

Dr. Ritchie Shoemaker developed the VCS diagnostic test to show evidence of a neurological deficit. A positive VCS result, in the presence of biotoxin exposure potential, and a symptom complex involving multiple systems, and in the absence of other historical, medical or treatment conditions that likely explain the symptoms, provide a basis for a credible diagnosis of probable biotoxin-mediated illness. Toxins from Lyme Disease organisms may remain in the body long after the spirochetes or intracellular protozoa have been killed by antibiotics. The Shoemaker treatment protocol is helpful for CFS and Fibromyalgia, and uses Questran/cholestyramine.[92]

Endnotes and continuing research on topics in Chapter 6 can be found at www.RA-Infection-Connection.com

7. NATURAL METHODS TO REVITALIZE THE IMMUNE SYSTEM

A well-known relationship exists between poor health among Americans and our sugar- and starch-laden diet combined with a sedentary lifestyle. However, the medical community asserts that if poor diet and lack of exercise were causative factors of disease, they would have discovered it a long time ago.[1] In fact, some of the causes of poor health are known, but there are far too many of them. Prevailing medical philosophy tends to prefer the single solution and simple answer to the complex one. This Occam's Razor[2] approach will not work for a problem as complicated and intricate as a dysfunctional immune system. Without a holistic view of their patients, the result is a simplistic pain-reducing prescription for pills that provide short-term relief with long-term effects.

While no vitamin, mineral, or supplement can fulfill all the advertising promises made by their suppliers, scientific studies are increasingly showing that arthritis sufferers can benefit from certain nutrients. In some cases, supplements may be necessary because the individual cannot absorb or use nutrients directly from natural foods, or may be taking a medication that interferes with normal nutrient absorption, or the body's chemical processes may block beneficial enzymes.

AEROBIC EXERCISE

Exercise is essential to keep the lymph system flowing and to keep blood circulating. Lymph channels remove toxic waste molecules from cells and tissues. Blood brings nutrients to cells throughout the body, but exercise in an inflamed state can be harmful. Inflammation can increase blockage of already constricted coronary arteries, as shown in autopsies of athletes like fitness guru Jim Fixx (1932-1984) and baseball pitcher Daryl Kile (1968-2002).[3] Stamina is enhanced and discomfort reduced with high levels of Coenzyme Q_{10}. Ascorbate (vitamin C) in levels of 3-6 grams per day per 100 lbs of body weight may reduce the pain that exercise causes in an inflamed state. It is best to consult with one's doctor before embarking on an exercise regimen.

Jogging and running are not helpful to arthritics since these exercises increase the pressure of gravity, compressing vertebrae and leading to wear and tear on ankle, knee and hip joints. Jogging and running consist of a series of sudden, severe, downward shocks to the joints. Brisk walking, water therapy, and gentle dancing[4] can be just as effective without the danger of impact damage. For those arthritics whose lower limbs are affected, the slow, gentle stretching of yoga, accompanied by deep breathing, can provide significant aerobic benefit. Movement, but not vigorous exercise or strain, is what is important to produce endorphins, the hormones that improve pain tolerance.[5]

Fatigue is a common symptom of chronic disease. Taking a nap may be tempting, but low impact exercise in conjunction with deep breathing may have the same restful effect while simultaneously reviving energy. Deep breathing exercises while lying prone on a slant board can enhance circulation, oxygenate cells, and relieve gravitational pressure on joints. By oxygenating cells, we make it more difficult for harmful anaerobic organisms to live and grow. Oxygen is catabolic (destructive) as well as cleansing by breaking down complex substances into more simple compounds. Oxygen destroys the by-products, or metabolites, of anabolism, the constructive processes of the body. The body is a dynamic balance of anabolic and catabolic processes.

Great benefits can also be found in range-of-motion exercises done in the buoyancy of water. Swimming is an excellent way to loosen stiff joints and to stop muscles from becoming weak. Daily exercise in a heated pool or spa will provide remarkable relief. Others find that alternating heat treatment with cool compresses or ice packs keeps pain and swelling symptoms in check.

Strength training to increase muscle tone in order to support the skeletal system may require specific gymnasium equipment, but can also be done with simple isometric exercises. Although joint movement is often accompanied by pain, arthritics must learn to do mild and gradual exercises with joints lightly loaded in order to keep them limber, lest their joints become immobilized and muscles atrophy from disuse. A strength training exercise regimen is also helpful in preventing osteoporosis.

STRESS REDUCTION AND PAIN MANAGEMENT

Short-term stress is actually beneficial for arthritics. The adrenal glands secrete the hormone cortisol (natural cortisone) into circulation several times daily, most of it around 8 a.m. to provide energy to start the day. Cortisol levels decline naturally from then on, but can spike if the body is abnormally stressed, by an event or by chronic infection, as discussed in Chapter 3.

Cortisol plays an important role in the body, controlling salt and water balance as well as regulating carbohydrate, fat, and protein metabolism. When the brain needs glucose (blood sugar), cortisol takes glucose from the cells of the muscles and liver, routing it to the brain. Our muscles need insulin to produce energy and to recover from the effects of exercise. Inflammation is a major cause of Insulin Resistance Syndrome, where muscles are unable to burn glucose circulating in the blood, so blood sugar level rises. Cortisol further raises blood sugar. The pancreas responds by releasing more insulin in an effort to lower the level. When resistance exceeds production, Type 2 diabetes occurs. High insulin levels prevent cells from breaking down fat, making it difficult to lose weight.[6] In addition, kidneys retain more fluid, raising blood pressure and creating a bloated, swollen feeling.

Stress-induced demand for cortisol may far exceed the body's normal daily production. Deficient cortisol levels during stress could lead to fever, low blood pressure, mood swings, and/or depression. If one becomes accustomed to supplemental synthetic cortisol in the form of an anti-inflammatory drug like prednisone, the body's adrenal glands will become lazy about producing cortisol on their own and become dependent on the drug. Prednisone has some serious side effects including immune system suppression, increased risk of infection, elevated blood sugar, gastritis, steroid-induced osteoporosis, anxiety, agitation, and insomnia.[7]

Dealing with a stressful event can be challenging but can provide some measure of distraction from the symptoms of joint pain and stiffness. However, long-term mental stress without compensating physical exercise can be taxing on the heart and immune system. Reducing stress can be done in a variety of ways besides exercise—some simple (taking a few minutes each day for quiet meditation), or comparatively extreme (finding a new, different career or relocating to another geographic area).

Studies have shown that quiet activities such as knitting or listening to soothing music can trigger a "relaxation response" manifested in the release of endorphins, the body's natural painkillers. Measurably high levels of endorphins in synovial fluid have been found in RA patients who had a joyful outlook on life and coped well with their symptoms compared to those patients who complained about joint pain.[8]

The American Academy of Pain Medicine reported in 2006 that chronic pain affects more Americans than heart disease, diabetes, and cancer combined.[9] Chronic pain is an enormous national epidemic, reflected in the numbers of pain control facilities springing up across the country. The cost, in terms of physical suffering as well as burden to taxpayers through Workers' Compensation claims, is staggering—in the hundreds of millions of dollars annually.[10] However, these pain control facilities are able to deal with patients more effectively and at lower cost than hospitals because nearly all treatments are done in one place, reducing the patient's work time loss and travel time. Also, the staff usually takes a comprehensive, holistic approach to the patients' health problems.

However, it is difficult to obtain valid assessments and accurate diagnostic data when many patients submit fraudulent claims. Studies have revealed learned pain syndromes, where the single most common reinforcing factor for illness behavior was the excused escape from everyday responsibilities.[11] This may explain why those legitimately suffering from Chronic Fatigue Syndrome or Fibromyalgia are often accused of "faking it" or being "lazy." Fatigue is a result of the cellular dysfunction caused by the cell-invading microbes.[12] CoQ_{10} can help restore energy.

Most acute pain involves tissue damage traced to an etiological (infection, allergy) and/or mechanical (injury, repetitive stress) cause. Neurophysiologists typically use duration of pain as a way to differentiate between etiological and mechanical causes. However, determining this distinction can be difficult, especially in cases of recurrent acute pain experienced by arthritics during flare-ups. Patients often become depressed and emotionally disabled by the chronic pain they experience, and may develop an inability to cope.[13]

Meditation and Self-Hypnosis

Using the mind's own ability to focus on positive goals and imagine peaceful settings is a powerful tool in pain control and stress management. There are many self-help guidebooks, audiotapes, and DVDs available to aid in learning meditation techniques.[14] A few sessions with a professional hypnotherapist can teach any highly motivated individual how to achieve relaxation and manage pain. The author can attest to the value of self-hypnosis from personal experience. Guided imagery is proven to be very effective in combating stress, coping with the discomfort of RA symptoms, helping to get a full night's sleep, and promoting a general feeling of well-being. Self-hypnosis—a form of deep meditation—is a drug-free and costless method of distraction therapy with no harmful side effects.

It is unlikely that an insurer will reimburse for lessons in self-hypnosis because it is not viewed as a "real procedure" and is considered a nonscientific approach. However, documented evidence[15] shows that hypnosis has great value as a therapeutic tool to control self-destructive habits (e.g., overeating, smoking), cope with pain, reduce stress, conquer fear, manage anxiety, overcome depression, and deal with emotional loss. Hypnosis is most often valuable not as a treatment but as a facilitator of other therapies. Hypnotic analgesia, or mastering pain, works by disciplined control of attention. The technique has been used as general anesthesia for surgery on patients who are unable to accept traditional anesthetics. It can also be very helpful with stroke patients to strengthen muscles required for motor control.[16]

Researchers in 1998 evaluated the effects of meditation on psoriasis.[17] Patients practiced guided imagery while listening to relaxation tapes and visualizing the ultraviolet (UV) light healing their skin. The control group received regular UV treatment without the tapes. The meditating group's lesions healed four times faster than the control group's, illustrating the mind's influence on the healing process. The study was repeated with two different groups to confirm the dramatic results.

Find a qualified hypnotherapist through the American Society of Clinical Hypnosis[18] or the Society for Clinical and Experimental Hypnosis.[19]

Energy Psychology

Under this broad heading are techniques combining needle-less acupuncture with psychology to obtain some of the most profoundly powerful tools in combating stress. Of these, the most popular method is called Emotional Freedom Technique (EFT). Dr. Mercola asserts that this is one of best ways to overcome stress and in turn, physical discomfort. It is one of the first things he prescribes for new patients with mild RA. The fundamental premise is that all negative emotions are disruptions in one's bioenergy system. These stress-induced imbalances often manifest themselves as physical symptoms such as joint pain, fatigue, headache, and other characteristics of chronic illness.[20]

Massage

Massage is not only soothing to the psyche, but has tangible effects in stimulating the activity of the lymphatic system, approximately thirty percent of which lies near the surface of the skin in some areas of the body. Massaging the affected joints will facilitate the natural breakdown process that is needed before cell rebuilding can occur. Massage can improve circulation and reduce pain and swelling. Always massage in the direction of the heart, using the fingertips or the heel of the hand, using a little cream or oil as a lubricant. Rolling a clean tennis ball over the affected area provides the same effect.

The medical establishment looked down on massage therapy for a very long time, but modern medical experts generally accept the efficacy of massage. Today over 70% of American hospitals now offer massage therapy as a part of their treatments for chronic pain, in cancer cases, pregnancy, infant care, joint and muscle mobility, stress management and many other symptoms and disorders. New research suggests that massage therapy helps to boost the immune system, lower blood pressure, and manage pain.[21]

The same funds otherwise paid for pain-killing drugs could instead be spent on a professional massage without the harmful side effects. Basic techniques can be learned from self-help books[22] and tapes. Massage is very helpful for arthritic pets. It also works for arthritic spouses.

Emu oil, high in oleic acid, acts as a transport mechanism for medications into the body when massaged on the skin. It is anti-inflammatory, antifungal, and antibacterial. It reduces inflammatory pain, swelling and stiffness in joints, heals various skin conditions, reduces toenail fungus, and reduces pain of injuries and strains. It is stable, does not spoil, and does not support microbe growth on the shelf.[23]

Massage for Post-polio Syndrome (PPS)

Poliomyelitis ("polio") is a highly contagious, and sometimes fatal, viral infection that affects the nerves. It can produce permanent muscle weakness and often paralysis. Polio has been known since ancient times, but major epidemics were unknown until seen in Europe in the 1880s, and in the U.S. in the 1940s and 1950s. Despite two effective vaccines, polio remains a latent threat today.

PPS is a progressive, degenerative condition that affects polio survivors 10 to 40 years after recovery. PPS is characterized by a further weakening of muscles that were previously affected by the viral infection.[24] In 2008, a massage therapist worked with a client with PPS for nine weeks and reported a marked increase in energy, and a decrease in muscle spasms, joint and muscle pain, and overall fatigue.[25]

The Sister Kenny Rehabilitation Institute, established in 1940, advocated early activity, hydrotherapy, and massage to maximize the strength of unaffected muscle fibers. At the time, this method was at odds with the conventional treatment of rigid splints, plaster body casts, and iron lung confinement, where muscles continued to atrophy.[26] However, the Kenny approach is now accepted and used successfully today.

After a polio infection, some motor neurons have been destroyed and the muscle cells those neurons once controlled are prone to atrophy. Remaining functioning nerve cells have a tendency to develop new axon tips to support some muscle fibers. That is, the motor unit (a single functioning motor neuron and all the muscle fibers it supplies) becomes larger. As PPS develops, this condition can lead to cumulative fatigue, stress, and wear-and-tear both on the overworked motor neurons and on the under-stimulated muscle cells. A skilled clinician must apply gentle massage treatment to avoid damage to motor neurons.

Massage won't eliminate PPS, but by directly taking the workload off the weakest muscles and supporting the strongest ones, bodywork can be part of a helpful coping strategy for an estimated 440,000 U.S. polio survivors.[27]

Granulomas are the hallmark of the host's response to mycobacterial infection. A 2005 study[28] showed that anti-TB treatment that includes massage to break up granuloma-like calcifications that both wall-off and protect bacteria from antibiotics has a better chance of success.

Neurostructural Therapy (NST) [29]

Also called Neurostructural Integration Technique, NST is performed by a trained practitioner in a sequence of movements designed to realign muscles, nerves and connective tissue. It combines key elements of massage, acupressure, and chiropractic for a gentle method of noninvasive healing. Originally developed in Australia by the late Tom Bowen in the 1950s, the method was called Total Body Modification (TBM). Several TBM websites provide detailed descriptions, lists of practitioners, and success stories.[30] This technique has given pain relief to many thousands of patients. Proponents have found that after a few NST sessions normal lymphatic flow is restored, the neuromuscular system resets tension levels, and scar tissue softens and shrinks.[31]

Tai Chi

This gentle, rhythmic exercise teaches balance, reduces stress, aids in blood circulation, and assists in cell building since it is an aerobic exercise. Tai Chi has been practiced in China for centuries as part of a daily physical fitness regimen. Groups of people can be seen early in the morning in public squares and parks, performing the specific sequence of moves called "forms." Intense concentration on exact body position and steady breathing while moving slowly give a meditative aspect to the exercise.

Because movement is slow and not strenuous, people of all ages can perform the exercise. It is ideal for arthritics and seniors, but not helpful if joints/tendons are badly inflamed. Tai Chi is the counterpart to the fast-moving martial art form of Kung Fu. Tai Chi is very popular in the United States. Classes are usually offered as part of city-sponsored adult education programs, health support groups, the local YMCA, or commercial gyms. Books and videotapes can assist with home study.[32]

Pilates Method

On a par with Yoga and Tai Chi is the Pilates Method for strengthening weak muscles and stretching tight ones. Pilates moves can correct muscle imbalances, increase range of motion, reduce pain, and improve mobility and joint stability by building up supporting muscles.[33] Arthritics with pain and inflammation in the spine, knees, or hips may have trouble getting up and down from floor mats. The maxim "No pain, no gain" should never be followed for any exercise.

Minimal movement therapies

When even the thought of exercise is painful, consider programs such as the Alexander Technique, the Feldenkrais Method, and the Trager Approach.[34] Each of these is named for its developer, and each offers maximum benefit for minimal movement. They offer relief of joint stress by retraining the body to balance and distribute weight more evenly, thus reducing wear and tear on the joints.

Physical therapists who work with stroke patients and those recovering from joint replacement surgery recommend these gentle techniques, but are quick to admit that they are also popular with athletes and performers at the peak of physical health.

Poor posture is an important contributing factor to pain as certain muscles tighten, spasm, or put pressure on nerves. Correcting the position of the head and neck can dramatically influence pressure on the spine and the nerves associated with it. As posture, mobility, and flexibility improve, organs realign and breathing capacity increases, in turn oxygenating cells throughout the body.

These techniques do not rebuild damaged cartilage, reverse joint deformities, or remove the disease, but they can decrease the need for medication. They can reduce pain while increasing mobility, personal confidence, and comfort. One's doctor is the best judge of the particular exercise therapy tailored to the patient's condition. Cost for treatments is comparable to physical therapy, but may not be covered by insurance unless a doctor recommends them.

Some HMOs offer one or more of these methods in the form of low-cost classes for patients with chronic pain. Kaiser Permanente in California, for instance, sponsors Feldenkrais exercise classes.

DIET ADJUSTMENTS

The typical American diet is high in refined foods, certain fats, and sugars—all of which undermine the efficiency of our bodies' various systems and functions. To strengthen the immune system, one must make an effort to eat raw, whole foods, i.e., not processed or refined, and reduce consumption of harmful fats and sugars whenever possible. Dr. Andrew Weil's Anti-inflammatory Food Pyramid is an excellent starting point.[35]

The practices of adding pesticides to fruit and vegetable cultivation and chemicals to animal feed are designed to produce cosmetically appealing food products as they make their way from farms to grocery display shelves. These additives may have long-term cumulative and detrimental effects as residual toxins in our bodies. Toxins associated with infectious pathogens and their elimination are discussed in Chapter 3.

Simple refined carbohydrates are found in unexpected places, so it behooves the arthritic to become an avid label reader to discover hidden sugar, honey, corn syrup, fructose, and other sweeteners in processed foods.[36] This is difficult in American society where we have been conditioned to ask, "Which pill should I take?" rather than "What should I eat?"

Maintaining a normal weight is also beneficial to the arthritis sufferer by allowing the circulatory system and lymph system to function more efficiently. Body weight is not a factor except for pain-caused physical gravitational pressure on inflamed, swollen joints in the lower extremities. In fact, underweight people have been reported to have a significantly higher risk of severe arthritis.[37]

The question of which diet is best for arthritis sufferers, found in many self-help books, has no consistent answer. An arthritic may religiously follow a diet that has proved to help others similarly afflicted, only to find that s/he is worse off than before. What has been ignored is not only the concurrent removal of toxins but also the possibility that the proposed diet contains a substance like gluten that can produce a severe allergic reaction in some individuals. A particular food sensitivity, pollen allergy, or chemical substance can initiate a Herxheimer reaction. Salmonella or botulism (food poisoning) can be such a trigger.[38]

One size does *not* fit all when it comes to diet. For instance, a corn, gluten, sugar, or milk allergy will cause a severe flare-up of arthritic symptoms in one person but will have no effect on another following the identical diet. Milk allergy may just be insufficient lactic acid bacteria in the gut flora. This is easy to fix with probiotic supplements.[39] An important personal step in countering arthritis is determining which particular foods are friend or foe. The typical physician's vague ("just eat a healthy diet") or no-comment stance on nutrition leaves the patient in a quandary.

It is advantageous to obtain a food allergy profile developed by a qualified specialist in both allergies and nutrition. The results of allergy testing may be the key to any progress in recovery if arthritis symptoms are severe. Allergy testing is discussed in Chapter 6. Analysis such as in-depth immunoglobulin (ELISA IgE and/or IgG) blood testing and applied kinesiology techniques in the hands of a skilled practitioner can determine specific allergens. However, it may be difficult to convince some HMOs to pay for such tests and/or the medical staff may reject the request because they do not have the training to interpret test results.

The closest one can come to a comprehensive set of guidelines for diet and lifestyle changes is that developed by Dr. Mercola over nearly a decade of treating thousands of patients in his clinic as well as hundreds of thousands over the Internet. The latest detailed version of this regimen can be found on his website[40] and in his 2004 book, *The No-Grain Diet*. Additional nutritional advice by Dr. Garth Nicolson is given on his www.immed.org website.

Some popular diets in self-help books advocate eliminating nightshade vegetables, which contain solanine, a natural toxin that is usually destroyed by a robust and healthy digestive system. A marginally functional digestive system cannot counter the nightshade neurotoxins (scopolamine, atropine, solanine, nicotine, and others), and the residues remain in the body. Another reason for avoiding the Solanum genus is that potatoes are one of the worst crops for retaining pesticide and fungicide residues. It is best to buy organically grown potatoes. Many people test positive for allergies to tomatoes. This is one of the first items to try on an experimental food-elimination diet.[41, 42, 43]

Importance of Water in the Diet

A "sure thing" part of any diet regimen designed to benefit arthritis sufferers (second only to avoiding sugar in all forms) is consumption of at least one quart of pure water (not tap water or distilled water[44]) daily for every fifty pounds of body weight. Some people find it convenient to fill 2-3 one-quart sports bottles in the morning and keep them accessible throughout the day. Many of us are chronically dehydrated. On average, food provides only 20% of our required total water intake.[45] Hunger can be a signal that the body needs water. We unconsciously seek water through chewing food that releases liquid and also through saliva generated. This doesn't slake thirst—it just increases calorie intake.

Water lubricates the body, thins the blood, transports nutrients to cells, reduces constipation, improves digestion, reduces the risk of kidney stones and certain cancers, assists the lymphatic system to excrete toxins, and relieves Fibromyalgia symptoms.[46] Pure water is essential for a healthy immune system. Unless your drinking water comes from a clean well or aquifer, invest in a good quality reverse osmosis filter to remove the fluoride in most cities' water supply.[47]

Fiber [48]

In the United States, our diet often consists largely of processed foods and little fiber or roughage. For this reason diverticulosis is one of the most common colon conditions affecting Americans. Diverticula are pea- to marble-sized pouches formed in weakened areas of the colon wall, usually in the sigmoid section on the left side of the abdomen. These diverticula develop as we age. They cause few problems—one is a vitamin B_{12} deficiency—unless they become inflamed or infected. If a pouch containing bacteria bursts, spilling its contents into the abdominal cavity, peritonitis can result. The bacteria seeps from the bowel through the pouch's thin cell walls and food molecules can enter the blood stream. Tetracycline antibiotics work to metabolize and destroy the pathogens in diverticula.

Too many diverticula can constrict the sigmoid area of the colon even more than its normal narrow state. Constipation, diarrhea, and/or spasms are the result. Prevention is simple: drink lots of pure water daily and eat 25-35 grams of fiber per day—whole wheat or oat bran, oatmeal, whole grains, fruits such as apples and berries, and fibrous vegetables like asparagus, broccoli, carrots, and squash. If your body is not used to fiber intake, introduce it very gradually to avoid gastric distress (e.g., gas, cramps).

Individuals whose health profile is characterized by high insulin levels, high blood pressure, excess weight, high cholesterol, and/or diabetes should minimize all grains. They will likely benefit from eating some animal protein. The main issues with meat (i.e., fat content, antibiotics, hormones, and pesticides) are avoided if one eats meat only from grass-fed livestock.[49]

Fiber helps to lower cholesterol intake and to stabilize blood sugar levels. It gives bulk to stools and speeds the passage of waste through the intestines. More than 50% of people over 60 in the U.S. have diverticulosis, but there may be few or no symptoms. If a diverticulum pouch ruptures and infection sets in around it, diverticulitis develops, with symptoms of abdominal pain and tenderness, and fever.[50]

Because diverticulosis is endemic to seniors, it is tempting to speculate that this condition may actually be infectious and that fiber intake is perhaps only palliative. Researchers should explore the following connections:

- Diverticulosis implies a leaky gut condition;
- A leaky gut implies food particles in the blood;
- Food in the blood implies an immune system allergic reaction;
- An allergic reaction implies a flare-up of arthritis symptoms.

Arterial Plaque

There is one instance where nutritionists and medical professionals agree: that diet plays a major role in many cases of myocardial infarction (interruption of blood and oxygen supply to the heart). Blockage may be due to an accretion of low-density lipoprotein (LDL, or "bad" cholesterol) deposited on artery walls. A cholesterol plaque can suddenly rupture. The sudden blood clot that forms over the rupture then causes a heart attack or stroke. A vitamin C deficiency leads to scurvy and also to atherosclerotic plaque deposits.

A heart disease risk assessment panel concluded that atherosclerosis could have an infectious origin requiring antibiotic therapy as a treatment option.[51] Their finding was based on observations of *Chlamydia pneumoniae* (Cpn) in the presence of oxidized LDL as macrophage engulfment of the pathogen creates a foam cell. Oxidized LDL, Cpn, and foam cells are major constituents of arterial plaque. Another hypothesis is that plaque is formed as a result of bacterial L-forms adhering to healthy cell walls and building cholesterol coats to camouflage themselves from the immune system's hunter/killer T-cells. The infectious aspect of Cpn is detailed in Chapter 3.

METALS: BENEFITS AND DRAWBACKS

Certain metal atoms provide molecular stability for enzymes. Elements considered are: Sodium (Na); Calcium (Ca); Zinc (Zn); Copper (Cu); Magnesium (Mg); Manganese (Mn); Tin (Sn); Silver (Ag); Gold (Au); Aluminum (Al); Cadmium (Cd); Iron (Fe); Nickel (Ni); Chromium (Cr); Cobalt (Co); Selenium (Se); Mercury (Hg); Lead (Pb); and Silicon (Si).

Some metals are needed in trace amounts but at higher levels they are toxic: Mn, Se, Ni, Co, Cr, Hg, Pb, micro-Si. Intake can be environmental through medical injections (aluminum adjuvants in vaccines), contaminants or traces in medicines, supplements, water, mineral dust, food intake (such as Hg in fish), or smoke and air pollution.

Metalloenzymes [52, 53]

Metals play roles in approximately one-third of the known enzymes as a co-factor or by forming a bond when incorporated into an enzyme molecule, where they assist in electron transfer. An exciting new area of research in antibiotic molecules is the study of the many metalloenzymes using both copper and zinc.

Metalloenzymes are incredibly diverse proteins. They function in a number of important physiological processes. One example is iron. Hemoglobin transports oxygen from the lungs to capillaries. In enzymes where a metal is an integral part of the structure of the molecule, the metal cannot be removed without destroying the structure.

Another example is zinc. The source is almost entirely through diet (vegetable protein), but could be through exposure to metal particles as part of one's work in the metal handling, battery, and semiconductor industries. The recommended daily intake is 15 mg but this should be increased to 20-25 mg during pregnancy and lactation.

Zinc deficiency can result in stunted growth, enlarged liver and spleen, and underdeveloped sex organs. Zinc can be lost through perspiration. It is well known that parasitic infections cause zinc depletion.[54] It is also known that antibiotics beneficially change the activity of certain metalloenzymes.[55]

Dental Fillings [56]

Amalgam tooth fillings are an alloy of 50 percent mercury, 35 percent silver, 13 percent tin, 2 percent copper, and a bit of zinc. Four consumer and dental groups claimed in late 2010 that the FDA used flawed science when it set the guidelines for mercury amalgam safety levels in 2009.[57] Dr. Mark Geier, epidemiologist and founder of ASD centers, published a study[58] that examined the effects of mercury, a known neurotoxin, on children with autism. According to Geier, "When we examined children with mothers who had zero to six fillings, we saw no significant effect. But when mothers had over six fillings, we found their children had a higher severity of autism than children whose mothers had fewer fillings." Dr. Mercola is highly opposed to mercury fillings and offers a mercury detox protocol on his website.[59] Find additional information by Dr. Nicolson in Appendix III.

Copper, Gold, Zinc, and Iron

Copper jewelry is often advertised as an arthritis pain reducer. The way copper works is similar to gold. Skin acid dissolves the copper into Cu++ ions in sulfate and chloride forms. The green color visible on the skin after contact with copper or gold indicates the presence of sulfate. A very small amount of the cupric ions are absorbed through the skin and pass into the blood and tissue near the point of contact. Copper in concentrations higher than 10 mg,[60] like gold salts, can be poisonous, but a more diluted amount can suppress Mycoplasmas and the L-form metamorphosed *Streptococcus pneumoniae.* Copper (2mg) as an amino acid chelate is sold in health food stores as a mineral supplement. High doses of vitamin C protect against copper toxicity.[61]

Copper serves as a co-factor in enzymes involved in cellular energy generation, connective tissue production, free radical detoxification, iron mobilization, and neuro-transmission. Copper is also required for normal embryonic development and the growth of new blood vessels. Using copper chelators, researchers have shown copper affects the production of many cellular growth factors, interleukins, and pro-inflammatory cytokines, such as TNF-α. Reduction of intracellular copper by chelation leads to a decrease of these growth factors, interleukins, and cytokines.[62]

When zinc is deficient, copper tends to accumulate in various organs—liver, brain, and the reproductive organs.

Copper toxicity is often overlooked as a contributor to many health problems including allergies, anorexia, anxiety, depression, fatigue, migraine headaches, premenstrual syndrome, atherosclerosis, childhood hyperactivity and learning disorders. [63]

There are two primary types of iron toxicity: inherited and acquired.[64] Iron accumulates over time in various organs—the heart, liver, brain, pancreas, and joints—leading to premature aging and death. Iron can accumulate in the synovial membrane of joints, interfering with zinc and copper metabolism, which are needed to maintain the integrity of the joint surfaces.

Suspicion of iron toxicity is often based on symptoms of joint pain, absence of a menstrual period, or sudden onset of shortness of breath. Iron toxicity is also linked with personality characteristics of a strong ego, rigidity, tenaciousness, hostility, stubbornness, and irritability. Excess iron can deplete vitamins B_6 and C, and can also cause a deficiency of essential minerals. Lab tests[65] and hair analysis[66] can determine iron (and other metals') levels. The fiber in whole grains and nuts and tannic acid in tea will bind with iron and inhibit absorption so the excess can be excreted.[67]

DANGERS IN FOODS AND DRUGS [68]

We don't like to think that our government would allow harmful substances to appear in the foods and drugs we consume. However, these hazards are on our stores' shelves. The thoroughness of enforcement of the Food and Drug Administration (FDA) and U.S. Department of Agriculture (USDA) regulations, as well as the rules themselves, are far from complete. Let the buyer and consumer beware, especially those who suffer from diabetes.

Processed (Cured, Smoked) Meats

Nearly all cured meats contain nitrates and nitrites. Processed (cured or smoked) meats, such as beef jerky, pastrami, bacon, luncheon meats, corned beef, hot dogs, and sausage may also contain oxidized (i.e., rancid) cholesterol, which can damage the nervous system and the cardiovascular system. Both turn into carcinogenic nitrosamines during the digestion process. While these carcinogens can be neutralized by either drinking several cups of green tea with each meal or making sure that intestinal flora is adequate by using acidophilus supplements, it is doubtful that the average consumer takes these conscientious measures.

In 2009, researchers found that cured or smoked meat and fish have been directly linked to childhood leukemia.[69] Some studies have found a link between highly processed meats with colorectal and stomach cancers.[70]

Pickles, Anchovies, and Other Salt-cured Foods [71]

The risk for nasopharyngeal cancer is more common in communities where people eat a lot of cured, salted, or pickled foods.[72] These toxins can be made harmless in the same manner as with processed meats, but the best approach is severe limitation or complete avoidance.

Those with risk of yeast infection should avoid fermented foods such as alcohol, vinegar, salad dressings, pickles, olives, or other pickled foods. Since yeast organisms feed on sugar, a low-sugar diet should also be adopted. Add yogurt, acidophilus, or probiotic supplements to maintain the "good" bacteria necessary for gut balance. Garlic has been shown to have natural antifungal properties, and should be used liberally to fight yeast overgrowth.[73]

Not all fermented foods are bad. Yogurt is made by fermenting milk with friendly bacteria, mainly *Lactobacillus bulgaricus, Streptococcus lactis, and S. thermophilus.* Lactic acid fermentation gives the sour taste to kefir, some cheeses, sauerkraut, and pickles. The sugars in the basic ingredients are converted into lactic acid that serves as a preservative.[74] Yogurt with sugary flavorings added is not healthy.

Food Coloring

Dr. Andrew Weil's books target artificial coloring substances as cancer-causing agents. Caramel coloring/flavor is merely burnt sugar—a carcinogen and immunosuppressive substance.[75]

Canned Fruit Juices

Here is a classic example of the consumer's need to read labels carefully. The list of ingredients usually begins with "water" followed by "high fructose corn syrup." Then we find the actual fruit puree. There is a 200-calorie and high carbohydrate price to pay for this sugar-laden, fruit-flavored water. Vitamin C is usually shown as 100% because the manufacturer has added 50-100 mg of ascorbic acid to the ingredient list. Some add traces of other vitamins as a sales gimmick. Better to skip the sugar eat a piece of fresh fruit (including the peel, if appropriate), and drink a glass of fresh water. Slicing the fruit into thin pieces increases the flavor and allows a smaller amount to satisfy hunger.

Parents and caregivers of very young children are quick to give fruit juice when water would be much better for them. Recommendations offered by a panel of doctors speaking for the American Academy of Pediatrics in 2001 set limits on the amount of juice children should consume.[76] The concern is that kids less than six months of age who drink too much juice run the risk of being too full to get adequate nourishment from breast milk or formula. There is also the risk of chronic diarrhea, since their immature intestines cannot digest so much sugar.

For older children given no-spill containers of juice with a small drinking spout, there is the danger of tooth decay and enamel destruction as the juice's sugar washes over their teeth all day. The juice cups also train kids to turn to sweet food for comfort, leading to overeating and bad nutrition habits in the future. Pure water flavored with a very small amount of juice or honey is an alternative to consider.

The Academy's guidelines state that children aged one to six should drink no more than six ounces of juice per day. Those aged 7 to 18 should consume no more than 12 ounces per day. Whole fruits are much better, since fruit contains nutrients and fiber in the form of pulp lost during juice processing. V8 vegetable juice is much more nutritious than fruit juice.

Milk

For decades Americans have been conditioned by advertising to believe that pasteurized, homogenized cow's milk is the perfect food for humans, especially children. The U.S. dairy industry is a multi-billion dollar business, and milk is its chief product. Celebrities with "milk mustaches" are paid for their endorsements.

Raw milk contains beneficial bacteria such as *Lactobacillus acidophilus*, which balances and controls the putrefactive bacteria that make milk curdle and turn sour. The pasteurization process destroys valuable enzymes and vitamins along with harmful bacteria. Some critics assert that pasteurization, like beef irradiation, allows the farmer to evade FDA standards of cleanliness; the standards imposed on farms producing raw milk are considerably higher. Pasteurization offers another benefit to the industry—the extension of shelf life of dairy products.[77]

Vitamin D is added to nearly all milk to facilitate calcium absorption. Dr. Mercola has written extensively on the importance of vitamin D in its various forms.[78] Some infections, like Sarcoidosis, increase vitamin D production to toxic levels where the active form of the vitamin triggers an immune cytokine cascade that appears to be an allergic reaction. Sun sensitivity is one symptom of excess vitamin D linked to an infection.[79]

When calcium absorption is inhibited, mineral imbalances cause toxins to accrue in tissues and joints, further aggravating arthritis symptoms. Calcium inhibitors include:[80]

- alcohol consumption;
- tobacco;
- lack of exercise;
- stress, excitement, or depression;
- excess salt;
- excess caffeine in foods and beverages;
- white sugar;
- certain drugs: aspirin, cortisone, corticosteroids, tetracycline, thyroid medication, blood pressure drugs, diuretics, laxatives, anticonvulsant medications;
- foods that contain oxalates (rhubarb, beets, okra, spinach, Swiss chard, sweet potatoes, chocolate, tea, and soy products);
- foods rich in phytates (wheat bran, beans, seeds, nuts, and soy isolates);
- excess protein (meat and milk).

The human body does not store protein. Any excess is broken down into ammonia and amino acids and excreted. However, for every molecule of these by-products cleansed from the blood, the kidneys lose an atom of calcium through the urine in a process called "protein-induced hypercalcuria."

Ironically, drinking pasteurized milk does <u>not</u> increase calcium—the mineral necessary to neutralize the acid formed when digesting animal protein—but instead depletes it. The body will take calcium from the bones in order to keep calcium levels in the blood within normal range and to be in balance with other minerals such as potassium and phosphorus. Calcium loss resulting from protein excess over the years is a major contributing factor in osteoporosis.

Far from being the "perfect food," milk can be the source of serious health problems. Consumption of processed milk and dairy products has been associated with iron deficiency anemia, allergies, diarrhea, heart disease, colic, cramps, gastrointestinal bleeding, sinusitis, skin rashes, acne, arthritis, diabetes, ear infections, osteoporosis, asthma, autoimmune diseases, atherosclerosis, multiple sclerosis, non-Hodgkin's lymphoma, and possibly lung cancer.[81]

Studies[82] show a possible link between unusually high heat-resistant *Mycobacterium avium paratuberculosis* and a variety of autoimmune illnesses, including TB, leprosy, and Crohn's disease. This cell wall-deficient mycobacterium is associated with Johne's disease, which afflicts cattle and contaminates their milk. The chronic fatigue and joint pain characterizing Crohn's disease are similar to RA symptoms.

The milk of mammals is species-specific, designed to protect the young of that species. Alteration of that milk by sterilization or pasteurization destroys that protection. Human breast milk contains high contents of oleic and palmitic acids and also antimicrobial lauric and capric acids. Cow's milk contains up to 20 times more of the protein casein than human milk. This makes the nutrients in cow's milk difficult (if not impossible) for humans to assimilate.[83] Processed milk and dairy products prompt the human digestive system to form unnecessary acid and mucous. Cows are usually injected with recombinant bovine growth hormone (rBGH) to artificially increase their milk production. Dr. Mercola warns against consuming any dairy products that contain rBGH as a cancer risk.[84] Organic milk has no rBGH.[85]

Most individuals are unable to digest significant amounts of lactose, the predominant sugar in milk. This is because there is a genetically programmed decline in lactase levels after the first year or two of life. Lactase deficiency is not the same as lactose intolerance. Problems arise when undigested milk sugar is transported to the large intestine where it ferments under bacterial action, producing short-chain fatty acids and gastrointestinal symptoms such as gas, bloating, or diarrhea. A physician should be able to diagnose incomplete absorption of lactose.

When total lactose intake is eight ounces or less per day, symptoms should be negligible.[86] Lactose-intolerant individuals should be careful to read labels on processed foods to avoid those containing whey, milk solids, or other hidden dairy substances which may push the total past eight ounces. Nonfat milk and yogurt pose no problems for the lactose-intolerant. The live active cultures in yogurt create lactase, the enzyme needed to digest lactose.[87]

If the reason for drinking milk is to keep calcium at normal level, one should consider other sources containing zero lactose: sardines, tofu, salmon, kale, cooked collard greens or broccoli.[88] Ripened cheese may contain up to 95 percent less lactose than whole milk.[89] Lactase supplements that allow proper assimilation of some dairy products are readily available. Find information on the Internet.[90]

Skim milk lacks the fat and enzymes necessary for proper calcium absorption and is high in lactose. More nutritious is plain, fermented, unflavored yogurt.

Heavy milk drinkers with *Chlamydophila pneumoniae* (Cpn) infections and low vitamin C and vitamin A levels will have arteries covered by cholesterol patches and plaque.[91] If this buildup is too thick, the artery becomes too constricted to sustain normal blood flow, leading to heart attack, low brain oxygen levels, and/or blockage strokes.

Sugar

For 6-8 hours after sugar from any source hits the bloodstream, body chemistry is thrown into biochemical chaos: hormone, fat, carbohydrate, and protein metabolism are greatly disrupted and the immune system is suppressed. Refined sugar is rapidly absorbed by the body and immediately enters the blood. The pancreas reacts by increasing the production of insulin, which signals cells to absorb the sugar. If the body's cells already have enough sugar, they turn it into fat and cholesterol. The fat is deposited in cells and organs, resulting in atherosclerosis, fatty liver and kidneys, and obesity. These fats cause blood cells to become sticky, thereby increasing the chances of blood clots, strokes, and heart attacks. Excess sugar raises adrenaline levels ten times, while increasing both cholesterol and cortisol.[92]

During the digestion process, pancreatic juices containing digestive enzymes flow to the stomach and small intestine where starchy carbohydrates are broken down into maltose or sucrose. These sugars are then absorbed into the lining of the intestine to be converted into glucose, which floods into the bloodstream, traveling to different tissues in the body where it can either be stored or used immediately as energy. The nerves and the brain depend on normal glucose levels for energy and to function properly.

Hyperglycemia (high blood sugar) increases the risk for impaired mental function and Alzheimer's disease among the elderly and diabetics.[93] Chronic hyperglycemia can have serious complications over a period of years, including damage to the kidneys, retina, legs, and feet. Diabetic neuropathy, as well as cardiovascular and/or neurological damage may be the result of long-term hyperglycemia. Treatment requires elimination of the underlying cause(s), which may be infection and inflammation.[94]

If insulin levels are too high, the body will crave sugar. The result is hypoglycemia (low blood sugar) with symptoms including weakness, dizziness, crying spells, insomnia, aggression, and depression. The adrenal glands secrete hormones that try to increase blood sugar levels to balance the insulin. If this cycle happens routinely, the overworked adrenal glands are unable to respond to stress and the immune system is less able to fight infectious pathogens. Adrenal exhaustion is a common problem for those with chronic illness. The sugar in one 12-ounce can of soda can suppress the immune system for up to six hours.

In 2011, the American Diabetes Association reported that 25.8 million children and adults in the U.S.—8.3% of the population—have diabetes. 1.9 million new cases of diabetes were diagnosed in people aged 20 years and older in 2010. Adults with diabetes have heart disease death rates about 2 to 4 times higher than those for adults without diabetes.[95] A healthy-eating plan using guidelines in Appendix III can help keep blood sugar under control.[96]

Stevia *(Stevia rebaudiana Bertoni)* is an herbal substitute for sugar taken from a shrub native to Paraguay. Sugar has 16 calories per teaspoon while Stevia has zero calories and is 200-300 times sweeter than sugar. It is sold in the U.S. as a dietary supplement, not as a sweetener (food product) because limited studies showed one of the glycosides to contain a component (steviol) that causes cell mutation in laboratory animals.

The FDA ruling denying GRAS (generally recognized as safe) status to Stevia is puzzling when one considers that caffeine and saccharin are FDA-approved but are potentially mutagenic substances.[97] In 2000, President Clinton signed a bill to remove the warning label from sweetener products containing saccharin, but sodium saccharin (a salt derivative) remains on the list of carcinogens and still requires warning labels.

Reducing sugar does not mean avoiding natural sugars found in fruits, vegetables, and grains. It means shunning *added* sugar, common in processed foods and beverages as high-fructose corn syrup, as well as honey, maple syrup, and white table sugar. Scientists have proved that fructose, a cheap form of sugar derived from corn, used in thousands of food products and soft drinks, can damage human metabolism and is a major cause of the U.S. obesity crisis.[98]

Beware sugar alcohols with names that end in -ol, such as sorbitol, mannitol, xylitol and maltitol. These sweeteners are chemically related to alcohol, but without the alcoholic effects. They are carbohydrates that are converted to ordinary sugar during digestion. Sugar alcohols are used in many products labeled as "low carb," "low sugar" or "sugar free."

One should consume no more than 10 teaspoons of sugar in any form per day. Labels often list sugars in terms of grams. To convert to teaspoons, divide grams by 4.2. For example, one 12-ounce can of soda contains an average of 38 to 46 total grams of sugars, equivalent to roughly 10 teaspoons.

Another way to view sugar intake is to visualize each 3 grams as one sugar packet served at restaurants. Thus, a can of soda would be equivalent to about 13 sugar packets. Keep a food diary for a week. It may be a shock to see how much added sugar is being consumed. There are 47 grams of carbohydrates in one medium order of French fries, which converts to (47/4.2) = about 10 teaspoons of sugar.

Just ¼ teaspoon of sugar is enough to tip the balance between normal and diabetic blood sugar. This means 10 teaspoons would be equivalent to 40 teaspoons for a person with diabetes. It is very hard work for the metabolic system to deal with the sugar load just from one order of fries. Imagine the stress on the system with a full fast food meal of a burger, fries, large soda or shake, and perhaps a dessert.

Oncologists know that cancer needs a sugar-rich environment to thrive, so it is puzzling why the American Cancer Society and some doctors give out cookies and Clinical Strength Ensure™ after chemotherapy. This drink contains extremely high levels of sugar (22 grams) as part of total carbohydrates (52 grams) in the form of sucrose, corn syrup, and corn-derived maltodextrin in a water base.[99] The cookies carry their own sugar and carb load.

In 1931, Dr. Otto Warburg won two Nobel Prizes for his cancer research. He discovered that cancer metabolizes through a process of fermentation, which requires sugar. Using Dr. Warburg's findings in 2004, University of Minnesota researchers experimented with a "smart bomb," an anti-cancer drug wrapped in a coating that makes it harmless until it finds a low-oxygen area in the body. Such a place is where cancer cells gather. Once settled, the "smart bomb" can release its deadly payload to kill the cancer cells.[100] University of San Diego, CA researchers have taken the "smart bomb" notion a step further using nanotechnology to direct low doses of drugs to cancerous tumors, slowing their spread throughout the body.[101]

According to Dr. Warburg, nutritional deficiencies are the cause of cancer. E.g., esophageal cancer can be healed by adding respiratory enzymes to the diet: iron salts, riboflavin (B_2), pantothenic acid (B_5), and nicotinamide (B_3).[102]

Salt

Public health experts estimate that Americans consume about 3400 milligrams of salt each day, exceeding the cautionary maximum of 2300 mg for adults and 1500 mg for those age 51 or older. They also note that most of this sodium intake comes from processed food, including items ordered from take-out eateries and restaurants.[103] Preparing meals at home isn't always practical or possible, but limiting salt is feasible. Including more fruits, vegetables and whole grains will not only offset the effects of salt, it will help to lower cholesterol and blood pressure.

Restricting salt should be done gradually, else one's taste buds will rebel. Salt substitutes like parsley, lemon, lime, pepper, or oregano add flavor. Check food labels for sodium content; choose products and brands that lower the risk of blood pressure and hypertension. Foods labeled "reduced sodium" or "sodium light" may still contain a lot of salt.[104] Avoid products with more than 200 mg of sodium per serving. Salt aggravates hypertension but does not cause it. Salt itself is not bad, but too much sodium upsets the body's optimal balance with calcium and potassium.

Antacids and Heartburn Drugs

Acid indigestion is caused by a *lack* of stomach acid, not a surplus of it. Without enough stomach acid to break down ingested food, the undigested mass ferments in the stomach.

The bubbles produced by fermentation make their way into the esophagus, bringing some stomach acid along. The result is the pain and discomfort of acid reflux. An antacid will end the painful symptoms but it will cause the partially digested food to enter the intestinal tract to wreak havoc on the already overburdened digestive system and in turn, on the immune system.

It is a simple matter to be tested for hypochlorhydria (low secretion of stomach acid). The remedy is also simple: supplement the diet with digestive enzymes or betaine HCl (a form of hydrochloric acid). Ask a qualified nutritionist to advise on additional and fish oil supplements.[105] Zinc is the required co-factor for the enzyme that produces natural hydrochloric acid in the stomach and aids in digestion.[106]

Allergies may play a role in heartburn if eczema is also a problem. Try eliminating known offenders from the diet: eggs, peanuts, soy foods, wheat, gluten, and dairy products.[107]

Aspirin

The claim that an aspirin per day prevents heart attacks and stroke has been discredited. Dr. James Howenstine, M.D. wrote in 2004, "Aspirin is a poison. The intake of 10 to 30 grams of aspirin can be fatal. Deaths directly related to aspirin usage are estimated to range from 7,600 to 14,000 annually in the United States."[108] He estimates that 20 million persons take aspirin daily for prevention of vascular accidents. Studies comparing buffered aspirin with plain aspirin have found that the latter can reduce heart attack risk. However, that turns out to be a false benefit since it does nothing to reduce the chance of actually dying from cardiovascular disease.[109, 110]

The main ingredient in buffered aspirin is magnesium, which dilates blood vessels, aids potassium absorption, acts as a natural blood thinner, and keeps blood cells from clumping together causing thrombosis (clotting).[111] Within 48 hours of a heart attack, the victim has a 63-88% chance of survival if injected with 50mmol of magnesium.[112] Nearly all autopsies on heart attack victims reveal a magnesium deficiency.[113]

For some individuals, continued use of aspirin can lead to peptic ulcers and bleeding of the stomach lining.[114] Another serious problem caused by long-term aspirin use is the significantly increased risk of macular degeneration with blindness and a 44% increased risk of cataracts.[115, 116]

Enteric coatings consist of plasticizers and pigments added to a polysaccharide (starch) and polymer base. The coating is applied to make the tablet smoother and easier to swallow, to control the release rate of the active ingredient as it moves through the acids in the gastrointestinal tract, to make it more resistant to the environment (extending its shelf life), or to enhance the tablet's appearance.

Randomized clinical trials testing aspirin usage by 5,011 elderly people, mean age 72 years, followed for a mean of 4.2 years, showed that use of aspirin caused a four-fold increase in hemorrhagic stroke and a 1.6- to 1.8-fold increase in ischemic stroke.[117]

Harvard Medical School studied 88,378 female cancer-free nurses in 1980 and tested them during the next 18 years of follow-up. By 1998, those who took two or more aspirin per week showed increased risk of developing pancreatic cancer by 58%. Taking daily aspirin raised the risk to 86%.[118] On the bright side, another major long-term study found in 2007 that the risk of colorectal cancer was reduced among those who take aspirin and NSAIDs regularly.[119] Rather than incurring pancreatic cancer risk from aspirin, it would be better to consider vitamin D with its anti-tumor effects.[120, 121] Fish oils high in dietary omega-3 fatty acids are also beneficial for cancer prevention.[122]

Aspirin is a proven vitamin antagonist, especially toward vitamin C, destroying huge quantities in the body. If aspirin is used for anti-inflammatory purposes, vitamin C supplements become extremely important. Vitamin C is also depleted by mental stress, oxidative stress, physical trauma, smoking, and caffeine. Appendix V discusses vitamin C.

According to the Mayo Clinic, there are important decisions to make regarding aspirin therapy that should be discussed with your doctor. E.g., abruptly stopping daily aspirin therapy can have a rebound effect that may trigger a blood clot, increasing the risk of heart attack or stroke. Also, taking aspirin with other anticoagulants, such as warfarin (Coumadin), could greatly increase the chance of bleeding.[123]

Ibuprofen

This over-the-counter (OTC) drug is often suggested for Rheumatoid Arthritis, Osteoarthritis, and flare-ups of chronic disease. Although physicians recommend that the smallest dose of ibuprofen that yields acceptable control should be used, individuals seeking pain relief routinely abuse this drug. Exceeding the suggested 3200 mg/day maximum dose can result in gastrointestinal toxicity, liver damage, blurred vision, edema (water retention), and renal (kidney) toxicity.[124]

FATS AND OILS

The following section contains assertions contrary to mainstream, conventional belief and practice, but they are confirmed by credible science. The published writings of a wide range of world-class experts are easily accessible in medical libraries and on the Internet. What follows is a summary of this considerable body of research.[125]

After prescribing powerful immunosuppressive drugs, the doctor may also suggest eating a "well-balanced diet high in fiber and low in saturated fats and cholesterol." This advice is based on decades of conditioning to perceive some essential fats as "bad" when they actually contribute to good health.[126]

Fats and oils are globally competitive agribusinesses, promoted by national agriculture departments. Fat nutrition studies are self-serving, designed to promote the consumption of each nation's oils and to take market share from other nations that also produce oils and fats.[127] Canola is one example.

Rapeseed (Canola) Oil and Cholesterol

This very cheap oil is used extensively in China and India for cooking but has very high emissions of potentially carcinogenic or mutagenic compounds. After genetic reformulation and processing in Canada to reduce toxins, it was fed exclusively to lab rats to prove its safety, but the rats developed fatty degeneration of the heart, kidney, adrenals, and thyroid gland. On withdrawing the rapeseed oil from their diets, the deposits dissolved but scar tissue remained on all vital organs. However, scientists found that rapeseed oil contained more cholesterol-lowering monounsaturated fat, second only to olive oil.[128] Renamed Canola oil in the U.S., it is promoted positively as a means to reduce cholesterol, but the consumer is unknowingly making an unhealthy choice.

Canola has high sulphur content and goes rancid easily. Baked goods using Canola develop mold quickly. Although marketed as a low fat hydrogenated or partially hydrogenated oil, it contains trans-fatty acids similar to those in margarine. Trans-fats have been linked to skin cancer.[129] Canola contains a long-chain fatty acid called erucic acid, which is especially irritating to mucous membranes. Canola consumption has been linked to development of fibrotic lesions of the heart, central nervous system degenerative disorders, constipation, lung cancer, prostate cancer, and anemia.[130, 131] Competitors with Canola include the much healthier but more expensive flax, borage, sunflower, peanut,[132] and olive oils.

Not all fats are responsible for cancer; some, like olive oil, actually fight the disease, according to the Mayo Clinic.[133] In the gut, lauric acid is converted to monoglyceride (monolaurin), the systemic antiviral agent that kills HIV.[134] Palmitic acid makes palmitoyl-oleoyl-phosphatidyl-glycerol (POPG) that fights RSV, pneumonia bacteria, and COPD.

The popular accepted view is that Canola oil is harmless because it is mono-unsaturated. However, during processing, chemical residues leach into the oil. Despite this fact, the USDA puts Canola first in its list of recommended oils.[135] Cottonseed oil may contain herbicides and pesticides since cotton is not considered a food and the USDA applies no rules regarding limits on levels of toxins. It behooves the consumer to read labels for the type of oil used to process any packaged food.

If a food label says "low cholesterol," beware. The FDA allows this wording for products with up to 20 mg cholesterol per serving. Whenever a "low fat" nutrition label lists 0g of a particular substance such as trans-fat, consumers assume that none of that nutrient is contained. However, the FDA allows a zero listing of trans-fat if the food contains less than 0.5 grams per serving. This becomes a problem when more than one serving is eaten.[136] E.g., each packet of microwaveable popcorn contains 2.5 servings, but most people assume that the whole bag of popped corn is a single serving.

The food industry uses trans-fats liberally because they are cheap flavor enhancers with a long shelf life. Trans-fats are found in most baked goods, margarine, shortening, potato chips, tortillas, nondairy coffee creamers, cocoas, cookies, crackers, bread, popcorn, French fries, and nearly all so-called "junk foods."[137]

By contrast, butter contains healthy palmitic acid and a small amount of lauric acid, both healthy saturated fats, while margarine has trans-fat. The harder the margarine, the more trans-fat (synthetic cholesterol) it contains, which may be converted to form defective cortisol. These synthetic oils change proteins in our bodies so that they reject insulin created by the pancreas.

Since the late 1970s, research has consistently linked these oils to heart disease, Metabolic Syndrome, and Type 2 diabetes. This variety of diabetes is characterized by the body's inability to use natural insulin. Diabetes reduces immune system actions, increases inflammation, depletes the body's reserves of essential vitamins, and blocks cellular energy use of glucose, turning that glucose into body fat.

When oils are oxidized, they become rancid, and in turn, carcinogenic. In the presence of low vitamin C (scurvy) and rampant ROS/NOS oxides, cholesterol can readily oxidize to become a neurotoxin. This may explain the scurvy-state neurotoxic effects of vaccinations associated with autism, as discussed in Chapter 5. It may be that oxidized, rancid oils could be the cause of cancer in pets. Many pet owners purchase large bags of dry food and keep them open for weeks. It is best to store food products containing oils in the refrigerator after opening to avoid spoilage. Naturally saturated tropical oils have long, stable shelf lives and do not turn rancid. Nor do they polymerize and cross-link to form sticky goo.

According to Dr. W. Vergil Brown, professor at Mount Sinai School of Medicine, hamburgers, cheeseburgers, meat loaf, whole milk and cheese, steaks, hot dogs, and eggs are the foods with the highest amount of cholesterol. One should severely limit these foods while supplementing with flax oil, which is high in Omega-3 and low in Omega-6 fatty acids that dissolve excess cholesterol. A diet plan called the Gerson Method clears the arteries of plaque, normalizes blood pressure, and prevents heart disease and stroke.[138]

The Misleading HDL/LDL Ratio

Healthy nutrition does not come through controlling statistical correlations with symptomatic measurements. It comes from understanding how human body chemistry works and making sure we eat what we need to properly feed the various molecule-making functional pathways that nourish our cells. Focusing on one symptom—lowering cholesterol—is a mistake. Cholesterol starvation shortens the lives of those who accept the false "saturated fats are bad" health propaganda.

Cholesterol is essential to tissue regeneration, nerve/brain health, and cell replacement.

One might postulate that microbes invading immune or epithelial cells are responsible for all diseases categorized as sclerotic (plaque-forming) and also the cause of all so-called "autoimmune" diseases with arthritis symptoms. To find "cures," we should concentrate on identifying and eliminating harmful microbes instead of optimizing statistical odds with fat ratios and risk factors that occasionally happen to correlate with symptoms. Changing the HDL/LDL ratio does nothing to combat the microbes that cause the disease.

Here is a good example of the functional medicine pathway: the probiotic *Lactobacillus rhamnosus* converts lecithin to TMA, a fishy smelling gas, that is converted in the liver to TMA oxide (TMAO), which is strongly linked to rapid growth of arterial plaques. But surprisingly, TMAO raises "good" cholesterol.[139] Although some strains of *L. rhamnosus* contribute to heart disease and atherosclerosis, this probiotic also protects against rotavirus, and enhances immune system function. *L. rhamnosus* is a required ingredient in Kefir, a probiotic used for centuries with many health benefits including reducing food allergies and atopic dermatitis, and helping to prevent colon cancer.[140, 141]

The worsening health statistics for COPD, obesity, and coronary heart disease (CHD) present clear evidence that there are serious errors in the consensus perception of "good" fats and "bad" fats. The abstract model of HDL versus LDL does not account for molecule-specific functions.[142] In 1998, the American Heart Association (AHA) removed their seal of approval from products containing partially hydrogenated oils, issuing a vague warning to minimize use of these items, but they continue to be marketed as "healthy" *only* because they lower cholesterol. In 2011, the AHA recommended eating 25-35% of one's daily calories as healthy fats but limiting trans-fats to less than 1%, and limiting cholesterol intake to under

200 mg per day for people who have CHD and to under 300 mg for those who do not.[143]

According to the National Heart, Lung, and Blood Institute (NHLBI), high cholesterol is one of the "major controllable risk factors" for coronary heart disease, heart attack and stroke.[144] Note that the NHLBI did not say that high cholesterol is a *cause* of these conditions.

Merely using statin drugs to reduce cholesterol, especially for older persons, and failing to treat the vitamin deficiencies and infection(s) has little or no real effect on heart deaths. Lowering one's cholesterol level is a mistake unless one is actually at risk for CHD. For those with small risk, drastically lowering cholesterol can in turn lower the serotonin levels, which may lead to insomnia, depression, the muscle weakness and stiffness of fibromyalgia,[145] and/or adoption of risky and/or aggressive behavior.[146]

In 2010, the NHLBI estimated that 102.2 million Americans are at risk from borderline-high to high cholesterol levels, up from 36 million in 2001. One person in eight with a chronic condition has high cholesterol.[147] However, they fail to point out that changes in diet, especially limiting saturated fats, and increasing exercise, are able to lower cholesterol without statin drugs. The Institute thus tacitly acknowledges that Americans prefer to let drugs do the work rather than give up unhealthy lifestyle habits.[148]

Excess cholesterol does not cause plaques. Plaques are associated with CWD polymicrobial infections and sub-clinical scurvy caused by deficiencies in vitamin C and certain unprocessed tropical saturated oils such as coconut (lauric),[149] palm kernel, and red palm oil. This is the opposite of what the "saturated fats are bad" lobby would have consumers believe. Statin drugs reduce normal cholesterol production, Heme, and CoQ_{10} levels[150], and increase age-related physical and mental deterioration.

The body produces LDL cholesterol naturally, but a few people have genes that cause them to make too much. The saturated fats that we use to make the HDL cholesterol also have systemic antibacterial and antiviral properties. Rats in Japanese and Canadian experiments were fed Canola oil exclusively to prove it reduced cholesterol. The experiment succeeded but the rats died because they needed the lauric and palmitic acids in saturated fats to survive.[151]

Cholesterol becomes soluble in the bloodstream when enough lecithin is present.[152] Lecithin is a phospholipid produced by a healthy liver and found throughout body cells and organs with a very high concentration in the brain and around nerve sheaths. It contains the B vitamin choline, important in building nerve transmitters. In the liver, lecithin metabolizes fat. In the bloodstream, lecithin emulsifies fats, preventing them from accumulating as plaque on the walls of arteries. In the intestinal tract, lecithin enhances the absorption of vitamins A, D, and possibly E and K.

However, while excess lecithin intake makes the HDL/LDL ratio measurably better, harmful plaques grow more rapidly. Intestinal bacteria normally metabolize choline and excrete it, but if transport systems for absorption of choline are overloaded, the result is a set of by-products causing atherosclerosis. The dramatic increase in the addition of choline into multi-vitamins over the past few years raises the daily safe limit and in turn introduces risk for CHD, plaques in the brain and in arteries.[153] Total choline intake from food and supplements (including lecithin) should not exceed 3.5g per day.[154, 155]

Lecithin is promoted as a quick weight loss product as well as providing various health benefits. These claims are unsupported. The only proven benefit and suggested use of lecithin or choline supplements is for those taking niacin (as nicotinic acid) to treat high cholesterol. In higher doses than 30g per day, lecithin supplements could cause weight gain, gastrointestinal problems, diarrhea, skin rash, dizziness, headache, vomiting, nausea, and/or a "fishy" body odor.[156]

Thus, we take a dramatically different view towards fats than is found in the consensus health dogma. Nutrition expert

Dr. Mary Enig has studied the global science on fats relative to diet. She has written extensively about the antiviral benefits of saturated monoglycerides found in coconut and palm oils.[157] The late Dr. Robert Atkins, trained as a cardiologist, refuted the simplistic model that a calorie of carbohydrates is equal nutritionally to a calorie of fats. He proved that only *carbohydrate* calorie intake leads to body fat generation and weight gain, while fats eaten with low carbohydrates are poorly absorbed and do not functionally increase body fat.[158]

At the root of the good-fat/bad-fat controversy is the claim that because cholesterol is found in plaques (a symptom), that by controlling this symptom, heart attack statistics can be improved. Later studies have falsified the assumption that reducing cholesterol and/or saturated fat is good. Yet this false premise is still taught in schools, featured in health publications, and promoted in the media, so those following low fat diets combined with vitamin C deficiency live shorter lives. Red palm oil makes more cholesterol but plaques diminish. Following Linus Pauling's nutrition rules (vitamin C, lysine, and proline), supplemented by palm oils that contain saturated fats, will result in plaques being controlled or even eliminated.[159]

Lower cost and the demonization of saturated fats has led most manufacturers to stop using safe, healthy oils like palm kernel, coconut, and lauric acid in favor of artificially saturated, hydrogenated soybean, corn, and cottonseed oils—the waste products of America's three biggest crops.[160]

Our approach is to trace the nutrient molecules through the body's systems to show how they are converted into the hormones and enzymes that need to be rebuilt and regulated. Thus, saturated fats are used to make cholesterol that is in turn used to make steroid and sex hormones in the adrenal glands and to normalize metabolic processes. Palm oil[161] is a precursor of POPG, a respiratory surfactant that eases breathing, fights respiratory infections like pneumonia and COPD, and moderates immune over-reactions. Low levels of vitamins A and C, or low cholesterol slow cellular replacement but speed the aging process and the progression of dementia. Sunlight on the skin converts cholesterol into vitamin D, so the amount of cholesterol in the blood goes down naturally.[162]

A low fat diet only causes hunger feelings to persist. Proper cortisol production depends on intake of tropical fats that are the foundation molecules required for "good" cholesterol. Gently processed natural oils are a rich supply of these essential, beneficial fat molecules and a source of systemically antiviral saturated fats. They contain lauric, palmitic, myristic and capric acid fat molecules, CoQ_{10},[163] and vitamin molecule complexes called A's, E's, and tocotrienols. Most other oils are not essential except fish oil (with Omega-3 and −6). Only tropical oils provide lauric acid, an essential precursor to adrenal hormone generation.

The French eat rich, fatty meals but their wines contain salicylic acid (the main metabolite in aspirin), which may explain why their incidence of cardiovascular disease is 30% lower than the U.S. Their Mediterranean diet probably decreases the inflammatory reaction in arteries, which is thought to play an important role in causing heart disease.[164]

NATURAL METHODS TO ELIMINATE TOXINS

Some of the toxins resident in our bodies are inadvertently consumed along with the foods we eat. Exposure to pesticides can be by ingestion, the most common method, or by tactile contact with chemicals found in household and garden products, or inhalation. Another source is aerial spraying and roadside pest/weed abatement spraying. Although individual exposure may be low, the effect can be cumulative over years.

Some pesticides like chlordane, DDT and hexachloro-cyclohexane (HCH, commonly called lindane) alter or disrupt the early development of the immune system's T-cells, reducing resistance to infection.[165] HCH has been found in soil and surface water near hazardous waste sites. It can accumulate in the fatty tissue of fish. Forms of HCH can vaporize and attach to small airborne particles like pollen or dust, so exposure can be through direct inhalation or absorbed through the skin when mixed with shampoo or lotion containing medication to treat lice or scabies.[166]

Buying organically grown fruits, vegetables, and meats, as well as organically produced dairy products, may minimize toxin intake. The USDA has excluded irradiated foods, crops fertilized with solid waste, and genetically manipulated foods from the "organic" category. There is little scientific evidence to prove more health benefits from organic food, with the exception of milk.[167] The buyer may be protected from exposure to potential carcinogens, but bacteria in manure-based fertilizers present other risks. Wash all produce thoroughly in a light peroxide or bleach solution, no matter the source.[168] Wear gloves and wash hands thoroughly after handling garden fertilizers and soil amendments.

Toxins that are natural by-products of infection must also be flushed from the body, else they will take up residence and cause problems later. As cells take in nutrients and begin the repair process, they in turn discharge waste chemicals. The circulatory and lymphatic systems must be in tip-top working order to convey these unwanted materials to the filtering, excretory organs (liver and kidneys). If antioxidants (e.g., vitamins A, C, E, and glutathione) are lacking and toxin exposure is high, these waste chemicals become far more dangerous. Amino acids and the B-complex group of vitamins are essential for optimum detoxification.[169] The herb Silymarin is very effective against liver damage as well as cancer.[170] Chlorella is a powerful detoxifier.[171]

Researchers have confirmed the existence of a long-suspected natural system the body uses to block the cancer-causing effects of toxic chemicals in food and the environment. When the immune system senses toxins, it increases production of phase II enzymes to neutralize them before they can damage DNA and trigger cancer. When a specific protein called Nrf2 is in short supply because the immune system is not working properly, the phase II enzymes cannot in turn be generated to reduce one's sensitivity to carcinogens.[172]

Specific anti-toxins have been developed for life-threatening toxins such as tetanus, diptheria, botulism, spider bites, snakebites, and box jellyfish stings.[173] Doctors Klenner and Cathcart, and others, have achieved dramatic results with buffered sodium ascorbate (SA), a form of vitamin C, given intravenously, and by injections, as a universal anti-toxin treatment. See Appendix V for details.[174]

SA works to neutralize all bacterial toxins if given in amounts high enough to neutralize both the toxin and the huge amounts of oxides in the ROS/RNS and histamine chain reaction. Several hundred grams of sodium ascorbate may be necessary. Recovery from toxic shock lethargy is remarkably rapid.

Other ways to expel these accumulated toxins are localized massage, herbs that stimulate circulation and eliminate toxins, increased water intake, and daily gentle low-impact aerobic exercise followed by elevation of the lower legs to above-heart level several times per day using a slant board. The toxins will be loosened and drain into the bloodstream to be eliminated by the kidneys, skin, and lymphatic system. Topical application of DMSO helps to reduce pain and swelling, in combination with topical oil of wintergreen (this is methyl salicylate, or "liquid aspirin").

The body depends on proper circulation for oxygen and nutrition as well as toxin removal. Fresh blood allows oxidation to occur in tissues. Blood leaving an area carries with it the waste products of oxidation and metabolism. As fresh blood flows to the muscles, lungs, brain, and heart, healthy cells are renewed. Daily consumption of at least two quarts of pure, filtered or spring water is essential to facilitate this process. Certain herbs that aid in oxygen transport are discussed in Appendix I. Vitamins and minerals that are key to good health are described in the next subsection.

VITAMIN AND MINERAL SUPPLEMENTS

The fewer vitamins and minerals we consume on a regular basis, the more fragile our health becomes. Although theoretically all our nutritional needs can be supplied by the foods we eat, only some of us consistently follow a strict dietary regimen that ensures proper intake of these elements. Also, it is doubtful that we come close to satisfying our true daily requirements because much of our food is so highly processed before reaching the grocery store shelves.

In 1943 the FDA published the first list of Recommended Dietary Allowances (RDAs) to be used as standards for nutrition labeling of foods. The latest edition of this list was published in 1989, updated in 2010.[175] What was the RDA is now called Reference Daily Intake (RDI). The guide is intended to be the accepted source of nutrient allowances for "healthy people" but the criteria for this term are not clear since individual differences in the need for, and intake of, vitamins and minerals are difficult and time-consuming to determine. The RDI is used to determine the Daily Value (DV) that appears on the "nutrition facts" part of a label on processed foods.

RDIs are in part incorrect, incomplete, or understated as not essential, especially regarding fats, as seen in a previous section of this chapter. Only Omega-3 and Omega-6 oils are mentioned. The RDI applies to those in generally good health, but during illness or infection, there is a much greater need for additional supplements (antibacterial, antioxidant, and antiviral). This need varies with the severity of the condition to avoid deficiencies. The RDI for vitamin C at 60 to 90 mg is just barely enough to avoid a scurvy state. Throughout this book are references to the importance of this vitamin, with multi-gram dosage supported by credible studies. A much higher RDI for vitamin C would contribute to the prevention of chronic illness and benign relief of a wide range of symptoms. We devote Appendix V to this topic.[176]

Sadly, the critical role of key nutrients is sometimes ignored in traditional medical treatment. This is where a qualified nutritionist or chiropractor can advise on medical conditions requiring a higher need for specific nutrients. Also, many Internet resources allow mapping specific disorders to helpful vitamin, mineral, and herbal supplements.[177] A new online database devoted entirely to dietary supplements has been created by the National Institutes of Health.[178]

Some supplements interact with prescription drugs.[179] Calcium can interact with heart medicine, thyroid medicine, tetracycline antibiotics, certain diuretics, and aluminum- and magnesium-containing antacids. Vitamin K can interact with blood thinners like Coumadin. Magnesium can interact with certain diuretics, some cancer drugs, and magnesium-containing antacids. St. John's Wort is known to adversely affect the antidepressant class selective serotonin reuptake inhibitors (SSRIs) and birth control pills. It is always best to inform your physician about any herbal supplements and vitamins you are taking.

Individuals using an antibiotic regimen should not take calcium supplements at the same time of day because these may interfere with antibiotic uptake and/or transport.[180]

Over 200 million Americans routinely consume dietary supplements of some kind, but many fail to discuss the matter with their doctors.[181] A 2010 AARP survey found that 69 of the 100 men and women interviewed used supplements. The five most popular included multi-vitamins; individual vitamins; fish oil; glucosamine, condroitin or a combination of the two; and CoQ_{10}. Only one-third of the group said their doctors questioned them about supplement use, yet almost all reported that they would admit it if asked. About half did not feel that supplements were drugs and a majority did not consult their doctor or pharmacist before taking them.[182]

Despite FDA rules requiring a facts panel on supplement labels, the Dietary Supplement Health and Education Act of 1994[183] actually requires and prohibits very little in terms of processing. Manufacturers and marketers still have considerable leeway. Although labels cannot claim to cure, treat, diagnose, mitigate, or prevent a disease, they can legally make "structure" or "function" claims.[184] For example, the phrase "reduces joint pain" is illegal but "supports healthy joints" is not. A label stating "lowers cholesterol" is not allowed but one reading "helps to maintain healthy cholesterol levels" is permitted. Under the law, skillful ad writers may use vague words and phrases to infer relief and to suggest hope for a cure, but they may not make specific claims.

The FDA mandates "good manufacturing practices" for makers of prescription drugs, OTC drugs, and food products. However, these rules do not apply to supplement producers. With no pre-market regulatory power, the FDA can act to solve a problem or recall a supplement only after the fact. Thus, consumers are relying on the technical capabilities and the ethics of the manufacturer to deliver a quality product.

CoQ_{10} is one of the most popular products and can be quite expensive. For this reason, it is one of the most synthesized items on the market. Kaneka Q_{10}™ is 100% pure, naturally fermented from a yeast (trans-isomer) ingredient. Synthetic CoQ_{10} (the CIS form) is chemically processed using tobacco and while cheaper, it is considered to be impure and difficult to absorb. Most Naturopaths and nutritional M.D.'s will normally recommend standard ubiquinone CoQ_{10} over the biologically active ubiquinol for their patients taking CoQ_{10} as a supplement for overall health enhancement.[185] Ubiquinol is usually reserved for serious therapeutic purposes such as angina, high blood pressure, high cholesterol, poor circulation, cancer, immune support, fibromyalgia, and others.

Health food store sales personnel are no substitute for credentialed nutritionists or medical doctors. The sales clerk's job is to sell the store's products, though some come close to diagnosing and prescribing by strongly recommending a "best seller." Until recently, most pharmacists knew little or nothing about dietary supplements, as this topic was not taught to them in school. An admirable policy by Rite Aid, one of the United States' largest drugstore chains, is to train its ten thousand pharmacists on natural medications so they can in turn confidently and credibly counsel customers.[186]

The list of vitamins and minerals in the next section are purposely unaccompanied by suggested daily amounts since specific dosages should be tailored to the individual's needs. Some substances in high doses may be toxic. The reader should research the precise amount necessary for his/her biochemical profile ideally with the assistance of a nutritionist or dietitian. Consumerlab.com offers online access (for a subscription fee) to product review reports that evaluate specific brands of supplements.

The Linus Pauling Institute for Nutrition Bioscience at Oregon State University offers an excellent free online resource for vitamins, minerals, diseases, and cognitive functions.[187] Another useful site is ActualCures.com.[188]

Immune System Boosters

Detailed information about supplements that are especially valuable in promoting a vigorous immune system are readily found on interactive medical websites like WebMD or mercola.com using the search window. A brief list is as follows:

- Vitamin A, a powerful antioxidant and antiviral; so vital that we devote a special section in Chapter 8;
- B-complex vitamins, needed to produce red blood cells, B-cells, T-cells, and antibodies. Vitamin B_6 helps metabolize protein and amino acids, and maintains the central nervous system (CNS). Vitamin B_{12} helps build and maintain myelin—a protective sheath found around the nerves; essential to DNA synthesis. Caution: Doses

of vitamin B_6 and B_{12} greater than DRI levels are contraindicated in conditions involving infections, as they may interfere with immune system reactions;

- Bioflavonoids help build resistance to infection, help maintain the walls of small blood vessels, and facilitating vitamin C absorption;

- Vitamin C (ascorbic acid), so vital that it could, by itself, restore and maintain health for nearly all human beings. Find more detail in Appendix V;

- Calcium builds and maintains strong bones and teeth; plays a role in nerve transmission, blood clotting, and smooth muscle contraction, which helps regulate heart rhythm; entraps and envelops harmful invaders. Caution: calcium in any form may interfere with the some prescription medications;

- Chlorophyll, which helps to remove toxins from the bloodstream;

- Coenzyme Q_{10} (CoQ_{10}), an important antioxidant and rejuvenator for cells that target and destroy harmful bacteria; [189] protection against cancer;[190] as the "spark plug" for all muscular contractions, CoQ_{10} helps the heart pump blood effectively;

- Copper, needed for COX-2 enzyme function; helps create red blood cells and collagen; facilitates iron absorption and transport;

- Vitamin D, second only to vitamin C in importance; See Dr. Mercola's resource page.[191]

- Vitamin E, a key antioxidant potentiated by extra vitamin C under conditions of oxidative stress; d-alpha is the natural form but dl-alpha is synthetic;

- Folic Acid (or Folate), a B-vitamin (B9) necessary for red blood cell production, growth, and reproduction; forms the nucleic acids for DNA and RNA;

- Iron, needed for hemoglobin formation and oxygen transfer from the lungs to every cell of the body;

- Vitamin K works with vitamin D to prevent/reverse bone loss; influences insulin balance and diabetes; helps good gut bacteria thrive; high levels of vitamin E reduce K levels;

- Magnesium is key to proper functioning of nerves and muscles and maintaining healthy bones; essential for blood vessel health; helps metabolize carbohydrates and proteins; aids in enzyme activation; enhances the absorption and use of calcium; prevents and treats heart attacks;

- Manganese helps metabolize glucose; synthesizes cholesterol and fatty acids; builds strong bones;

- Niacin breaks down carbohydrates, fats and proteins; keeps the skin, digestive tract, and nervous system functioning; helps in the production of red blood cells; reverses cholesterol plaque formation[192];

- Pantothenic acid (calcium pantothenate), a water-soluble B_5 vitamin that helps in cell building (especially antibody synthesis); supports adrenal gland function and CNS development; essential to connective tissue formation; usually deficient in persons with RA;[193]

- Phosphorus is essential for cell growth, maintenance, and repair; but excess prevents other minerals from being assimilated;

- Potassium helps metabolize carbohydrates and synthesize protein, and to transmit nerve impulses; works with sodium to maintain the body's fluid balance;

- Selenium stimulates lymphocytes to produce more antibodies and encourage the activity of phagocytes; protects cell membranes from free radicals;

- Zinc is an antiviral that heals and develops new cells; helps the liver detoxify alcohol; needed to insure normal insulin activity; aids in protein digestion; helps mitigate colds, flu, and respiratory infections.

A diet including several daily portions of legumes, protein, green leafy vegetables, and fruit will supply many of these essential vitamins and minerals. Specific food sources can be found online at many natural health websites such as RealAge.com[194] and interactive medical sites like WebMD.[195] A list is shown in Appendix VI.

Some extremely beneficial supplements, such as CoQ_{10}, are not yet part of the FDA's list of RDIs.[196] Biochemists and nutritionists caution against excessive supplement use.[197, 198] Potassium deficiency has been suggested as either causing or exacerbating RA.[199] However, metabolite testing is usually part of any routine physical exam and can reveal assorted nutrient deficiencies.

Some vitamins and minerals are not water-soluble and remain in the system, many helping, but some potentially causing harm. Exceeding selenium limits, for instance, can lead to hair loss and brittle nails. Zinc lozenges, which can mitigate the symptoms and duration of a cold, should be used in moderation. Too much zinc can drive other essential metals out of the body and cause anemia. Excess zinc inhibits motility of phagocytes. Aluminum is a component of injected vaccines and may accrue to toxic levels. This can lead to serious conditions such as Alzheimer's disease, liver and skin diseases, gastrointestinal distress, heartburn, learning disorders and disabilities, and chronic fatigue.[200]

Fortunately, metals detoxing is easy. Vitamin C has a chelating effect, so a tablespoon of lemon juice in a cup of warm water twice daily helps move the metals out of the cells and tissues and back into the body's elimination system. An alternative is apple pectin, which also binds with metals and prevents absorption by tissues. For nearly all metals, chelation is recommended.[201] Dr. Mercola lauds chlorella as a natural detoxifier as part of a general nutrition program.[202]

Strict vegetarians ("vegans") may require protein supplements, although many insist that the full range of requirements are satisfied through consumption of a range of fruits and vegetables rich in protein.[203] Vegans may be missing essential vitamin B_{12}, not available from plant foods. Since B_{12} deficiencies can cause anemia and nerve disorders, supplements are strongly suggested.[204]

Although cell structure is standard among human beings, every individual's physiology is admittedly different. The manner in which Mycoplasmas form and migrate to joints is standard among humans and similar among the other mammals. Individual metabolic profile, age, blood sugar balance, and many other factors must be considered when trying to understand why some people respond well to vitamin supplements and others do not.[205] For example, enzymes are essential to proper digestion and metabolism of food intake. Those who do not respond to vitamin therapy may be consuming, but not assimilating, the supplements they take. The undigested material passes through the digestive system and is wasted.

Some vitamin pill formulations do not dissolve properly because of the binding material used, and are not released in time to be useful. Some supplements should be taken alone. That is, they either inhibit or enhance the action of other vitamins or minerals, so allow at least ½-hour delay before ingesting other supplements for optimum effect. An online supplement/herb interaction checker can be found at www.DoctorOz.com. Some examples are:

- Iron should not be combined with calcium (pills or dairy products).
- Vitamin B_6 in combination with magnesium is effective for significant reductions in premenstrual anxiety
- These are more effective when taken together: Vitamins C and E; selenium and E; Vitamins B_6, B_{12} and folic acid; Calcium and magnesium.

Improper digestion is aggravated by consumption of caffeine in coffee, tea, and soft drinks. Alcohol and tobacco are detrimental as well. These substances dilute and may even cancel the efficacy of some vitamin supplements. A particular dilemma for arthritics is that they seek a "pick-me-up" from beverages containing caffeine to offset the fatigue and energy loss that is symptomatic of an infection. They then incur the harmful effects of caffeine consumption. CoQ_{10} is a much better energy booster and fatigue fighter.

Women, especially those with thyroid conditions, should seriously consider calcium supplements to prevent osteoporosis, alleviate PMS, and potentially help maintain hormonal balances.[206] Noting that caffeine causes urinary excretion of calcium, increasing the risk of osteoporosis, one should consider eliminating or severely restricting caffeine intake.[207] Caffeine also influences the adrenal gland's production of the hormone cortisol, which is essential to efficient thyroid function and balance.[208]

Switching to decaffeinated coffee presents some drawbacks. A 6-ounce cup of decaf coffee could contain up to 5 mg of caffeine.[209] Better to abstain or severely limit <u>all</u> coffee intake to no more than two cups daily.

Glucosamine and Chondroitin

Glucosamine sulfate, an amino sugar and a component of proteoglycans, occurs naturally in the body. It is responsible for the synthesis of hyaluronic acid and glycosaminoglycans within the joint, used to grow new cartilage. Glucosamine helps to generate chondroitin, a complex carbohydrate that helps cartilage retain water; both substances are important components of connective tissue. Chondroitin is essential to keep cartilage strong and flexible, and also acts to inhibit breakdown by destructive enzymes. Glucosamine and chondroitin supplements are thought to stimulate the production of hyaluronic acid or reverse its depletion, and in turn to restore mobility to the joints.

Hyaluronic acid is responsible for the high viscosity of synovial fluid and its lubricating, shock-absorbing properties.

Osteoarthritis develops when aging cartilage breaks down, accompanied by metabolic changes including the secretion of corrosive enzymes like hyaluronidase that erode cartilage by destroying collagen and proteoglycans. Hyaluronic acid is the proteoglycan that is depleted more than any other. Vitamin C disables the hyaluronidase that infectious bacteria generate. Vitamins A and C help to stabilize and regenerate collagen, a primary protein used to build cartilage. Both supplements were tested in a major two-year clinical trial showing that either 1,200 mg of chondroitin or 1,500 mg of glucosamine (or both) taken daily could relieve moderate to severe arthritis pain more effectively than a placebo, but not significantly.[210]

It may more effective to take hyaluronic acid supplements directly. Western, especially American, diets do not include gristle and cartilage as do many foreign dishes. One Asian recipe calls for boiling down a whole chicken to extract the cartilage, then drinking the liquid. This practice could perhaps prove to be as beneficial as supplements such as unflavored gelatin granules (two teaspoons daily dissolved in water or juice), hyaluronic acid, pectin, glucosamine sulfate, and chondroitin sulfate. Natural sources of hyaluronic acid are Japanese vegetables, available in Asian supermarkets. A 1-inch slice eaten raw daily has the same effect but is inexpensive and non-invasive. Look for satsumaimo, a type of sweet potato; yamaimo (also called nagaimo), a sticky white yam; konyaku, a prepared gelatinous root vegetable product; and imoji, a potato root.

Proteoglycan structures use large volumes of water, organizing it in multiple interacting layers or shells during formation of protein chains. Additional water is trapped in the interstices of the chondrocytes' extracellular matrix. The resilience of cartilage depends on this water-structuring activity. Nourishment of cartilage in the joints does not come from blood vessels—there are none in cartilage—but from the liquid brought there by the physical compressions and relaxations during bodily movement. This makes the strong case for daily intake of water and regular exercise.[211] Long periods of inactivity dry out and weaken joint cartilage, making it thin and fragile. Ligaments and muscles also atrophy quickly.[212]

Since the 1970s there has been a popular FDA-approved procedure called "viscosupplementation" where synthetic hyaluronic acid is injected into the knee joint(s) over several weeks.[213] The product does not repair damage or stop the disease's progression. It provides temporary cushioning and can reduce pain for up to eight months.

CHOOSING A NUTRITIONIST/DIETICIAN

There are many publications, websites, and media resources offering helpful nutritional advice, but at some point the individual with chronic illness may need a personal consultation with a professional nutritionist or dietician. The usual starting point is a "detox" regimen for clearing accumulated toxins from the body. Often the cravings for allergy-producing foods will disappear along with symptoms of fatigue, low energy, depression and other signs of toxicity.

A growing number of enlightened registered dietitians are practicing integrative nutrition, which takes the best of modern science to detect deficiencies and to use the results construct a profile of the patient's dietary needs. They may be clinical researchers as well as consultants to physicians who use therapeutic nutrition as part of their treatments.

A qualified nutritionist should be a member of the American Society for Nutritional Sciences (ASNS) in addition to having an academic degree. At the doctoral level, the American Board of Nutrition offers certification in clinical nutrition (M.D. only) and human nutritional sciences (M.D. and PhD).[214] Most board-certified nutritionists are affiliated with medical schools and hospitals. Some acupuncturists and chiropractors have a diet/nutrition subspecialty.

Nutritionists will often have experience in a specific area based on their work in a particular health environment, e.g., gerontology or diabetes. Credentials are not as important as clinical experience, advanced education, and success rate. Beware of nutritionists who suggest that disease is caused by faulty diet alone. Be skeptical of those who sell one particular line of vitamins in their offices or who offer a one-size-fits-all diet plan.

Do not hesitate to interview several nutritional counselors in advance. Ask key questions such as: (a) What degrees and credentials do you have? (b) What sort of diets do you design? (c) What diagnostic tests do you recommend? (d) May I call a few of your clients for references?

Choose a practitioner with whom you feel comfortable discussing every aspect of your lifestyle. Ask for the reasons behind the nutritionist's recommendations for dietary adjustments. If you understand the explanation and agree with it, you will be more readily motivated to take an active role in reaching your health goals.

Endnotes and continuing research on topics in Chapter 7 can be found at www.RA-Infection-Connection.com

8. TRENDS IN INFECTION RESEARCH

During the past ten years since the first edition of this book, many investigations have confirmed that cell wall-deficient (CWD) bacterial forms play a significant role in suppressing the immune system by invading immune system cells. Not just Mycoplasmas, but many other bacterial species and viruses do this.[1] Infection research has made important strides toward our understanding of microbes, antivirals, and antibiotics, and has achieved groundbreaking results in immune system sensors and DNA indicators. But scientists have not made much progress in defining drug delivery systems.

An important breakthrough in 2011 described the development of a broad-spectrum antiviral approach that selectively induces apoptosis in cells containing viral double-stranded RNA, rapidly killing infected cells without harming healthy cells.[2] The approach is nontoxic *in vitro* and *in vivo*, potentially suitable for either prophylactic or therapeutic administration. The method applies to many viral pathogens, including clinical viruses (HIV, hepatitis viruses, etc.), natural emerging viruses (avian and swine influenza strains, SARS, etc.), and those relevant to bioterrorism (Ebola, smallpox, etc.).

Scientists continue striving to fully understand the immune system and polymicrobial infections. The following research areas have shown promise to unravel long-hidden scientific mysteries related to chronic disease.

The Human Genome Project

The international Human Genome Project, launched in 1990 to perform detailed mapping of the complete set of human genes, has achieved astounding results. However, this is only the beginning of the real medical challenge: to understand the structure, activity, and complex interactions of the two million or more proteins in the human body using a new scientific approach called "proteomics."[3]

Unlike the genome, which is relatively static, the proteome changes constantly in response to tens of thousands of intra- and extra-cellular environmental signals. The proteome varies with health or disease, the nature of each tissue, the stage of cell development, and effects of drug treatments.

Every chemical reaction essential to life depends on proteins. They are the hormones and enzymes that direct all movement and action in organisms from bacteria to humans. In living cells, the DNA contains the pattern used to make RNA molecules that are templates/catalysts for assembling target molecules. As various component molecules encounter the template, they fit into the shapes of the template and the target molecule self-assembles. In this way, ingested food molecule components are used to make proteins, hormones, enzymes, etc. Even entire cells are made from the DNA patterns in the cells' nuclei and mitochondria.

"Genomics" starts with the gene and makes inferences about its products (proteins), whereas proteomics begins with the functionally modified protein and works back to the gene responsible for its production. Medications based on genomics and molecular biology have been developed. Treatment of disease by gene therapy is expected to be commonplace by the year 2020.[4] The Project foresees the development of new, more effective drugs to treat arthritis symptoms in the short term, suggesting that some day gene therapy may be able to stop RA at the cellular level.[5]

In 1989, scientists discovered the cystic fibrosis gene. In 2000, a gene for one form of arthritis characterized by recurrent fevers was mapped. As of 2009, at least twelve genes have been found for Lupus, but it is unknown how many remain.[6] A sizable international team found five genes that convincingly show an increased risk of developing RA.[7]

Ongoing details of the Human Genome Project can be found online.[8] A complete archive of all *Human Genome News* newsletters (1995-2002) is provided through the U.S. Department of Energy.[9]

The genomes of microbes have also been sequenced, revealing their capacity to make both useful and harmful molecules. This opens the way to make artificial microbes, first to prove that we can assemble a microbe from components, and later to make designed microbes with only useful genes and leaving out the harmful genetic elements.

THE IMMUNE SYSTEM AND INFLAMMATION

Inflammation is an essential tissue-adaptive immune response that enables survival during infection or trauma, to restore the body to balance. However, excessive inflammation causes a decline in normal tissue function, which can contribute to persistent, continuous imbalance and disease. This probably explains chronic inflammatory conditions that are associated with Type 2 diabetes, cardiovascular and neurodegenerative diseases, obesity, cancer, and asthma.[10] Infection and/or trauma have been shown to trigger the inflammatory response in rheumatic conditions, as explained in this book.

Understanding how the critical balance is maintained between tolerance and protective immunity is a key challenge for immunologists. Research shows that both diet and medicines influence gut flora in ways that can upset immune system balance, increase the growth of pathogenic microbes, and promote inflammation.[11] In one experiment,[12] after just one day on the Western diet (high fat and sugar), laboratory mice usually fed a diet low in fat and high in plant polysaccharides showed changes in their microbial composition, metabolic pathways, and gene expression.

The implications of this lab result are profound. It means that variations in past experiment results can perhaps be traced to the <u>diet</u> of the experimental animals, not to the experimental <u>agent</u> being tested. Many study results may have been falsely positive or negative due to inappropriate diet controls for lab animals. Subtle differences in results may have been lost or tainted because they were influenced in gene expression by the food. The conclusion is that certain gut microbes are necessary for the regulation of human immune responses, and some mixtures of microbes are more beneficial than others.[13]

Stated simply, poor diet is a major factor leading to chronic inflammatory disease. Rather than develop new anti-inflammatory drugs, it seems more efficient and cost-effective to devote more attention to proper diet with the goal of maintaining immune system balance. Managing nutrients and food intake and avoiding sugar is an important first step, as advocated by Dr. Mercola for over a decade.[14]

The Role of Vitamin A

The availability of vitamin A in our food is a key factor in a tolerant, highly functional immune system, starting with the mucosal gut lining. Vitamin A cannot be synthesized by the human body; it must be absorbed by the intestine from what we consume.[15]

Vitamin A is a group of about 8 active molecules out of a complex of some 300 related retinoid molecules, most of which are inactive. It is fat-soluble and is stored and processed in the liver. It plays an essential role in stem cell differentiation. As these cells mature to become target-cells, they replace cells that are at the end of their useful lifetime or that have been induced to die off by toxins or cellular invader-microbes.

Immune system cell production depends on vitamin A. Mucosal (epithelial) cells that line the respiratory, digestive, and urinary tracts act as a barrier against viral infection.

Retinol or its metabolites maintain the integrity of these cells. Vitamin A and retinoic acid effect development, differentiation, and activation of white blood cells called T-lymphocytes. The need for vitamin A depends on genetic factors as well as the presence of certain viral gut infections. If vitamin A storage in the liver is nearly depleted, a few days of very high dosage (about 400,000 IU daily) can recharge the liver and allow it to resume using vitamin A in a normal manner. This approach is proposed as the only specific effective antiviral treatment for children with active acute measles. Caution: any dosage this extreme must be supervised carefully by a physician to avoid toxicity.[16,17]

Vitamin A deficiency can be considered a nutritionally acquired immunodeficiency disease.[18] Deficiency leads to anemia—a failure to develop red blood cells and to charge them with iron. Vitamin A has antiviral actions. Along with vitamin C, it can reduce the severity of childhood viral gut infections or live virus MMR vaccine reactions. Vitamin A deficiency increases the severity and incidence of deaths from diarrhea and measles in developing countries. HIV-infected women are three to four times more likely to transmit HIV to their infants if they are Vitamin A deficient.[19] A major cause of blindness in developing children is vitamin A deficiency, which is common in Africa. Vitamin A helps to reverse age-related macular degeneration.

Red palm oil is very rich in vitamin A, CoQ_{10}, vitamin K, vitamin E, and tocotrienols as well as saturated palmitic acids. Palm kernel oil and coconut oil can increase metabolism and in turn reduce obesity.[20] These oils contain saturated, antiviral lauric acid. Chapter 7 has shown that tropical oils and their vitamins work systemically against viral infections, help maintain proper blood pressure, keep inflammation under control, reduce total and LDL cholesterols in the blood, slow the growth of many cancers, stop neural/brain damage caused by oxidative stress, and increase induced heart attack survivability. Vitamin A regenerates endothelial cells, repairing plaque sites cleared by vitamin C plus lysine and red palm oil.

Basal metabolism rate is the steady-state rate the body uses to burn energy. Metabolic rate is controlled by thyroxin. Vitamin A and iodine are necessary diet components used by the thyroid to make thyroxin. A deficiency in either vitamin A or iodine can result in low thyroxin, a lower basal temperature, and lower rates of food energy use. Both thyroxin and CoQ_{10} production decline with age, leading to lower energy and a tendency to gain weight. Kelp supplements are superior to inorganic sources of iodine.[21]

New Immunology Models [22]

Immunologists today are questioning the "self/non-self" model that has dominated thinking for over 60 years. Antigen-presenting cells (APCs) are the messenger cells that communicate to other immune cells, telling them what to do (tolerate or defend) and where to act. The new Infectious-Nonself model holds that APCs can discriminate between "infectious nonself" and "noninfectious self." Under this model, invading pathogens elicit an inflammatory response, but innocuous microbes like probiotics elicit anti-inflammatory reactions. This model is too simplistic. We are beginning to understand that microbes both stimulate and reduce immune functions opportunistically in time-varying amounts, using many complex mechanisms.

In April 1994, National Institutes of Health (NIH) researcher Dr. Polly Matzinger, head of the T-cell Tolerance and Memory section at the NIH's National Institute of Allergy and Infectious Diseases (NIAID) proposed that what spurs the immune system to action is a distress call from dying cells. Dr. Matzinger contended that T-cells require a signal from critical white blood cells (dendritic cells, which inhabit every tissue of the body) to initiate action. The dendritic cells lie dormant until cells nearby call out in shock. A specific example would be the general description by Dr. Brown for the reaction of microbes to antibiotics and the resulting Herxheimer flare.

Dr. Matzinger's nontraditional point of view about the immune response became the famous "Danger Model."[23] Her observation that T-cells don't attack *all* "foreign-looking" substances, e.g., milk proteins from newly lactating breasts in pubescent females, led her to question the central "self/nonself" metaphor of immunology held since the early 1900s. She claims that immunosuppressive drugs such as cyclosporine are often ineffective because they block signals between T-cells and transplants but don't block the alarm that cells in shock send to dendritic cells.

Taking it one step further, the Danger Model proposes that APCs are activated by alarm signals from injured cells, whether these cells are exposed to pathogens, toxins, trauma, or other distress.[24] But even this model needs updating to reflect a systems approach to immunology where the APC response is tailored to fit the tissue in which the alarm occurs rather than just being tailored to fit the pathogen triggering the alarm.[25] By a "systems approach" we mean: holistic, more complete, contextual, and one that describes the total host/microbe(s) interaction process, including side effects.

The new models describe how microbes don't fall neatly into good/bad categories but rather how they interact with the host symbiotically and dynamically under conditions that can change with time, tissue viability, genetic predisposition, and other factors. It is almost as if some microbes can negotiate an equilibrium state that establishes a tolerated guest/parasite relationship as long as the host is not killed. The equilibrium sought between host and microbes can generate a Superorganism: a collection of co-located cells (host and microbes) that can act in concert to produce a mutually acceptable situation whose aim is efficient digestion, detoxification, nutrient synthesis, defense, etc.[26]

Although the body needs to eliminate some pathogens (or at least keep them under control) we need to maintain healthy tissues with special attention to the commensal flora in the mouth. APCs are necessary for oral mucosal tolerance, and in turn, systemic (body-wide) tolerance. As migratory dendritic cells, APCs can initiate an immune response in the lymph nodes. Gut-resident APCs trigger the proliferation of regulatory T-cells throughout the body to suppress adaptive immune responses quickly in their initial stages.[27] Epithelial cells in the gut lining train the APCs so that digested food molecules are not considered dangerous invaders. Food allergies are the result if the gut lining is a dysfunctional, weak filter, passing along food molecules for which no APC "safe" training has occurred.

Recent research has made a compelling case that intestinal microbiota profoundly influence the body's metabolic and immune pathways, and participate directly in both balanced health and systemic immune diseases, especially gastrointestinal inflammatory diseases, from autism to cancer. Research continues to determine the impact of gut dysbiosis on immunological "diseases" (i.e., dysfunctions) outside the gut.[28] The interaction of a complex community of trillions of bacteria in the gut exerts both pro- and anti-inflammatory reactions as it constantly seeks equilibrium (i.e., mucosal balance, discussed in Chapter 3).

Cancer [29]

For decades, genetic mutations were assumed to be the primary cause of cancer. Since the 1980's it has been widely accepted that cancer is caused by specific infections, e.g., the causal linkages between human papilloma virus (HPV) and cervical cancer; *Helicobacter pylori* and gastric cancer; HPV and oropharyngeal cancer; Hepatitis B/C and liver cancer. The WHO stated on World Cancer Day 2006 in Geneva that one-fifth of cancers worldwide are due to chronic infections. Recent findings in the fields of molecular and evolutionary biology have proved viral infections to be the initiating causes of cancer, with mutations at later stages of the disease's development. Based on this revolutionary research direction there will be new options available to clinicians for cancer treatments and prevention.

The new thinking about cancer is to understand how viruses have evolved in order to persist after compromising barriers against cancer in the host. The challenge to science is to determine at what stage cancer-causing viruses are present. One strategy is to compare different cancer patients' histories, looking for viral genomes at every stage. Another approach is to see what specific pathogens are disproportionately involved in each group of patients with a particular type of cancer.

The prediction is that during the next 20 years candidate viruses Epstein-Barr (EPV), HPV, Simian Virus #40 (SV40), cytomegalovirus (CMV), xenotropic murine leukemia virus–related virus (XMRV retrovirus), and the John Cunningham virus (JCV, a type of human polyomavirus), will figure prominently in cancer research. These viruses perhaps have evolved to persist in humans because opportunities for infection (e.g., sexual transmission) are relatively infrequent, and we should expect to see these viruses in higher proportions associated with cancer.[30]

A new hypothesis[31] is that the acute and chronic adverse effects of cancer chemotherapy can be reduced by molecular replacement of membrane lipids and enzymatic co-factors, such as Coenzyme Q_{10}. Tests are underway to determine—by administering nutritional supplements with replacement molecules and antioxidants—whether oxidative membrane damage and reductions of co-factors in normal tissues can be reversed, thereby protecting and restoring mitochondrial and other cellular functions.

Lipid replacement therapy is the natural replacement of oxidized or damaged cells using lipid supplements that are protected from oxidation/damage. These supplements have been shown to significantly reduce fatigue symptoms within one week.[32] Examples of dietary lipid supplements are oils—

notably sunflower seed oil, palm kernel oil, fish oil, fat-soluble vitamins, sterols, cholesterol, phospholipids, monoglycerides, diglycerides, and triglycerides (fats). [33]

Diagnosis Challenges

Cell wall-deficient bacteria can change shape and form to adapt to their environment. Under the microscope, they can appear to have fungal forms (e.g., filamentous structure, budding) and shift to coccal/rod forms. They can break into pieces, capable of reproduction, filterable through micropores. This explains why a condition such as Lyme Disease (LD) can have a different set of symptoms at different times of testing.

Physical symptoms of LD can include:[34]

- *Erythema chronicum migrans* rash;
- recurrent joint swelling/pain;
- cardiac conduction defects;
- interstitial cystitis;
- Irritable Bowel Syndrome (IBS);
- conjunctivitis;
- neurological symptoms such as cranial neuritis (Bell's Palsy), optic neuritis and atrophy, aseptic meningitis, and many more;
- presence of various Mycoplasma strains, mold toxins, EBV, CMV, HHV-6 as well as Borrelia, Babesia, Bartonella; and/or
- persistence of attenuated measles leading to immune depression.

Psychological LD symptoms can include:

- depression
- excessive daytime sleep
- extreme irritability
- word-finding difficulties
- memory loss
- fatigue (mild to severe)

- sensitivity to everyday sounds (hyperacusis)
- spatial disorientation
- light and sound sensitivity
- mood swings
- phobias and obsessive-compulsive actions

It is not surprising that LD is so hard to diagnose with this wide variety of symptoms. Biotoxin exposure symptoms overlap those of LD and Chronic Fatigue Syndrome.

All cell-invading microbes (fungal, bacterial, viral, amoebic) can induce profound metabolic abnormalities that target muscles or nerves and set the stage for replication. Retroviruses like HIV and mouse-related viruses (e.g., XMRV) illustrate this general principle. The effects of these microbes' metabolic activity include: elevated oxidative stress (e.g., by induction of hydrogen peroxide), glutathione depletion (which also increases oxidative stress), and a decrease in the type of DNA modification (methylation) needed to suppress viral genes and nearly all types of cancer.[35] These reactions can be induced by intact (i.e., infectious) viral particles or viral proteins (especially envelope proteins) that are found in vaccines. Live pathogenic viruses or Mycoplasmas have been found to contaminate live vaccines in the rush to market them. It seems our safety processes continue to be corrupted by false urgency. Do you really need a flu shot if extra vitamin C can help your immune system resist pathogens?

According to Dr. Niel Nathan, one can reduce the above metabolic impacts by nutritional support, immune modulation through specific targeted drugs and stem cell therapy, depleting viral reservoirs using GcMAF (Gc protein-derived macrophage activating factor), and in turn decreasing viral replication to maintain the virus in a latent state. These proven, successful approaches to complex, chronic illnesses are described in his excellent 2010 book, *On Hope and Healing.*[36]

BIOFILMS AS MICROBIOMES [37]

Some microorganisms "hibernate"—sometimes for centuries, in rocks, soil, or water—until conditions are optimal for them to become active. Biologists are deterred from studying such microbes because of false positive results that have tainted their efforts to recover ancient DNA. During their state of suspended animation, these microbes can adapt to their environment (e.g., plaque on teeth) and assume different forms, often in moist clusters called "biofilm communities" or simply "biofilms."

More than 99 percent of all bacteria types can live in biofilm communities.[38] Some are beneficial, such as those used in sewage treatment plants to remove contaminants. Biofilms are found wherever surfaces are in contact with water. Examples are slime on river stones, insides of household water pipes, swimming pool walls, and water filters. These colonies are the source of much of the free-floating bacteria found in drinking water. The common *Pseudomonas aeruginosa* biofilm bacteria can infect immunosuppressed animals.[39]

Mostly anaerobic, these bacteria can adhere to clean stainless steel within 30 seconds of exposure. Biofilms have been found to cause the rejection of medical implants. They can colonize on feeding tubes, orthopedic and prosthetic devices (e.g., heart valves), and catheters. Nine specific pathogens were detected in a particular 2005 experiment analyzing microbial communities during overgrowth in feeding tube patients. The highest prevalence were *E. coli*, corynebacterium, Enterococcus, and Candida.[40]

Most research has focused on bacteria, but scientists are learning that biofilms can contain a mix of bacteria, viruses, and fungi, and that many (if not most) chronic biofilm infections are polymicrobial. *Shigella dysenteriae* and *S. sonnei* have been found surviving inside amoebae, serving as a transmission reservoir for Shigella in water.[41]

Although a biofilm cluster can spread by ordinary cell division, it will also shed cells with the express purpose of starting new colonies. Some other microorganisms within a colony, such as Lactobacillus, act symbiotically with (and may regulate) harmful microbes in the biofilm, sharing nutrients and providing mutual protection for community survival. Biofilms have been called "communal slime cities." The resident organisms can "wake up" from hibernation at any time to reinfect, start a new biofilm community, and challenge the immune system. The colony can either emit small numbers of bacteria or release a fragment of the biofilm.

The use of water purification systems causes bacteria to alter their cell wall structure in order to increase their ability to adhere to surfaces. Biofilm resistance to biocides is remarkable according to CDC experiments.[42] The biofilm colony surrounds itself with a protective shield of polysaccharides and polymers. A disinfectant's oxidizing power is depleted before it reaches the interior cell responsible for forming the biofilm. Free-floating, fluid-borne planktonic organisms are more vulnerable. Because biofilm bacteria anchor themselves to surfaces with exuded sticky polymers, simple flushing is inadequate to remove them. Chlorinated reverse osmosis water systems, copper piping, and water filters on all house taps (including ice makers) can limit biofilm contamination of drinking water.

The human body is about 60% water. The bacteria in our bodies' organic "pipes" exhibit the same behavior as biofilms. The protective coating secreted by biofilm bacteria on metal or plastic pipes to ward off attack from disinfectants is analogous to the way antigens try to thwart the immune system's antibodies in the human gut. Pathogens like *Escherichia coli* can adhere to intestinal epithelial cells and form biofilms that shield the colony from immune system attack.[43] On the other hand, beneficial intestinal biofilms may enhance the uptake of nutrients from food, and thus extend the reach of the intestinal epithelial cells for the body's overall health.[44]

One could consider lymph fluid as one big biofilm stew—impeding flow, increasing viscosity, and narrowing the "pipes" leading to conditions like Fibromyalgia and high blood pressure and perhaps even cancer.[45]

Although biofilms have been with us for eons, their behavior suddenly became a topic of intensive research in the early 1990s. Bacteriologists had persistently assumed that bacteria are simple unicellular microbes. This was because the hunt for disease-causing organisms traditionally began by isolating a single cell of the suspected pathogen. Many existing theories of bacterial behavior are based on extrapolations made from this early research. Scientists have developed a database describing these elusive bacteria not only as a resource for evolutionary research but also to study the potential for using these ancient organisms in the industrial production of chemicals.[46]

Studies have revealed that bacteria build complex communities, differentiate into various colony-specific cell types, act cooperatively in groups, and secrete chemical trails to direct movement of others in the colony. Antimicrobials often fail to penetrate the surface layers of the biofilm because bacteria have learned to alter their micro-environments.[47] A new chemical compound developed in 2010 shows promise to destroy biofilms harboring acinetobacter and MRSA, and re-sensitizes those bacteria to antibiotics.[48] One might add: "For now, at least."

Microbes are essential components of our biochemical structure. Researchers are speculating that some diseases may be caused by a change in the body's internal microbial balance rather than invasion by a single pathogenic microorganism. It may become evident that there are other specific relationships to consider: e.g., the biochemical catalyst-to-enzyme ratio and the toxin-to-anti-toxin ratio.

With newly developed molecular methods (e.g., cloning, gene sequencing, *in situ* hybridization and tissue preservation), researchers can make advanced observations. However, due to the difficulty in obtaining samples, information on gut biofilms is limited. Tests usually require the patient to use laxatives, which destroy biofilms in the area of the large bowel where Crohn's disease, ulcerative colitis, or colorectal cancer could be detected.[49] There are new diagnostic methods for assessing the composition of biofilms. PathoGenius and Innovotech are two companies making headway in this area. They are identifying both bacterial and non-bacterial elements of biofilms.[50]

Haemophilus influenzae is a recognized cause of acute *Otitis media* in children and chronic obstructive pulmonary disease (COPD) in adults. Studies suggest that the bacterium grows as a biofilm colony in the lower respiratory tract.[51]

Microbes living in biofilms in the mouth represent a potentially deadly mix of infectious pathogens.[52, 53, 54] Dental infections are discussed in Chapter 3.

Mining Microbes

Previously unknown and unstudied bacteria in ordinary soil may be the starting point for specialized genomic research. The proteins produced by these organisms could have beneficial properties unlike any other currently exploited substances. Most of the antibiotics used in medicine today come from soil-based microbes.[55] Two examples are streptomycin, the first treatment for tuberculosis, and vancomycin, considered the last resort for serious infections. However, intravenous vancomycin treatment is very painful, and can cause two types of allergic reactions: red man syndrome and anaphylaxis.[56]

Recent advances in technology have sparked a resurgence in the discovery of natural product antibiotics from bacterial sources.[57] Rising testing costs and delays in obtaining approval is causing the production of new drugs to decline. Since 1998, the FDA has approved only ten new antibiotics, only two of which were truly novel. In 2002, among 89 new medicines emerging on the market, none was an antibiotic.[58] Of concern is that there is no antibiotic class for which some level of bacterial resistance does not already exist. New antibiotics are needed to treat chronic diseases caused by microbial pathogens that are becoming increasingly resistant to existing drugs. Progress is being made using microbial sources and also from chemical modification of antibiotic classes other than those now in clinical use.[59]

Researchers are experimenting with DNA samples from biofilms, seawater, sediment, and lichens.[60] The DNA strings must be long enough to extract and isolate a complete set of genes for study. This is a delicate and painstaking process, complicated by the fact that most of the unknown organisms cannot be grown in the laboratory.

By 2006, progress in decoding of the human genome had revealed hundreds of gene sequences that come from bacteria and ancient viruses.[61] In 2010, a genome research team produced the first bacteria strain using a man-made collection of genes originating with *Mycoplasma mycoides*. Team leader Craig Venter said, "We refer to such a cell controlled by a genome assembled from chemically synthesized pieces of DNA as a 'synthetic cell,' even though the cytoplasm of the recipient cell is not synthetic."[62, 63]

MICROCHIP TECHNOLOGY

Radio Frequency Identification (RFID) chips are already being used as implants to identify pets, keep track of livestock on farms, and as a means to thwart kidnapping. Exciting new applications for medical diagnosis and testing are being developed using semiconductor industry technology merged with chemical sensors on the chip.

Biochip Testing

Testing for allergens is an excellent application for biochip technology. Antibodies in the blood bind to allergens prepositioned on the chip. By amplifying the fluorescence for sensing by a chip-reading instrument, the existence and severity of particular allergens can be determined at the same time.[64] Conventional allergy tests require either watching for reactions after injections of suspect substances or sending blood samples to a lab for testing. Both methods are costly and time-consuming, but as many as 100 different allergens at once may be tested using a single drop of blood smeared on a biochip.

Biochip technology was developed in 1987 in Germany as a testing mechanism for autoimmune and infectious diseases and as a screen for monoclonal antibodies. The biochip testing method combines three usually distinct micro-analytical techniques: ELISA, Blot, and indirect immunoflourescence techniques. Classical ELISA by itself is limited and does not identify specific microbes linked to RA or other chronic disease.

Immunofluorescence works by joining antibodies to fluorescent molecules. The antibody clusters around the component of the serum to be analyzed. Each cell has a different antibody mapped by coordinates in a computer. Programmed scans find coordinates of hot cells and look up the matching antibody in the list.

The biochip product is a mosaic that permits effective miniaturization and standardization of serological analyses. An autonomous, small, cheap, portable "lab-on-a-chip" has been developed by U.C. Berkeley scientists.[65] The device simultaneously processes five separate whole-blood samples by separating the plasma from the blood cells and detecting the presence of biotin (vitamin B7). The conventional "moisture chamber" and other incubation methods are superfluous as the liquids are maintained in an enclosed area and the exact height and position of the droplets are precisely defined by the geometry of the system.

Companies are using competing methods to make state-of-the-art probes, transferring pieces of cell DNA or RNA or proteins onto half-inch glass squares (one company has more than a million squares on its chip's checkerboard) or filter paper. An assortment of masks superimposed on the pattern builds up variations of probes in the millions. Based on proven ELISA principles, an innovative feature of immunoassay biochips is simultaneous multi-analyte testing. Each biochip can have dozens of individual test paths. These comprehensive biochip panels can do diagnostic testing for clinical use, drug abuse screening, private and public sector research, forensic applications, pharmaceutical drug development, veterinary testing, and DNA analysis.[66]

Microarrays

The first DNA microarray (genome chip) test was approved by the FDA in 2007. Biochips continue to be tested for use in disease diagnostics to: 1) identify infectious microorganisms at the genetic level; 2) categorize cancers at the genetic and molecular level. Much of the technology used in the manufacture and test analysis of biochips is labor-intensive and expensive. But better methods are being developed, e.g., direct detection of hybridization by electric current, based on the fact that single-stranded DNA conducts electrons at a different rate than double-stranded DNA.

This remarkable multi-testing approach could be the optimal means to identify swiftly evolving pathogens and microorganisms. Such a test method gives physicians a valuable wide scope tool for disease identification. Despite temporary manufacturing drawbacks, biochips are an important enabling technology of the future and will some day be as common as x-rays as a diagnostic technique, yet without the risks that x-rays pose. Test results would also be available almost immediately.

DNA microarrays are about the size of a credit card. Single-stranded DNA segments called "probes" coat the surface. The microarrays help biologists define a cell's genetic makeup and determine which parts of the cell are active under particular conditions. Numerous websites document DNA microarray research being done worldwide. One of the most comprehensive and detailed is the Massachusetts Institute of Technology's site developed by Dr. Leming Shi at www.Gene-Chips.com.[67]

Microbeads and Nanobarcodes

Scientists are leveraging semiconductor technology to detect pathogens and disease agents using microbeads and microscopic barcodes. Collections of metalized polymer beads contain unique barcodes to identify associated assay targets.[68] Synthesized crystals called "quantum dots" use the optical properties of semiconductors to measure emitted light when electrons in the crystal are excited. Combinations of the crystals are blended into tiny polystyrene capsules called "microbeads."

Each microbead is uniquely cataloged based on color mix and intensity (i.e., the number of quantum dots), analogous to a bar code. The microbeads are chemically attached to the DNA probes. Fluorescent dye is attached to selected single strands of DNA and these treated strands are mixed with the microbeaded probes. The interreactions using spectroscopic analysis allow researchers to discover which genes are present in an unknown DNA sample.

Barcodes are used to identify and quantify molecules in fluid samples taken as part of standard medical diagnostic tests. These "nanobarcodes" are microscopic rods striped with gold, silver, or other metal. Varying the width, number, and order of the stripes can generate hundreds of thousands of unique identifier rods. These rods could be attached to probes that bind to specific biological molecules, allowing retrieval and computer analysis of thousands of different tagged samples.

Today's biological tests use analog measurement of fluorescent tags in microarrays, which let researchers analyze only a few types of molecules at a time. Emerging nanobarcode technology will help scientists detect patterns of behavior and molecular signatures of various diseases in different stages of severity and progression, and to trace them back to the genes responsible.[69] Researchers are using nanobarcodes to examine molecular patterns in diabetics' blood and Alzheimer's patients' brain fluid.[70]

A quantum dot-based analysis tool developed by Indiana University researchers has the potential to identify some 40,000 genes in ten minutes, compared to 24 hours required by gene chip testing. Detection of proteins is also possible by replacing DNA probes with antibodies.

Research into microchip-based devices, called biological microelectromechanical systems, or bioMEMS, is currently much further along than studies using quantum dots, just now being tested in academic labs as a means for delivering drugs. In this approach, bioMEMS would be implanted in the body as a drug delivery system. So far, only a few studies have appeared in the literature but several companies are developing such systems.[71]

Protein Chips

Some scientists theorize that most of the million proteins are just variations on a few basic designs, and that there may be as few as 5,000 distinct shapes to catalog definitively. But identification is much simpler than understanding how these shapes are formed and how they behave. Several high tech companies are producing biochips as two-dimensional grids of proteins as a microarray. When this protein chip is exposed to biochemicals or protein solutions, the molecules adhering to the microarray can be identified and tagged with various markers. The binding ability of molecules is what makes pharmaceuticals effective.

The chips can be used as diagnostic tools, measuring abnormally high or low amounts of blood proteins in a given sample. Biochips could be the key to early detection of serious diseases such as heart disorders and cancer.[72, 73]

Microchip Implants

The idea of medical implants began in the early 1990s with a polymer wafer used to treat brain cancer. This innovation, developed by Dr. Richard Langer at MIT in 2001, may be an effective alternative to traditional chemotherapy.[74] After surgery has been performed to remove the tumor, the gradually dissolving wafer releases drugs directly to the site. The blood/brain barrier keeps the medications from traveling to other parts of the body.

A colleague of Dr. Langer, Dr. John T. Santini, Jr., is developing a variety of devices made of silicon and having circuitry. These chips have tiny etched electronic channels, each containing a minute amount of a drug, usually a protein. The channels, sealed with a fine layer of gold, can be selectively hit with an electric charge that dissolves the gold to release the drug. A companion chip implant acts as a controller to deliver the charge on a programmed schedule, or perhaps could be activated remotely on an as-needed basis. Dr. Santini's research group is experimenting with a sensor chip implant that would monitor the bloodstream to determine when and where drugs should be released.[75]

Carl Grove, president of iMEDD in Columbus, Ohio, is leading his company to develop a similar microchip with a polymer coating that could treat heart disease, diabetes, and various forms of cancer.[76] These targeted, specific drug applications avoid the traditional problems of long-term treatment, for example:

- injected drugs break down too quickly on their way to the site of the tumor, infection, or trauma;
- like vancomycin, the drug doesn't get past the gut lining to the target site;[77]
- ingested drugs either can't fully survive the digestive system or react adversely to produce negative side effects;
- there is a risk of overdosing to be sure enough of the drug eventually reaches the intended site;
- scheduled lab visits for treatments are inconvenient and time-consuming for both patients and medical staff;
- indigent or transient patients are not apt to maintain a regular treatment schedule; or
- elderly patients pose a major problem in terms of insuring compliance with a regimen.

According to Dr. Santini, in as little as five years microchips might replace injections as the preferred delivery method for cancer and Hepatitis C drugs.

The Dark Side of Biotechnology

Researchers estimate that in just a few years it will be possible to construct synthetic designed viruses and perhaps even individual, non-replicating, and/or replicating cells. Improved vaccines will benefit humanity, but creating deadly viruses as biological weapons is on the agenda of military planners in hostile nations. Many viral genomes have fewer than 10,000 DNA bases, i.e., letters in their genetic code. HIV is a viral genome. The largest DNA synthesized so far is the 582,970 base pair genome of *Mycoplasma genitalium*, although as of 2009 this synthetic DNA has not been "booted" to life.[78]

Biotech companies will soon be not just allowed but encouraged to perform their own in-house studies to determine whether their genetically modified agricultural seeds are environmentally safe. This means that companies like Monsanto, which provides about 90 percent of the world's transgenic crops, will help the government decide whether their own products should be approved. Furthermore, companies will be able to outsource the research to third parties and subsidize the cost.[79] Trusting agencies and manufacturers in developing countries can lead to health risks. Cost-saving means using fake ingredients and chemical additives in food and OTC supplements. China has a deplorable record of poor food safety. The FDA and private labs cannot keep up with the flood of incoming imports, but even domestic U.S. suppliers are guilty of taking shortcuts to increase profit margins.[80, 81, 82, 83] E.g., the absence of any actual pollen in honey sold in U.S. stores.[84]

NUTRITION TRENDS

As seen in Chapter 7, some key deficiencies exist today in our Western diet. Sometimes toxic, non-nutritious, refined fats have replaced natural essential oils. Antioxidant foods are needed in greater quantities to destroy free radicals that cause oxidative stress and inflammation. We should look at the best ethnic diets and the best world tribal diets to understand how and why certain ingredients work.

Some current medical assumptions are potentially too risky, or have unintended negative outcomes, as shown in the discussion of statin drugs being used to force a desirable cholesterol ratio (Chapter 7) and vaccines (Chapter 4).

Nutritional and Diet Guidelines

Some of our health maladies are derived in part from faulty nutrition practices and lifestyle habits, e.g., obesity, Metabolic Syndrome, joint pain, heart disease, COPD, ASD, gut disorders, cancer, diabetes, etc. For decades, the commercial and agricultural interests have set our nutritional rules. We have compiled a list of the best nutrition websites and put them on our website.[85]

Mineral deficiencies such as magnesium and zinc need general supplementation. Toxic materials like aluminum (vaccine adjuvants) accrue in muscle and organ tissues. We need a critical re-evaluation of these adjuvants and other vaccine-related toxicities, to insure that we stop inadvertently poisoning our children.

Certain amino acids like lysine are needed by persons susceptible to heart disease[86] and herpes virus activity. Lysine suppresses HHV pathogenicity. Chocolate, nuts, and gelatin contain arginine,[87] which is needed by HHV viruses to thrive, so their intake should be minimized. Analysis of specific amino acids that inhibit/encourage pathogens is an area worthy of study and the results brought to the public's attention.[88, 89]

Diseases like MS, myasthenia gravis, and some ASD factors are examples of vitamin shortfalls. That is, for these individuals, intake levels far above the normal level are required to offset their conditions. E.g., Dr. Klenner has found dosages that are therapeutic for the B-complex (B_1, B_3, B_{12} applied to MS),[90] A-complex (applied to ASD impaired night vision genetics),[91] and vitamin C (general ROS oxidative stress).[92] The various forms of vitamin D, E-complex, CoQ_{10} and others (e.g., Coenzyme-A) need to be re-evaluated for dosage amounts using two different criteria: healthy persons for which vitamin deficiencies can be problematic, and those individuals with vitamin-dependent maladies for whom amounts can be as much as a thousand times greater than the FDA's daily recommended dietary guidelines.[93]

Drugs can induce nutrient unbalances. Two examples are CoQ_{10} depleted by statin drugs[94] and folic acid levels reduced by aspirin. Prescribing drugs that block immune functions with no concurrent antimicrobial treatment or nutrition supplementation can lead to long-term negative (sometimes tragic) outcomes. Drug-caused dysbiosis needs probiotic replacement. Microbe strains found in probiotics[95] need vetting to assure their safety.

We need to be well-informed regarding essential food molecules to insure that we eat them regularly. Much of this information is readily available on the Internet and in self-help books. A well-qualified nutritionist could assist. A test would be that person's familiarity with Dr. Klenner's work and an appreciation of the vitamins and oils described in Chapter 7.

Ketosis

Ketosis plus vitamin C (ascorbic acid, or AA) is a very effective adjuvant to the low-dose tetracycline antibiotic protocol.[96, 97] Benign ketosis is induced by drastic reduction of carbohydrate intake (fewer than 15 grams per day), as described by Dr. Robert Atkins in his diet induction stage.[98] The liver shifts from fat storage mode to fat extraction mode, leading to weight loss, as discussed in Dr. Mercola's 2003 book, *The No-Grain Diet*.[99] Fats are catabolized to acetyl Co-enzyme A to feed the Krebs cycle where ATP is made to supply energy to all the body cells. Body-cell sugar use shuts down. Hypoglycemic condition stops abruptly in ketosis mode. The ROS associated with the illness oxidizes the AA to the Dehydro Ascorbic Acid (DHA) form. Microbes, viruses, and microbe-infected cells (especially cancer cells) need sugar to survive, and ingest oxidized DHA instead. Inside the microbes and the infected cells, the DHA oxidizes the cells' mitochondria and induces apoptosis (cell death).[100]

Diet dramatically affects human health, partly by modulating gut microbiome composition. A 2011 study found that two organism categories play a major role in long-term diets: Prevotella (associated with carbohydrates) and Bacteroides (associated with protein and animal fat).[101] Keeping these in balance is the key to controlling obesity and the Metabolic Syndrome,[102, 103] discussed in Chapter 3.

Carbohydrate Intake and Chronic Illness

Dr. Joseph Brasco has provided scientific evidence on the link between carbohydrates (carbs) and a wide range of illnesses, including hypoglycemia, heart disease, high blood pressure, diabetes, and cancer.[104] Problems with added sugars to foods and beverages have brought about a global obesity epidemic, and with it the risk of Type 2 diabetes and heart disease, especially in children. The WHO estimated in 2005 that 1.6 billion adults worldwide were overweight and 400 million obese, with numbers steadily rising. In the U.S., diseases linked to obesity are calculated to be about 9% of total annual healthcare costs.[105]

The American Heart Association stated in 2009 that sugar-sweetened beverages are the primary culprit because these various forms of sugars, including high fructose corn syrup (HFCS), are readily absorbable carbs.[106] Between 1970 and 2005, average sugar intake increased by 19%, adding 76 calories to Americans' average daily count. Excessive consumption leads not just to metabolic dysfunctions but also shortfalls of essential nutrients calcium, magnesium, zinc, and vitamins A and D.

Substituting artificial sweeteners, especially in diet beverages, brings in another set of problems. Several epidemiological studies have suggested a positive association between diet soda consumption and weight gain, and the risk of Metabolic Syndrome.[107, 108] Because they have little nutritional benefit, intake of both sugar-sweetened and artificially sweetened beverages should be limited and replaced by healthy alternatives such as water and herbal tea.

Ketosis and Alzheimer's

In a recent study of patients with mild dementia, the group who ate a very low carb diet for 6 weeks did significantly better on memory tests than the control group who ate a normal diet.[109] Quoting from that article:

"Contemporaneous with the developing dementia epidemic is an epidemic of obesity and associated metabolic disturbance. Currently, 64% of the USA adult population is overweight and 34% obese.[110] It is projected that by the year 2030, 86% will be overweight and 51% obese.[111] Likewise, diabetes prevalence is accelerating, particularly in the aging population.[112] Hyperinsulinemia, which is a precursor to Type 2 diabetes, occurs in more than 40% of individuals aged 60 and older.[113]"

Dr. Mary Newport estimates that 15 million people in the U.S. will have Alzheimer's by the year 2050. This condition is very easily prevented with a ketogenic diet and coconut oil.[114] An additional benefit is weight control because beneficial gut microbes are nourished. The lauric acid in coconut oil is the active antiviral and antimicrobial agent at work.[115] The publishers of the online e-zines *Dementia Weekly* and *Alzheimer's Weekly*[116] recommend what they call the "Keto-Dementia Diet."[117] As our brain ages, it is less able to burn glucose efficiently. Since glucose is the brain's primary energy source, too little glucose will result in declining mental ability. Researchers found in 2008 that ketones are an alternative energy source to glucose.[118]

Antipsychotic drugs are commonly over-prescribed in patients with dementias such as Alzheimer's. Medicare often covers them in nursing homes, making them an easier, more profitable solution than healthier, milder non-drug therapies or nutritional supplements. Those with diets low in trans-fats and high in omega-3 fatty acids and in vitamins C, D, E, and the B vitamins also had higher scores on mental thinking tests than people with diets low in those nutrients.[119] Using antipsychotic drugs offers a quick fix to behavioral problems but at the expense of patients' good health and quality-of-life. The nonprofit group CANHR (Long Term Care Justice and Advocacy) offers a free guidebook on this topic.[120]

In 2006, researchers found that an enzyme called Pin1 blocks the formation of tangle-like lesions ("tau tangles") common in the Alzheimer's brain. Pin1[121] also helps protect against the development of amyloid peptide plaques, another kind of brain lesion characteristic of Alzheimer's.[122] <u>Caution</u>: increasing Pin1 in neurons effectively suppresses the disease development in cases of Alzheimer's, but it accelerates disease progression in other types of dementia and Parkinson's.[123] Pin1 is found in viruses like adult T-cell leukemia[124] and other types of cancers. Perhaps anti-Pin1 therapy might be effective against some cancers without creating a significant general toxicity to normal cells.[125]

Endnotes and continuing research on topics in Chapter 8 can be found at www.RA-Infection-Connection.com

9. REFLECTIONS ON METHODOLOGY

During our 14 years of medical reading and over 50 years of life experience and (hopefully) wisdom, the authors have encountered passionate, almost religious, fervor that precludes debate and stifles scientific investigation. In our engineering careers we have seen science and statistics manipulated to suit commercial interests, politics, personal face-saving agendas, and emotion-driven causes.

This book presents our in-depth research and thoughtful analysis. Some points may be controversial, but our goal is fact-based, rational advocacy without critical omissions, bias, rhetoric, or prejudice. This chapter illustrates some of the obstacles to progress in solving the puzzle of chronic illness. We put our trust in government health programs that are based on "science." But what if the science process is broken?

HOW WE THINK

An influential philosophy that has guided the research and diagnoses of mid-20th century scientists was popularized by Karl Popper (1902-94). According to Popper, a scientist proposes a hypothesis, then designs experiments to either verify or disprove the hypothesis. But philosophers, says Popper, are the driving force in determining what factors determine the validity of the experiment's scientific results. Furthermore, they even determine the nature of science itself and influence the direction of viable research. As one theory is falsified (i.e., disproved wholly or in part), another evolves to replace it and more reliably explains the new observations.

According to Popper, any scientific hypothesis and its experimental design should be given up as soon as it is falsified (shown to be erroneous by observation or experiment). Although his notion of "falsifiability" is not universally accepted, it is still the foundation of the majority of scientific experiments. Critics maintain that applying Popper's approach to the scientific method would have dismissed the theories of Darwin and Einstein at the outset. When these theories were first advanced, each of them was at odds with accepted available evidence at the time and deemed false by the scientific establishment. Only later did evidence emerge that gave their theories deserved attention and endorsement.

This leads to a consideration of a basic law of forensics, first stated by astronomer Carl Sagan: ***Absence of evidence is not evidence of absence.*** Corollary: any number of incompetent failures to duplicate an experiment's results cannot refute a competently produced result. They just delay the progress of science, sometimes for decades.

E.g., Dr. Albert Sabin was asked to duplicate an experiment evaluating the efficacy of vitamin C on viral diseases like polio.[1] Because he did not follow Dr. Claus Jungeblut's 1937 carefully documented procedure (Sabin incorrectly used oral instead of injected, and just one dose instead of frequently repeated doses) Sabin's result was seen to be a "falsification" of Dr. Jungeblut's positive conclusions. Dr. Sabin was faced with a dilemma. If vitamin C were found to be useful, his own polio vaccine work would be questioned as unnecessary, more costly, and risky.

With his future career at stake in 1939, Dr. Sabin made a public statement as to the dubious value of vitamin C, which he claimed falsified the hypothesis that "large dosages" (actually, he used small dosages) of the vitamin could be therapeutic. So powerful was Sabin's reputation that his skeptical view of vitamin C has persisted for over seventy years. Despite countless vitamin C experiments, successful documented therapies, and credible double-blind studies, vitamin C is still considered "controversial."[2]

Popper's philosophy has merit in an ideal world where no investigators are biased or incompetent, and where particular scientific views are not politicized or agenda-driven. However, in a world with pharmaceutical advertising and scientifically incorrect health propaganda, commercial interests repeatedly overwhelm competitive inexpensive treatment modalities. The public is the victim while the powerful commercial interests have deliberately suppressed publication of competing benign, cheaper methods, treatments, and ideas for decades.

Validity and certainty can be the enemy of discovery. The way leading to discovery and insights is brainstorming, which leads to new ideas, hypotheses and possible associations. Of course, one must then apply objective analytical constraints in order to modify, validate, or invalidate the hypotheses about suggested linkages.

A problem arises either when analysis is applied too early in the process, suppressing new concepts and curtailing discovery, or when proposals for new research are turned down because the proposed direction is not in line with conventional wisdom or an approved political point of view.

An example is the National Cancer Institute's rejection of Linus Pauling's several proposals regarding vitamin C in 1977.[3] These self-serving rejections had truly tragic consequences by delaying the adoption of non-toxic, low cost, potentially life-saving treatment modalities.

Scientific progress depends on the validity of our model of the natural world and how we think about it. Two ways of thinking are given in Table 6. The approaches are complementary, not mutually exclusive. Each way of thinking is useful in its own time and place, and under prevailing circumstances. The truth is somewhere in-between the conventional view and the non-traditional approach.

Table 6. Ways of Thinking About the Natural World

Conventional Way to Validity & Certainty	Non-traditional Way to Discovery & Insights
Aristotelian logic: T/F Truth is absolute and unchanging Propositions are T/F (0=F, 1=T) Context change can invalidate.	Fuzzy Logic (Calculus of probabilities) Truth changes as a function of time, place, and situation Probability of Truth: $F=0 < P(t) < 1=T$
No exceptions or the rule is false. [Falsification criteria]	Explore exceptions and expand the model.
Seek a single/simple cause (Occam's razor).	Seek multiple factors, correlations, and intersects.
Exclude anecdotal data: --Restrict scope; --Discard outliers; --Disregard data not matching preconceptions/ prejudices; --Disregard data from sources that conflict with preferred theory and select only agreeing data; --Use rhetoric to persuade.	Look for patterns in anecdotal data: --Collect, correlate, and validate; --Find patterns in correlations; --Analyze, postulate, and synthesize; --Theorize, extrapolate, test and re-validate; --Analyze outliers for what may be overlooked.
Internet Search: Constrained You find less, but: --More relevant, but less data; --Seek consensus; --Consensus may be wrong.	Internet Search: Open You find more, but: --Less relevant, too much data; --Less certain relationships; --Seek new causes and correlations; --Question conditions, validate.

The website www.quackwatch.com operated by Dr. Stephen Barrett is notorious for eloquently defending the partly-failed status quo against the competition of ideas that present new solutions that very often actually work. His words apply standard validation criteria to unconventional medical concepts disseminated on the Internet.

Some, but not all, discussions on this website are thoughtfully written and collect a wide range of material from many different authoritative sources on a diverse assortment of topics. These are worth reading and thinking about in order to understand how medical scientists who lack analytical skills and/or wisdom view non-traditional medical concepts.[4]

For example, Dr. Barrett vehemently criticizes the Marshall Protocol, which recommends a regimen of several antibiotics, strict dietary restrictions, and avoiding vitamin D. The protocol has been proven to work. Dr. Barrett insists, rightly, that vitamin D is a very important supplement *for healthy people*. He fails to recognize that for someone with a chronic illness like Fibromyalgia or Sarcoidosis, colonies of microbe-invaded macrophages can manufacture excessive amounts of vitamin D (1,25-D), resulting in a surplus that is toxic and can paralyze muscles. The Marshall Protocol seeks to keep the D-ratio in balance for those with infected macrophages.[5, 6]

The prejudicial, negative tone in which Dr. Barrett describes some alternative medical treatments or procedures offends those who sincerely believe in those concepts and who have experienced positive results. For a balanced view, use a search engine to explore the Internet with keyword *iatrogenic* for some of the failures of conventional medicine.[7]

Koch's Postulates

For decades, researchers have tested the relationship between a specific pathogen and a disease by using rules developed by microbiologist Dr. Robert Koch in the late 1800s. The criteria have expanded over time, but the basic principles remain the same.[8] The microorganism must be:

- Observed in every case of the disease; not in healthy individuals;

- Isolated and grown in pure culture (within a short time);

- Reproducible when the pure culture is inoculated into a susceptible host animal; and

- Recovered from and observed in the experimentally inoculated, diseased host animal.

There are many exceptions to these rules that make them outdated today, but they still appear in medical textbooks. Many pathogenic microbes are persistent. The bacteria are pleomorphic (shape-changing). The invaders live part of their lives inside our cells. The target multiple cell-types include immune cells and epithelial cells everywhere in the body. The invaded target cells make disrupting bioactive molecules and stop making others, according to their dynamic survival needs. Koch's postulates represent a compelling intellectual simplicity: one bug = one disease = one medicine. This kind of constrained thinking cannot inadequately characterize multiple microbe complexes (e.g., biofilm and plaque colonies) associated with the human biome and chronic illness.[9]

RESEARCH RESOURCES

For the health researcher, the amount of data and useful information to be found on the Internet is amazing. A good place to start is the National Institutes of Health's NLM archive of free full text biomedical and life sciences journal literature. PubMed at this writing comprises more than 21 million citations for biomedical literature from MEDLINE, life science journals, and online books.[10]

Subscribers to <u>Medscape.com</u>'s free interactive online publications include physicians, nurses, naturopaths, medical students, and individual researchers. Medscape compiles articles and medical news from a variety of credible sources.

This new NLM and Internet information technology also brings chronic illness sufferers from all walks of life and from around the world in touch electronically. Non-medical people are able to discuss their courses of treatments with physicians, naturopaths, and fellow arthritics and to compare notes about success or failure of various approaches taken by each one's health care provider.

Synthesizing this knowledge enables the individual with a home computer to benefit by exploring new methods of diagnosis and treatment that can be discussed with one's physician. A well-informed patient is also better able to seek out and evaluate skilled medical support.

There are, unfortunately, medical information hoaxes as well as passionate, sincere but misguided, and unscientific nonsense placed on the Internet. When conducting research, it is important to seek information only from credible sources such as libraries of major universities, scientific publications by established medical journals, institutes operated by licensed physicians, and government agencies such as the CDC and the NIH/NLM. Blogs, for the most part, represent opinion. Some are very useful, if accompanied by references that the reader can check. Methods for researching health-related information online are shown in Appendix IV.

Most websites have identifiable sponsors. Those sites with unknown or hidden sponsors are suspect, especially those with a strong commercial orientation and without a medically trained staff.

Public access to medical knowledge on the Internet is akin to the revolution in literacy caused by the invention of the printing press. Ordinary people can gain easy access to the results of research previously unavailable to them, hidden away in obscure medical journals and dusty archives, ignored by medical school professors, accessible only through hard work or special permission or status.

An individual without affiliation to the medical community as either a practicing physician or medical student can now browse journal articles and scan the medical/scientific collection catalog of a major university from one's home computer. This was never before so easy to do. Nor was it possible to find, correlate, and discuss research findings openly—across different eras and across different disciplines—globally and electronically with ease, speed, accuracy, convenience, and usually without cost. An example is the valuable collection of articles by Dr. John Ely of the University of Washington, published in the *Journal of Orthomolecular Medicine.*[11]

Sadly, a sizable body of research work remains out of reach in a timely manner because one must be a paid member of the publishing organization to view specific journal articles. An example is the Infectious Diseases Society of America. Annual membership costs $1000. A non-member must pay a $40 fee per 24-hour access to the current IDSA journal. After one year, 880 organizations submit all journal articles but 1461 submit only selected articles or just abstracts to the NIH's public access collection of 2.2 million PubMed documents.[12] At this time, the IDSA does not choose to participate in this system.

It would behoove organizations that publish medical research to team with a commercial distributor to develop a means to gather together articles on a particular topic and make them available as a set for a flat fee. A researcher would thus be able to obtain a real time, dynamically-created "journal" from diverse sources.

The potential benefits to the medical research community are considerable: universities/societies would receive deserved recognition for providing worthwhile, timely data; journal authors would see their work presented to the wider medical community; and most importantly, medical advances could be made that might otherwise be undiscovered or delayed only because of high-cost access. In the meantime, use search engine Scholar.Google.com to find unusual publications not in the popular domain.

THE QUEST FOR A CURE

For decades, media articles have ended with vague statements such as "In the next few years there will probably be dramatic changes in our approach to RA." The U.S. Pharmacopoeia and the Arthritis Foundation have only tentatively accepted tetracycline treatment for Lyme Disease[13] and for over 60 years still consider Dr. Brown's antibiotic protocol for RA to be "controversial."[14]

The conclusion they would have the public draw is that these treatments are still experimental when in fact they are both available now and proven to be effective through numerous credible and sizable scientific studies. The term "controversial" seems to imply that the drug companies are working against these treatments being used since the only organizations advocating informing the public of low cost curative treatment protocols are nonprofits such as the Road Back Foundation and The Arthritis Trust. They have no funds to place competing full-page ads in national magazines or to run educational TV spots.

For years advertisers have conditioned us to take a pill at the first sign of discomfort, so it is no surprise that our society is looking for a single magical cure for diseases like arthritis that acts almost immediately, without altering one's lifestyle. After all, if aspirin can "cure" a headache within a few minutes, why not a similar drug to "cure" arthritis?

Unlike a physical trauma injury where tissue or bone is suddenly destroyed, arthritis is slowly degenerative. We can hardly expect a single drug or herb to effect a complete, rapid cure for a disease that has developed over years and has so many complex organisms that can cause it. Yet new, marginally effective products continue to vie for market share on the promise of a pain cure or at least dramatic symptom relief. The 50 million arthritis sufferers in the U.S. form a large and highly motivated customer base for marketing over-the-counter drugs and natural health products. Of that total, 2 million RA patients are the target buyer base for costly prescription drugs.

The 1998 FDA-approved drug Enbrel is a genetically engineered medication that works by absorbing the tumor-killing cytokine called "tumor necrosis factor" (TNF) before it can signal immune cells to multiply unnecessarily. Other drugs in this TNF category are Humira, Remicade, Cinzia, and Simponi. In 2009 the FDA issued stronger warnings about the risks linked to TNF blockers: tuberculosis (including re-activation of latent TB), MS, Hepatitis B re-activation, myelitis, potentially deadly fungal infections, (especially histoplasmosis), optic neuritis, lymphoma, pancytopeni, aplastic anemia, sepsis, central nervous system disorders, psoriasis, and opportunistic infections. The FDA has receives ongoing annual reports of seriously adverse reactions. Class action lawsuits are pending.[15, 16]

The category of non-steroidal anti-inflammatory drugs (NSAIDs) called COX-2 inhibitors is designed to target prostaglandin production. Two examples are Bextra and Celebrex. Vioxx was removed from the market in 2004. None of these drugs cures the disease, but may slow its progress with fewer known side effects than other medications currently prescribed. However, there are concerns about the risk of heart attacks and strokes for users of COX-2 inhibiting drugs. Enter the drug name in the search window at www.fda.gov to find details.

The insurance company AARP's magazine and *Arthritis Today,* the publication of the Arthritis Foundation, routinely carry articles on coping with painful arthritis symptoms, asserting that science is "moving closer to a cure for arthritis" and describes "the latest breakthrough" but this seems to be merely a prelude to announcing the latest palliative drug. Most of their full-page TV and magazine ads are paid for or subsidized by major pharmaceutical companies.

The agenda appears to be a search for a *revenue-generating* "cure." Off-patent, older drugs are not profitable, so they are not promoted in favor of costly new drugs that may or may not have equivalent effectiveness. E.g., tetracycline is in the common domain, it is cheap to manufacture for human treatments and available in various formulations, but it is not promoted because its profit margin is low. As seen in Chapter 4, more money can be made in producing tetracycline antibiotics for livestock feed.

The global market for arthritis drugs in 2008 was worth $35 billion, out of which TNFα inhibitors accounted for sale of $18 billion. Branded NSAIDs, OTC drugs and generics generated sales of $10 billion, COXIBs at $3.7 billion and DMARDs $3 billion in 2008. Enbrel with sales of $7.4 billion was the market leader followed by Remicade with sales of $6.5 billion and Humira at $4.5 billion. Enbrel, Remicade, and Humira all showed annual gains of over $1 billion in 2009.[17]

The cost of Enbrel or Humira for one month (without insurance) is about $2,000. By contrast, a supply of minocycline taken 3 times per week for one year costs about $600. Tetracycline and doxycycline, which are often substituted for minocycline, cost about $90 per year.[18]

Following the nutritional advice described in Appendix II in conjunction with the antibiotic protocol not only relieves symptoms in many cases but also may lead to remission or at least help immune inhibitors to work better.

In the words of the late Dr. Harold Clark,[19] "A major financial consequence of a debilitating and costly disease like arthritis in a majority of senior citizens has been the serious erosion of our Social Security system." Expensive drugs, treatments, and operations also sap Medicaid and Medicare funds (which are a portion of Social Security tax income), and increase private insurance premiums.

The Pathway to Restoring Health

The approach to remission from chronic infectious diseases like Rheumatoid Arthritis involves a coordinated strategy involving several steps:

- identify, understand, attack, and remove the cause(s) of the infection;
- neutralize toxins and destructive enzymes;
- flush toxins from the body;
- avoid artificial (processed) foods, environmental toxins, and unhealthful food additives (e.g., sugar, Canola oil, MSG);
- consume the proper mix of essential natural and antimicrobial foods;
- give up unhealthy lifestyle habits (e.g., drugs, smoking, alcohol to excess);
- identify vitamin/mineral deficiencies and take appropriate supplements;
- seek benign, natural methods to reduce stress and pain, and in turn, reduce dependency on toxic drugs.

Attempting to achieve one step without the others is useless. Our physicians must be part of the first step—to identify and eliminate the multiple systemic infections through the sophisticated testing methods at their disposal. Guessing at a diagnosis and/or prescribing only immuno-suppressing NSAIDs or DMARDs without the right antibiotic(s) protocol is not the best or optimal answer, nor is it good science. Long term, it is harmful and shortens life.

Should the multi-infection hypothesis be universally accepted to be correct and useful, the treatment of RA will need to be slightly revised, but the consequences for the pharmaceutical industry will be enormous. It could become unethical to use only steroids or agents that block prostaglandin synthesis, as we cannot be sure they do not promote the proliferation of other harmful organism(s), and so eventually will lead to more severe disease. Alternative benign regimens and immuno-therapeutic protocols will need to be developed for other rheumatic and so-called "autoimmune" illnesses caused by, or triggered by, infections.

When one's health is undermined by improper lifestyle habits, the dysfunctional condition cannot be fixed solely by wonder drugs. The body has the potential to heal itself, but it may take time, insightful treatments, and a conscientious effort to retrain all systems to work together in a balanced manner, e.g., Dr. Klenner's protocol for MS treatment.[20]

RA and other chronic diseases will occur if any or all of the following factors are present, which correspond to the four kinds of stress (biochemical, environmental, spiritual, behavioral). The following are examples.

Biochemical stress:
- There is a gradual buildup of polymicrobial parasite(s) populations and toxins in the body without sustained antimicrobial immune defense;

- The cause(s) of the infection is/are not identified, suppressed or removed;
- Toxins, heavy metals, and harmful enzymes are not eliminated but remain and cluster in the body;
- Vaccine adjuvant toxins[21] remain in the body for a long time, persistently exciting the immune system;
- Vaccines cause adverse long-term immune system hyperactivity against central nervous system molecules that are similar to the virus envelope;
- Mineral deficiencies or imbalances (e.g., calcium, potassium, magnesium, phosphorus, zinc, copper) lead to immune system dysfunction; and/or
- Cardiovascular systems have deteriorated through poor circulation, plaque, blockages, low CoQ_{10} levels, and degraded oxygen transport.

Environmental Stress:

- Prolonged exposure to contaminated air/water/food, pollens, dust mites, mold spores/toxins, MTBE, inorganic (chromium, nickel, mercury, aluminum, lead, cadmium, selenium) residues, and pesticides affect many bodily systems, especially the immune system;
- Excess heat/cold or wet clothes increase the stress of outdoor activities.

Spiritual stress:

- Mental stress causes faster pulse rate, headaches, high blood pressure, anxiety, depression;
- Psychological, financial, career, and/or family discord factors can increase chemical stress levels.

Behavioral stress:

* The immune system is weakened by months or years of drugs, improper diet, alcohol, smoking, lifestyle-stress, allergies, and chronic infection(s);
* Joint capsules are damaged by extreme exercise or sports injuries;
* Poor dietary habits include foods that overtax the immune system and rob cells of nourishment to grow, maintain, and repair;
* Muscle tone is soft and circulation (especially lymph system function) is poor because the body lacks exercise;
* Excess weight puts strain on joints, organs, and the skeletal system; and/or
* Lungs are weak through habitual shallow breathing, COPD, or heavy smoking.

When joints, especially load-bearing joints, are surrounded by weak muscles, it does not take a significant motion out of the normal range of the joint (or long term repetitive motion) to cause serious tissue damage to the area. The pressure of inflamed tissue on the joints and nerves can be both painful and harmful.

Maintaining normal weight, adopting good nutrition habits, and staying physically fit can be a challenging but achievable goal, one worth targeting to be free of the pain and immobility of arthritis. Adopting a healthy regimen requires some work and persistence, especially if the body has been out of shape for a long time. It could take as much as one full year of proper diet and gentle exercise to achieve effective total body functioning after removing the infection(s).[22]

Reducing the four kinds of stress is an important step to attaining a healthy lifestyle. Stress depletes vitamin C. Countless studies have shown that high levels of ascorbate significantly increase stress tolerance.

Foreign Medical Systems

Medical professionals in foreign nations have a longer history of different medical traditions, admitting a variety of approaches and philosophies of life, proven traditional plant medicines, alternative therapies, and theories of how the body works and reacts to chemical substances. Physicians in Europe, India, and Asia often prescribe herbal remedies, enzyme treatments, physical therapies (e.g., acupuncture, yoga and massage), and also nutritional supplements as well as standard pharmaceuticals.

Foreign medicine systems do not have, nor do they claim to have, any magical cures for the various and complex forms of arthritis and rheumatic diseases. But they seem much more open to consideration of a wider range of treatment options than their U.S. counterparts.

There are exceptions, of course. An example is the story[23, 24] of brilliant French-Canadian microbiologist Gaston Naessens who in the 1940s developed a microscope with enlargement at 30,000X. This device used ultraviolet and light technology, and was much better than the classical optical microscope (1,800X) but certainly not as powerful as the electron microscope (400,000X). The 714X compound he developed as a cancer treatment consists of a mixture of camphor, ammonium chloride and nitrate, sodium chloride, ethanol, and water. It must be injected into a lymph node in the groin. Three series of 21 daily injections are the minimum treatment.

Naessens asserted that 714X was successful in reversing the disease in over 75% of 1,000 cases of cancer and more than 30 cases of AIDS. 714X is designed to reinforce and strengthen a weakened, dysfunctional immune system by making lymph channels more efficient and directing nitrogen to the cancer and lymph cells in order to stop their toxic secretions.

His findings were publicly ridiculed and the medical bureaucracy arranged to have him deported from France. Naessens continued his research in Quebec, Canada. In 1989, he was again arrested and ostracized when another physician misused his 714X formulation, resulting in the death of a patient. Naessens was tried, but acquitted.

Naessens hypothesized that there are microscopic, dense particles he called "somatas" that energize the cells of all living beings. These somatids are living organisms, distinctly different forms from cell wall bacteria and viruses, with their own life cycle observable with his high-powered "Somatoscope." He asserted that if somatids are exposed to an assault (such as trauma, pollution, or radiation) they begin an uncontrolled growth cycle leading to cancer. A somatid is a tiny shape-changing (pleomorphic) cell invading organism responsible for cancer and many other degenerative diseases. 714X injections supposedly return the somatids to a normal state.

Could it be that Naessens' somatids are actually CWD bacteria,[25] L-forms, or Mycoplasmas? His theories concerning the etiopathogenesis of cancer were then, and still are, not consistent with prevailing mainstream medical and scientific opinion. *Mycoplasma fermentans* invades healthy cells, disrupting their ability to function. The failure of cells to auto-destruct (apoptosis) may be the root cause of cancer.

Currently 714X, an apoptosis enhancer, is available in Canada, Mexico, and Western Europe but not in the U.S., where it is still (after 10 years) under investigation but not approved by the FDA.[26] Do not look for approval any time soon. This low cost alternative treatment competes with a multi-billion dollar cancer drug "industry."[27]

The Somatoscope (UV microscope) is now finally recognized as an indispensable instrument for precise measurement of living and moving microbial life forms in some research laboratories and in industry.[28] These microscopes are available to researchers in some facilities to visualize Mycoplasmas and other small microbes in the blood, cerebral spinal fluid, lymph, and synovial joint fluids.

With UV microscopy, a size/shape taxonomy could conceivably be developed to permit identification of ultra-tiny microorganisms and immune system components characteristic of viral and microbial infections. Computer image input would permit shape recognition algorithms to classify categories of shapes and compute frequency/population histograms of the most common shapes. Some population patterns are normal but others indicate pathogenic conditions.[29]

As new electromagnetic (EM) frequency bands have opened up for both irradiation and detection it now becomes possible to create UV and other band spectroscopes, scanners, and molecule-resonance exciters and detectors. Science is finally catching up to the inventions of Doctor Royal Rife and Gaston Naessens.

The U.S. Medical System

The needless suffering of Lyme Disease (LD) patients for the last two decades is an indication of the failure of medical science to look beyond current dogma to develop new and more dependable testing methods for alternate strains of LD-causing organisms.

It is also a failure of insurance companies and the government medical bureaucracy to protect the public health by yielding to pressure from lobbyists and corporations to approve new symptom-relieving drugs for individuals desperate to get pain relief.

The active opposition to long-term multi-antibiotic LD treatment protocols is a parallel to the politicization of the search to find root causes of chronic disease as described in the late Dr. Clark's insightful book *Why Arthritis?*.

The problem is not that doctors are insensitive and uncaring. Access to health care has become so ineffectual and frustrating that most patients don't bother seeking help until they are in dire distress. Managed care has become a system of bureaucrats requiring authorizations to perform even the most basic health care procedures.

Patients pay a $10-$30 co-payment for an office visit but are blocked from seeing the right kind of doctor at any time. One cannot see a specialist without a referral from the assigned primary care physician. The wait for these two appointments may take months. There are severe restrictions on particular tests, therapies, and medications allowed by the patient's HMO based on negotiations with the insurance company gatekeepers.

Denial of medical services is not always apparent, but delay is typical. One of the more common means of withholding services is "rationing by omission." This means that patients are simply not told all of the possible options for their medical condition. They are only informed of those treatments covered by their insurance.[30] The doctor receives only about 30% of the fees charged, with a large percentage of the remainder going to overhead and to the multiple layers of insurance administrators.[31]

To avoid being a victim of this sort of rationing, the patient must research his/her medical condition as deeply as possible and come prepared to discuss alternatives. When the patient or the doctor requests a particular service, and the health plan denies the request, the reason is usually that the requested service is not "medically necessary"—a subjective term often based on the cost of the procedure. In some instances, doctors hamstrung by contractual commitments to perform only insurance carrier-specified procedures will quietly send their patients to physicians who do offer the required treatment, but the cost must be borne by the patient.

Admittedly, the multi-dimensional nature of testing for the cause of a complex chronic infection is difficult and expensive. However, the cost of incomplete testing is reflected in an increasing number of chronic illness patients putting a strain on all prepaid health care funds. Managed care was sold to the public as a means to control the rising cost of health care, but it has evolved into a huge administration with a growing bureaucracy of its own to support. HMOs circumvent some of this insurance overhead.

Today's U.S. medical system is dysfunctional:

- Patients are not counseled by their doctors in detail on proper nutrition or about antimicrobial supplements;

- HMOs may provide nutrition courses[32] that merely teach marketing propaganda and leave out important ideas such as vitamin C as an anti-stress supplement, or the benefits of natural/essential oils (seen in Chapter 3);

- Vaccines (described in Chapter 4) can be contaminated and flu shots often fail to match mutated strains;

- Existing diagnostic tests are unreliable, and unnecessary surgeries are often performed based on those tests;

- Many blockbuster drugs (e.g., statins[33]) have harmful side effects and cause symptoms that require other drugs to offset;

- Patients are forced to fend for themselves, researching their own conditions using the library or the Internet or, in some cases, self-medicating or seeking treatment or lower cost drugs outside the United States.

Those patients who are aggressive about presenting documented evidence to their doctors have a much better chance of obtaining effective treatments that will not only relieve their symptoms but also achieve long-term success.

The primary goal of this book is to educate patients in ways to approach their physicians with substantial evidence of proven treatments.

Persecution of "Maverick" Doctors

In 1988 Dr. Brown, a successful rheumatologist and physician of last resort for arthritis, was encouraged that the medical community had begun to recognize the risks associated with conventional arthritis treatments using toxic drugs. He was hopeful that researchers would revisit the neglected but successful methods of the early 1950s, before what he called the "cortisone revolution." However, he was dismayed that fewer than a dozen of the several hundred grants awarded to pursue arthritis research were looking at an infection connection to chronic illness.[34]

Dr. Brown was not the first physician whose findings upset the medical community's status quo. As seen in the accounts of Gaston Naessens and Doctors Blount, Prosch, and Rife, acceptance of new theories is glacially slow. Scientific skepticism is laudable, but when hundreds of documented experiments and studies are ignored and their authors branded as "mavericks" or worse, it calls into question the scientific pretenses and arrogance of some medical skeptics.

Another example illustrates the point. Dr. Laszlo K. Csatary of the United Cancer Research Institute has been publishing clinical observations on viral oncotherapy in major medical journals for three decades. Dr. Csatary first used a viral vaccine to treat cancer patients with "apathogenic" (i.e., "friendly") viruses in 1968. However, this technique has only gained attention in 2001 as a new and innovative approach.[35] Note that at one time, Mycoplasmas used to be apathogenic.

Why does it take so long for the medical intelligentsia to recognize techniques that are proven to work? One reason is that they apply a different standard of proof to so-called "controversial" treatments: (a) they only accept as proven those studies done by a small subset of researchers from certain universities or laboratories; (b) those in control of awarding grants refuse to approve studies they deem to be unworthy according to dubious (agenda-driven) standards.

Medical journals contain countless articles on the failure of current drug therapies for RA as well as credible studies advancing the theory of infectious organisms as the cause. Those doctors who ignore these studies usually are convinced only when they (or someone close to them) become ill and they find that conventional therapies fail to help. U.S. doctors and dentists who seek alternative treatments that they would not prescribe for their own patients routinely visit Mexico's clinics.[36]

Rheumatologists who are especially critical of Dr. Brown's work seem to be the first to denounce any new alternative to symptomatic treatment. They are reluctant to consider any therapy that does not conform to the prevailing medical community's mindset or to their own medical school training, which may be decades old. They seem curiously defensive and protective of their assumed role as the only appointed purveyors of treatments for rheumatic conditions.[37] Many do not work with support groups.

A good example: Dr. Robert A. Greenwald of the American Council on Science and Health roundly criticized *The Road Back* on the Internet and put Dr. Brown's regimen in the category of 'Worst of the Worst." Rheumatologist Greenwald claimed that the only effect of minocycline is to reduce the action of collagenase, and that for arthritis symptom reduction it has no more effect than a mild NSAID or even a placebo, when it actually does much more.

The 1985 study that Dr. Greenwald cited[38] was requested by Dr. Brown and funded by the Arthritis Institute of the National Hospital, Arlington, VA and Johns Hopkins. Unfortunately, the study was done incorrectly. It was carried out by an incompetent statistical organization that was solely responsible for its design, the abstraction of primary medical records, and the summarization and analysis of patient data reported in the final manuscript. Dr. Brown was too ill to correct the conclusions and it stands, erroneous, as published. After Dr. Brown's death in 1989, team researchers offered to redo the study and to correct the mistakes. However, there was no money available to fund the work.

There have been several important, subsequent studies— much more controlled and with many more participants— that should nullify the faulty 1985 study. However, this flawed study continues to be cited worldwide, doing a great disservice to RA sufferers and also to Dr. Brown's important contribution to rheumatology.

Obstacles to Antibiotic Treatment

Physicians may be reluctant to use the Marshall Protocol or the long-term, low-dose antibiotic regimen as advocated by Dr. Brown for any of several psychological or economic reasons, including:[39]

- Many physicians are not familiar with the appropriate administration protocols for long-term treatment with combinations of antibiotics;[40, 41]

- The Herxheimer reaction may be mistaken for an allergic reaction to the antibiotic and the patient is ordered to stop using the protocol;

- Candidiasis and other gut disorders may develop if probiotics are not ordered as part of the treatment;

- Many patients are not disciplined enough to stay the course of a sustained treatment lasting months or years, even if it is clearly explained to be beneficial;

- Doctors may be reluctant to use antibiotics because they have been over-prescribed in the past;

- "Do no harm" has become "Take no risks" because of constricting malpractice insurance rules.

RESEARCH TOOLS ARE INCOMPLETE

The search for the root causes of disabling chronic diseases and polymicrobial infections should be among the top issues of our government's national health policy. If our war against pathogenic microbes is to be given a priority on a par with national defense, we need to enlist the resources of the CDC, the National Academy of Science, and the NIH to develop research tools, machines, and capabilities such as:

- Complete online library of genetic codes, recipes, and shapes linked to sub-libraries of:
    - microorganism genetics and taxonomy
    - pathogenic microbe database (i.e., the FDA's "Bad Bug Book" of pathogens, diseases, tests, symptoms, etc.)[42]
    - organic genetic specialty associations
    - DNA-PCR markers and gene associations

- Antigen/molecule test marker design
- Classification tools for microbiological taxonomy and molecular recipe taxonomy
- Molecular EM spectroscopes and analyzers
- Molecule-shape library and recipes for molecule fabrication (either organic synthesis or via DNA-RNA templates to make useful molecules and enzymes via template-building and replication or by fermentation using gene-tailored microbes)
- UV and other band microscopes with video shape recognition image analysis software and pattern matching/recognition algorithms

Organizing such an enormous body of data is a huge effort requiring both a logical data framework and a professional staff with medical, biochemistry, DNA analysis, computer science, and database management skills. These data must be accurately cataloged and organized according to retrieval and presentation standards that facilitate use.

Security of the data may become an issue based on the rights of the owner, and on the possibility of terrorist misuse. Access control will require knowing the identity, affiliation, and location of each person granted access, and time and extent of access to each sensitive item in a library of protected data. This type of access record-keeping is quite feasible to implement.[43] Similar methods track viewing of Internet ads, gathering data to determine future purchases based on demographics.

A Suggested Testing Approach

One of the disturbing aspects of chronic illness is that it can be the result of complex polymicrobial infections. It is beyond the scope of this book to document and describe all chronic illnesses and so-called autoimmune disorders.

However, there appear to be categories of chronic diseases clearly attributable to identified sources such as Mycoplasma, insect-borne spirochetes, mycotoxins, molds, inhaled bacteria, and viruses that cause respiratory infection followed by migration to invasion colonies (biofilms) where the microbes live inside and around epithelial cells.

The major obstacle to targeted treatment is a system of accurate testing and diagnosis. The Pareto chart in Figure 7 shows the scope of the pathogen classification problem in a hypothetical way.[44] The chart shows a large number of possible causative factors for rheumatic diseases, but many of these have very low actual occurrence rates. There is also an incubation period (weeks to months or even years) from initial infection until the arthritic symptoms appear, as reported by persons who have Lyme Disease.

Figure 7. Hypothetical Pareto Chart of RA Causative Agents

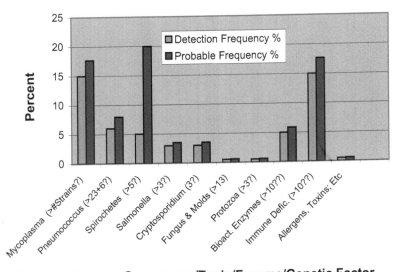

Possible Agents: Suppressor/Toxin/Enzyme/Genetic Factor

The numbers given in the chart are notional, and not derived from actual statistics. The chart shows what might be seen if data could be collected in a complete manner, and values varying by geographical region and with time.

The percentage values for each pathogen-factor charted show two bars. The first (light-shaded bar) is the hypothetical measured percentage of positive test results for the factor (i.e., the detection frequency). The second (dark bar) is based on the first bar value, divided by the test effectiveness. Effectiveness depends upon the number of false negatives. No false negatives means effectiveness is 1. False positives are not considered in this simplified model.

For many of these factors' currently-used test methods, a high level of false negatives exists due to unidentified factors in the category that are not tested for, so the effectiveness of the test may actually be near zero.

Measured percentages also are quite possibly near zero for significant factors, so the second bar reflects errors resulting from $(\sim 0) \div (\sim 0)$ values. Improvements in measures of test effectiveness are needed so that such a chart will depict meaningful relationships. Identifying as many causative organisms as possible, all their associated strains, and testing for all of them are necessary to make these improvements. This is a very tall order. But an added benefit of this kind of data collection would be that blood test results would be predictive of future donors' medical problems, since the growth of the organisms is very slow, and the harm they do is cumulative.

Until effective microchip screening tests are developed that are low cost, we will continue to be limited to testing for only the most significant likely diseases that have cost-effective tests available. HMOs, doctors, and insurance plans require some reasonable probability of a positive result. If tests are expensive and often have negative or borderline results, they will not be used.

Fortunately, the science of DNA testing is becoming more affordable and yields results that can tell if an infection is currently active as distinguished from the old serum tests that merely show a history of infection.[45]

Endnotes and continuing research on topics in Chapter 9 can be found at www.RA-Infection-Connection.com

10. CONCLUSIONS

Billions of years before humans appeared on the scene, bacteria were competing in the primordial soup. Today, our bodies contain them as their "soup"—i.e., their biome. We are the vehicles by which both helpful and harmful microbes transport themselves from one place to another in order to invade, transform, reproduce, abide, set seed, and expel their seeds.

Within the microbes' universe, either our immune system fights them successfully, or more commonly, an uneasy truce is established with persistent invaders. Microbes in the colony carry DNA-coded recipes to assemble molecules that add to and/or detract from our chemical processes and control our immune reactions.

The sum of these colonies' immunosuppressive actions degrades our immune system cumulatively. Colonies reside in our body cavities as biofilms where the microbes live together in a dynamic balance that is upset when a new colonist species or strain arrives, carrying possibly more pathogenic molecule-making recipes. Microbes that invade immune cells, tissues, organs and epithelial cells cause biochemical and energy-related dysfunctions in the cells' mitochondria.

Dr. Thomas McPherson Brown and his associates worked for over 40 years to understand the activity of Mycoplasmas and other cell wall-deficient (CWD) bacterial L-forms whose sizes and genetic complexity range in-between viruses and cell wall-bounded prokaryotes.[1] An accumulating body of evidence links these CWD microbes and their invaded-cell dysfunctions as primary and co-factors in chronic degenerative diseases such as Rheumatoid Arthritis, sclerotic pathologies, Sarcoidosis, CFIDS, Fibromyalgia, Scleroderma, ALS,[2] and Lupus.

It is likely that all invading pathogens (yeasts, bacteria, viruses, prions, fungi, protozoa, amoebas, protists, and worms) are persistent parasites that have CWD forms, re-seed forms, cysts, and other forms that invade the target host's blood, tissue, and/or epithelial cells for replication purposes. The malaria plasmodium microbe life cycle is typical of this multiplicity of shapes. More has been learned about infectious microorganisms in the last thirty years than was known in all previous recorded history but scientists have cataloged only a few of their forms and functions.

Microbes have pleomorphic forms inside their hosts because persistence and replication are necessary to be able to leave the host at the right season, with the right transport mechanism, and in quantities to be able to infect new hosts. Otherwise, the parasite species would die out.

The cell invaders siphon energy from the host cells, contributing to the host's lethargy, depression, fatigue, pain, and even psychological symptoms like schizophrenia. Some changes have the effect to increase or decrease the host's need for certain vitamins according to the invaders' needs.

We accumulate microbial parasites as we age. Invaded cells with their acquired mitochondrial dysfunctions are everywhere in the body and must die naturally or be killed-off and replaced. This process must be done slowly, because the cell renewal process from stem cells is slow. The more invaded cells there are, the more the inflammation and ROS, and the more antioxidants (vitamins A, B, C, E, and CoQ$_{10}$) we need. Leukemia viruses and some other microbes invade stem cells themselves.

Microscopic insects like mites, chiggers, no-see-ums, fleas, etc. are carriers associated with complex microbial colonization similar to Lyme arthritis.[3] The microbiome of these insect-borne pathogens remains a biological Terra Incognita with countless untracked strains.

NEW PARADIGMS FOR A NEW MILLENNIUM

Chronic illness takes far more than a physical toll. It translates to billions of dollars in health care costs and lost productivity. The scourge of chronic disease will not go away without functional medicine-based treatments of each of the parasite infections that are linked to the dysfunctions and the inflammations. Understanding of the *full* life cycle of every pathogenic microbe can lead to the targeting of points of vulnerability where its proliferation can be blocked. Adequate and sustained funding for basic research in this area needs to be targeted at filling in the gaps in our knowledge, starting with the most problematic strains.

A new NIH initiative called the Human Microbiome Project[4] akin to the Human Genome Project was launched in 2008 to characterize microbial communities. The five-year international Project will focus on five body sites: oral, skin, vaginal, gut, and nasal/lung. Some 3,000 genomic sequences of individual bacterial isolates are planned. This effort holds great promise for new discoveries that will open doors to our understanding the complexities of autoimmune disease and chronic illness and in turn, effective treatments.

Iatrogenic Health Problems

Faulty testing. The goal is to identify truly effective eradication protocols including tests that eliminate false negatives. We now know enough about pathogens to stop pretending that the causes of chronic illnesses are a mystery. We should get on with the job of killing the harmful microbes that infect most all of us humans using information, tools, and methods already available. In addition, we can more fully identify helpful probiotic microbes, their genetics, and catalog the bio-molecules that each strain makes.

Change the basis of nutrition from how to sell products and instead look at the *essential food elements* that we all need as a precursor to healthy molecular chemistry. Scientists should focus more attention on slow-growing infections that develop as a result of gut microbe imbalance, as shown in Chapter 3.

Ultrasound has been used with increasing power levels to the point where it can in certain circumstances be dangerous. Prenatal ultrasound exposure may cause later neural maturation dysfunction leading to Autism Spectrum Disorder symptoms, as discussed in Chapter 5. Appropriate safety standards must be updated and enforced.

Vaccines: Problems persist in the way[5] the U.S. has administered and approved vaccination programs in the past where negligent supervision and approvals without proof of safety[6] have been reported. Examples are live HIV in Hepatitis B[7] and SV-40 in live polio vaccines; Mycoplasmas found in many live virus vaccines. Years later, SV-40 appeared as a cancer co-factor due to widespread live polio vaccinations.[8] CDC vaccination guidelines have been published and followed but they have safety-gap loopholes that occasionally lead to preventable tragedies.[9]

In the UK, administrators approved an unsafe Japanese strain of mumps vaccine, banned in Canada, over expert objections. It proved to be a medical and political disaster. As seen in Chapter 5, the U.S. Vaccine Court system for autism-related claims is broken. Insurance funds are far too low[10] to cover the actual costs of the harm caused.[11]

Scurvy and illnesses coincident with vaccinations have led to Sudden Infant Death Syndrome (SIDS), Shaken Baby Syndrome (SBS), Munchausen's Syndrome By Proxy, and lasting neural injury.[12] Live vaccines are unsafe for those with infection-produced mitochondrial dysfunction, with impaired immune systems, with heart disease, and susceptible genetic subgroups.[13]

Diagnosis of Multiple Infections

The traditional search for a single cause of Gulf War Illness and other chronic diseases is indicative of a flawed mindset—oversimplification based on Occam's razor.[14] New testing methods and diagnostic tools have demonstrated that individuals can be afflicted with *polymicrobial* infections, needing a combination of antimicrobial treatments. It is only logical to believe that in a lifetime a person will become colonized with a multitude of microorganisms. The entrenched practice of seeking a single common pathological cause to explain a given disease is outmoded and overdue for revision. Co-infections are present in all of us. In the case of chronic illness, pathogenic microbes, genetics, and faulty nutrition combine to produce injurious results.

A new approach to the understanding of chronic rheumatic diseases like RA and Lyme Disease must be developed. To do so will involve knowledge from a variety of medical disciplines such as virology, microbiology, lymphology, bacteriology, immunology, epidemiology, and parasitology. These are currently considered separate fields with their own goals and methodologies.

Perhaps the new field of microbial ecology will unite rather than divide scientists, emphasizing links rather than differences. The Institute for Functional Medicine[15] has made great strides in presenting patient/clinician education programs that break down walls among medical disciplines to avoid insular research that stifles progress in diagnosis and treatment.

One goal of research is to understand and to map the genetic complexity of these microorganisms and then to relate this genetic map to harmful/beneficial effects on the host. The traditional two-dimensional matrix that maps antibiotic drug(s) to microorganism(s) has become five-dimensional as we add strains, the various pathogens' toxin/enzymes and the effects of the drugs on bioactive molecules/cells' physiology/organs/systems of the body. The same is true for antiviral drugs. These data need to be online for all to reference. Some data are beginning to appear on the Internet at NIH/NLM, but persistent searching must be done. Often only abstracts are visible, and sometimes access to important studies is deliberately blocked. (See Chapter 9).

Treatment of Multiple Infections

The conventional RA treatment with powerful steroids, antibiotics, antihistamines, interferon- and TNF-disablers, T-cell killers, and immunosuppressive drugs upset the immune system, sometimes facilitating the gradual proliferation of the invading colonies. Effective anti-mycoplasmal drugs intensify an inflammation (Herxheimer) reaction. Therefore, a treatment combining a specific anti-microbial antibiotic and an effective anti-inflammatory should be used.[16]

Tetracycline family (minocycline), quinine-based, and fluoroquinolone antibiotics such as Ciprofloxacin have shown strong effectiveness against the various strains of Mycoplasma and bacterial CWD L-forms.[17] Longer term, lower dosage use of certain tetracyclines, sometimes with short periods of on/off administration, often starts to become effective after just a few weeks or months. Treatments spanning eighteen months or more are frequently needed to avoid relapses.

There are many patients who do not improve on the single antibiotic protocol advocated by Dr. Thomas McPherson Brown. E.g., Lyme Disease patients also have chronic neuroborreliosis. These conditions require much higher doses of antibiotics in order to get the serum concentrations to levels high enough to penetrate the blood brain barrier. A wider range of antibiotics must be used, including anti-protozoal, anti-malarial drugs for Babesiosis.

Similarly, the Questran/cholestyramine protocol[18] advocated by Dr. Ritchie Shoemaker can be helpful in controlling some (not all) of the symptoms which result from the Herxheimer "die-off" effects of toxins that are released by the dead and dying spirochetes.[19]

The Marshall Protocol is another example of a successful multi-pronged antimicrobial treatment.[20] Sadly, the medical establishment has not fully appreciated or adopted long-term antibiotic protocols, as discussed in Chapter 9.

Passage of antibiotic pills through the gut provides opportunities for intestinal flora to develop resistance. Serum infusions (about $2,000 per series) or injected forms can avoid this problem but are not as convenient to administer, especially over a period of months or years.[21] Appropriate antibiotic delivery methods need to be developed, made affordable, used at the right stage of the disease, and administered for a time frame necessary to be effective.

GOVERNMENT ACTION

Many long-term treatment failures related to chronic infection include IBS, chronic cystitis, AIDS, COPD,[22] Autism/ASD, heart disease, cancers, Gulf War Illness, diabetes, hypoglycemia, Metabolic Syndrome, autoimmune diseases, tick-borne diseases, Mycoplasma infections, and many more. In addition to these, outbreaks of well-known diseases like tuberculosis and malaria are returning in potentially epidemic proportions. Insufficient resources have been spent in ineffective ways to understand, control, and treat these diseases.[23]

Funding for Chronic Illness Research

The events of September 11, 2001 shifted national priorities to bioterrorism attacks, civilian defense, hostile nations' ongoing development of biological weapons, and disease control. Nevertheless, our government agencies must also greatly improve their effectiveness in the interest of public health and safety as a part of national defense against indigenous microbial attacks.

In December 2001, Congress approved an FY2002 appropriations bill (HR 3061) that increased total funding for all institutes under the NIH almost 16 percent to $26.6 Billion. However, two-thirds of the increase was earmarked for construction to protect NIH facilities against terrorist attacks[24]—a priority of bricks and mortar over knowledge improvement. While $26.6 Billion may appear to be large, compare the mere 1.06% of the $3.55 Trillion total FY2010 budget allocated for health research ($35 Billion) with the 20.14% allocated to Medicare plus Medicaid ($710 Billion), or another 20.04% for Social Security ($710 Billion).[25]

With an estimated 40 million sufferers, arthritis in all its varieties, including RA, is this nation's number one crippling disease.[26] It is also one of the most costly major socioeconomic problems in the U.S., but arthritis takes a back seat to funding for AIDS with about 1 million people infected.[27][28]

To put this in perspective: the $528 Million total NIH/NIAMS (National Institute of Arthritis and Musculo-skeletal and Skin Diseases) 2010 research budget[29] was equivalent to $13.20 per person of the estimated 40 million stricken with arthritis, if all NIAMS research dollars were devoted to studying that particular disease. Domestic HIV/AIDS research is funded at $18.2 billion, or $18,200 per patient.

Our public health organizations (NIH, CDC, FDA, and others) are increasingly coming to terms with the hazards that pernicious pathogens represent on a global scale.[30] They should request and receive adequate funding for:

- Etiopathogenic research of organisms such as fungi and molds, Mycoplasma, protozoa, worms, and spirochetes;
- Improvements in UV and multispectral microscopy;

- Development of comprehensive DNA/antibody/ antigen/anti-toxin tests; and
- Development, testing, cautious approval, and distribution of <u>safe</u> multivalent vaccines, anti-toxins, anti-enzymes, and antigens.

If these efforts are not pursued, the cost of existing chronic infections will still be paid in the form of increased costs for the health maintenance of United States Medicare participants, in decreased productivity of the workforce, and in human suffering by the millions throughout the world. The CDC estimated that health care costs for chronic disease treatment in 2008 accounted for over 75% of national health expenditures and 7 out of 10 deaths.[31]

Attention to particular non-HIV organisms should be granted international project status—far more encompassing than the Human Genome/Microbiome Projects—for a multi-disciplinary effort to find ways to render those organisms ineffective as a bioterrorism threat or as a cause of widespread medical problems approaching epidemic status.

The government should also consider humane methods to quarantine and/or treat those contagious persons who pose a public health danger to society.

Congress should take a hard look at the outlay of tax dollars for fruitless research, and insist that NIH funds be allocated to finding the probable suspect organisms being discovered and already documented in scientific publications.

Fixing a Broken Health Care System

Conventional wisdom asserts that the U.S. healthcare system is superior. It is not. Key areas need to be fixed:

1. Access to care. Insurance companies and HMOs have come to terms with the financial realities of chronic illness. They are finding new ways to deny coverage for the high cost of treating the chronically ill patient. By refusing to authorize crucial diagnostic tests in the short term, they only delay later claims for disabilities brought about by chronic disease. The universal healthcare controversy regarding expanding the coverage base with no added funds available to support it is not feasible. Managed, rationed care does not work. We need to reduce demand and make treatment simpler and more efficient. Preventive measures such as upping the DRI for vitamin C would be a universal benefit.

2. Treatment authorization. Insisting that doctors prescribe only from a mandated list of therapies and particular drugs limits the physician's ability to treat the patient's condition properly and in a timely manner. It makes it difficult if not impossible for new treatments to be authorized and applied. Doctors should not be censured for their judgment in prescribing more effective (and perhaps alternative) treatments, especially if they work.

"Evidence based medicine" (EBM) is code for "cost-based treatment with prejudicial selection independent of the patients' circumstances." The so-called evidence is an evaluation of treatments in meta-studies where inputs are subject to editorial selection to produce the desired outcome, i.e., by stacking the deck. This methodology is thoroughly non-scientific at worst. EBM is a fraud against insured patients, enabling insurers to control treatment costs and increases the number and seriousness of treatment failures.

3. Drug costs. The multiple cost of a physician visit, delays, transaction costs, and a high-cost drug could all be minimized with many more medications allowed to be prescribed by a pharmacist with unified patient drug records reviewed by database software for history, condition, or conflicts, and with patient's primary care doctor's oversight.

Low-cost drugs for arthritis such as quinine sulfate, doxycycline, aureomycin, and topical salves are candidates for this category. In many foreign countries, the professional pharmacist has a much greater role in drug selection and customer assistance without a physician intermediary.[32] WalMart is positioning a medical doctor at its pharmacies to allow their customers to access to low-cost common drugs. The usual drug/treatment approval rules are too complex, too costly to follow, and approval times take much too long.

Government efforts to make more OTC medications available would shift costs from insurance to the patients.

4. Lack of effective tests. A wider variety of quick, dependable, comprehensive tests for infectious agents must be made available to doctors so that chronic infections can be reliably detected and suppressed. Currently too many tests yield false negatives or equivocal results, e.g., Lyme.

However, until databases matching organism strains to symptoms and to targeted treatments (drugs, anti-toxins, vaccines, etc) become routinely available to the physician, access to crucial diagnostic indicators will not be possible. Doctors will continue to depend on a minimal, constrained set of tests and guesswork. Wider use of ascorbic acid as an anti-toxin and antimicrobial using Dr. Cathcart's proven benign method with over 9,000 patients would obviate the need for specific test results.[33] This approach, described in Appendix V, could lower treatment costs substantially and reduce demand for more costly services.

5. Use of antibiotics. Dr. Brown's low-dose, long-term antibiotic regimen trains the RA patient's immune system to fight resident pathogens gradually, over several months, or in some cases, years. It does not introduce the harmful side effects usually associated with indiscriminately prescribed broad-spectrum antibiotics that suddenly suppress the immune system and leave the patient open to new assaults. This protocol is described in Appendix II and also at rheumatic.org and roadback.org. Dr. Trevor Marshall's multi-antibiotic protocol is found at mpkb.org.

326 *Arthritis and Autoimmune Disease:*
The Infection Connection

6. Availability of safe vaccines. Many more vaccines that are now proven to be effective on animal subjects need to be developed for human use and tested for safety before they are made available. Prevention of chronic illnesses caused by microbial parasites should be a priority. Without vaccines, pathogenic organisms have many opportunities to establish colonies before symptoms become evident. By that time, these pathogens are difficult to eradicate. Coordination of vaccination with ascorbate intake will have a great effect on reducing adverse events. (See Appendix V).

7. Failure of the Vaccine Court. Unsafe live virus vaccines, given too early, without checking family genetics and/or the patient's ascorbate blood levels have led to a tiny number of extremely adverse reaction cases. The level of claims far exceeds the insurance funds. Politics and a statutory diversion of "surplus" insurance tax funds have led to a mass denial of justice for those cases.[34]

8. Treatment approvals for alternative therapies, no matter how convincing the evidence for efficacy and safety, appear to be stalled or outright derailed by drug companies intent on promoting their own profit-making products. The approval process calls into question the motives and agenda of the FDA.[35] High drug prices are needed to cover the high cost of the cumbersome FDA drug approval process imposed by government bureaucracy. Streamlining drug approval mechanisms would save huge developmental costs, and make new drugs available sooner, but should not sacrifice long-term safety. In the case of vaccines, the rush to market is too fast and safety has been sacrificed. (See Chapter 4.)

9. An intriguing new business model. The "Clinic at WalMart" in-store program offers walk-in medical services, injections, and immediate access to their low cost ($4/30day $10/90day supply) formulary of ethical drugs. WalMart has the global reach to buy worldwide from low production cost sources, providing high quality pharmaceuticals. They take cash or insurance at 140+ clinics nationwide. They buy prepackaged drugs from Canada, India, and other centers of production excellence. This system eliminates much of the overhead from pill counting, insurance, delayed billing and accounting. Franchised clinics are independently owned.[36]

10. Improvements in nutrition. There should be more public education reflecting the need for essential vitamins and the dangers of deficiencies. An FDA priority should be more emphasis on good fats and oils rather than supporting manufacturers' propaganda to sell low-cost products e.g., Canola oil, discussed in Chapter 7.

11. Chronic, persistent infections eradication. Viral, bacterial, fungal, and other microbial infections are reaching epidemic levels but are not considered a national health priority. Examples are failure to deal with Autism Spectrum Disorder (ASD) and to recognize the causes of Gulf War Illness. Some key factors are:

- increased Lyme/insect-borne reported infections;
- inconclusive diagnostic tests;
- polymicrobial syndromes dismissively attributed to "old age": arthritis, sclerotic disease, urinary/respiratory tract conditions, Alzheimer's, and many more;
- antibiotic(s) protocols controversy.

12. Improved safety, problem analysis, and control for vaccines, ultrasound, and cholesterol-lowering statin drugs. Politics and profit seem to be corrupting the science.[37] E.g., there is an almost religious fervor characterizing those who hold that vaccines play a part in ASD. Instead of taking a hard analytical view of the statistics and science, superficial understanding is circulated as "fact" on the Internet.[38]

13. Reporting systems are broken: Microbe-presence testing, disease reporting, and drug/vaccine adverse incident reporting systems are inadequate, are often designed to minimize serious problems and deny claims, or they produce false negative results. Treatments fail, public health costs are huge from untreated infection conditions, and vaccine disasters occur.[39]

HEALTH CARE INDUSTRY'S ROLE

Large private organizations such as the Arthritis Foundation are part of the U.S. health care industry. They use collected funds to cover the costs of managing a sizable bureaucracy, promoting the Foundation, operating classes teaching arthritis sufferers how to cope with symptoms, publishing an informative magazine, and lobbying for research. The Foundation solicits funds from charitable contributions as well as from major pharmaceutical companies who advertise in their monthly magazine.

The Arthritis Foundation's persistent appeals for federally funded research have paid off, but not to the point of producing conclusive improvements in medical outcomes. The Foundation aggressively lobbies for increased funding for its programs in the annual duel for scarce federal funds. In 2010, the Foundation obtained nearly $20 Million in government grants, but only $10.7 Million of their $111.6 Million total income was allocated to research. By contrast, $13 Million was spent on fundraising and about $42 Million on "public health education" (code for ads and lobbying).[40] That is, they spend $5.50 to get $1 for research.

The number of competing medical technology research areas is huge, and interdependent NIAID funding is also related to arthritis and inflammation. For every specific chronic illness there is at least one private foundation appealing for donations to find a cure, but because their research funding process is uncoordinated and sometimes misdirected, their efforts have had little payoff. Meanwhile, the pharmaceutical industry continues to develop "improved, new" drugs to relieve symptoms but usually with associated serious long-term side effects. Combined anti-inflammatory and antimicrobial treatments are still rarely applied.

The question arises: "Will there ever be a cure for arthritis?" If a cure were found, the drug companies would suffer a huge loss of income. The business case is clear: producing drugs to treat arthritis symptoms is a billion-dollar industry—why seek a cure and kill the golden goose?

Government assumption of total health care regulation and cost limitations provide a motive either for a cure or for reducing the numbers of the cases to be treated.

Because of the immunosuppressive nature of symptom-reducing drugs, the FDA must do a better job of carefully reviewing their long-term safety vs. short-term effectiveness. Enbrel is a good example. (See Chapter 7).

THE NEAR TECHNOLOGICAL HORIZON

Biotechnology is now producing DNA-based tools for more precise identification of pathogenic microorganisms by type and strain. For conditions like Lyme Disease where identification does not correspond with ordinarily effective treatment, more research is required to match organisms' strains with targeted treatments and to find the right combination of antibiotic(s)/vaccine(s)/anti-toxin(s). New biotechnologies will enable a better understanding of how the body's complex interrelated systems deal with resident microbes (both harmful and beneficial) as well as invading organisms. The result will be effective ways to prevent disease rather than merely deal with symptoms. The next goal will be a giant step toward reducing the permanent damage and debilitating effects of powerful, toxic drugs.

To the extent that Mycoplasmas, malaria-like microbes, and viruses invade the body's cells, new ways to identify the invaded cells and kill them must be found. This calls for more research on the mechanisms of apoptosis; for example, how radiation and toxic medicines potentiate apoptosis, and why apoptosis genes fail to make an invaded cell destroy itself.

But drugs are not the only answer. Natural means to prevent and combat chronic illness need to be more actively promoted. As seen in Chapter 7 and Appendix V, vitamin C should be rediscovered as an essential factor to good health.

ADVANTAGES OF A HOLISTIC APPROACH

Bolstering the patient's immune system while working to suppress a relentless inflammatory infection requires a holistic view of the individual. We are each unique in terms of nutritional needs, physiological factors, emotional outlook, environmental stressors, gut microbiome, genetic inheritance, infections acquired and retained, and induced allergies. It is encouraging that a growing number of physicians are using "integrative" medicine (also called "complementary" or "functional" medicine) to better treat their chronically ill patients. This holistic approach combines the best of conventional diagnoses and clinically proven treatments with documented, effective alternative therapies.

Once the pathogens have been correctly identified, their destructive features suppressed or the organisms eliminated, after allergens and toxins have been neutralized or removed,[41] then naturopathic methods can be applied. These benign treatments can be very effective in revitalizing the body's collective system of systems—especially the immune system—to ward off future infections and to reduce the symptoms and spread of chronic disease.

The respiratory tract and gastrointestinal (GI) tract are the first lines of defense against systemic infections.

Individuals diagnosed with autoimmune diseases like RA show one or more symptoms of chronic fatigue, allergies, inflammation, ROS, COPD, and chronic stress. They have weakened immune systems that can be traced to RT and GI tract epithelial infections. Treating RT and GI dysbiosis with tools such as antibiotics, antifungals, antivirals, special diets featuring antimicrobial foods and nutrients, digestive enzymes, prebiotics/probiotics, and vitamin supplements can be extremely effective in getting one's health back on track.

Patient's Responsibility

Nutritional understanding is an essential first step. The more we understand about our body's cellular makeup, its functions, and its nutritional needs, the better we know how to keep our body's systems in balance. We are responsible to eat right and avoid intake of harmful substances. The next step is to seek out a health care provider who can do more than prescribe pills to relieve symptoms. The doctor-patient relationship is a team effort to identify the cause(s) of the infection(s) and remove it/them. Diligence and commitment are necessary for an effective course of treatment.

The patient must also make lifestyle adjustments to strengthen the immune system. These adjustments include improving one's eating habits, avoiding allergens, quitting harmful addictions to sugar, refined grains, cigarettes, alcohol, antidepressants, narcotics, etc., and adding vitamins and supplements to counter deficiencies and dependencies. Specific tests may be required to identify allergens. A nutritionist can help develop a personalized dietary profile. Counseling may be required to help conquer addictions, deal with stress, and control negative emotions.

Each chronically ill patient (or family caregiver) must take an active role in managing his/her health. This means learning as much as possible about the condition and using all available resources to find the root cause. Powerful search engines on the Internet with appropriate key words open a gigantic pool of information to the public. Appendix IV points to some of the best online health references and resources now available to research symptoms and treatments, find similar case histories, participate in blogs and condition-related support group websites. Share what you learn about therapies, nutrition, vitamins, etc. with your doctor. Regional medical libraries are federally funded, with computers available for public use in most major cities.

One should not expect magical results from any regimen. Improvement/remission rates vary depending on a combination of factors: how conscientiously the patient follows the protocol (especially dietary requirements), age of the patient, number/severity of co-infections, other medical conditions, status of the immune system, and so forth. Even in cases where remission appears to be complete, a relapse or re-infection may occur after months or years; the protocol that the patient/doctor team adopts may need to be resumed.

For some chronic illness sufferers with severe and/or recurring infection(s), the regimen becomes a permanent lifestyle adjustment. Heredity plays a role in the susceptibility of an individual to recurring infection(s). Stress and new environmental factors may bring on re-infection or vitamin depletion and, in turn, the need for resumption of the protocol and increase in vitamin intake.

With drug companies promising "success" by using a powerful short-term medication, it is tempting to settle for immediate relief from pain. However, the definition of "success" should be eradication of the root cause of that pain—the microbes responsible.

THE ROAD TO REMISSION

There have been many books written about arthritis. Typically, these books either describe coping techniques or they advocate a particular substance that will act as a magic bullet to relieve painful symptoms. This substance could be pectin or yucca root or olive leaf extract or some unique combination of herbs. The truth is, there is no magic bullet because each of us has a unique, complex, and dynamically changing biochemical microbiome. So many influential factors contribute to our physiology—diet, metabolism, allergens, environmental conditions, immune system genetics, level of exercise, the way we handle stress, past exposure to chemicals (especially insecticides) , accrued biotoxins, and interactions with other medications—that the idea of a single cure for chronic illness is preposterous.

Various strains of infectious organisms have different sensitivities to the substances that may be able to suppress their activities. They can also send a "stop doing that" signal to the host via allergic flare-ups such as the Herxheimer reaction when they are adversely threatened by an effective treatment. Antibiotics, anti-inflammatories, and antioxidant vitamins should be used together to control the "Herx" flare.

Proven antibiotic treatment for Mycoplasma infection has for too long been labeled as "not adequately tested in humans" by the "authorities" controlling research, who themselves have worked to deny funding for such testing or have established test criteria based on short-term tests when long-term studies are indicated. Dr. Clark calls this "one of the greatest failures in medical history."[42]

RA sufferers are faced with the problem of finding physicians who will not only agree to test for mycoplasmal infection but also monitor their progress through a course of antibiotic treatment over a long period of time. A starting point is Dr. Franco's website (thearthritiscenter.com), Dr. Nicolson's website for the Institute for Molecular Medicine (immed.org), and Dr. Mercola's website (mercola.com).[43] Dr. Nicolson's website also provides information on disease identification, testing (for humans and pets), and treatment in over 100 publications that can be downloaded at no cost.

Dr. Vojdani's facility (immunoscienceslab.com) is a significant testing and research resource in southern California. Other testing labs are listed in Appendix III.

The nonprofit Road Back Foundation and the Arthritis Trust of America keep a database of doctors willing to employ the antibiotic protocol, at least as a probe to test for infection. Their discussion groups offer increased odds of finding a physician who will be receptive to the idea of trying Dr. Brown's regimen.[44, 45] Reports of reduction in painful symptoms and even remission using the methods described in this book are significant and encouraging. This means that millions of individuals in the U.S. are eligible for, and deserving of, new hope for the future and restored health.

Endnotes and continuing research on topics in Chapter 10 can be found at www.RA-Infection-Connection.com

BIBLIOGRAPHY

Dozens of health books and hundreds of medical articles were referenced to support the research presented in this book. More entries to the bibliography will be added as our research continues. To avoid using pages in this 3rd edition for a dynamically changing list, it is more efficient to put the full list on our website for access by the interested reader.

However, as a convenience for those who do not use a computer, an excerpt of this sizable bibliography is printed on the following pages. For the most up-to-date list of books, see www.RA-Infection-Connection.com/Bibliography.

For specific numbered references to medical studies and articles (often with hot links) supporting each chapter's topics, visit www.RA-Infection-Connection.com/Endnotes. Printing over 1,000 endnotes would dramatically increase the size and weight of this book.

Bibliography Excerpt

Airola, Paavo. *How To Get Well*. Health Plus Publishers: Phoenix, AZ, 1974.

Anderson JW, Trivieri L, and Goldberg, B. *Alternative Medicine: The Definitive Guide* (2nd updated edition), Celestial Arts, 2002.

Anderson, B., Pearl, B., and Burke, E. *Getting in Shape: 32 Workout Programs for Lifelong Fitness*. 2nd ed. Shelter Publications: Bolinas, CA, 2002.

Atkins, Robert C.. *Dr. Atkins' Vita-Nutrient Solution*. Simon & Schuster: New York, 1998.

Baker, Sidney. *Detoxification & Healing: The Key to Optimum Health*. (2nd ed.) McGraw-Hill, 2003.

Berger, Stuart M., M.D. *How to Be Your Own Nutritionist*. Avon Books: New York, NY, 1987.

Bingham, Robert, M.D. *Fight Back Against Arthritis*, Desert Arthritis Medical Clinic: Desert Hot Springs, CA, 1984.

Bliznakov, Emile G., M.D., and Hunt, Gerald L. *The Miracle Nutrient: Coenzyme Q_{10}*. Bantam Books: New York, 1989.

Bock, Kenneth, M.D. and Sabin, Nellie. *The Road to Immunity: How to Survive and Thrive in a Toxic World*. Simon & Schuster: New York 1997.

Bremness, Lesley. *Herbs*. Dorling Kindersley: New York, 1994.

Bricklin, Mark. *The Practical Encyclopedia of Natural Healing*. Penguin, 1990.

Brown, Thomas McPherson, M.D., and Scammell, Henry. *The Road Back: Rheumatoid Arthritis—Its Cause and Its Treatment*. M Evans and Company, Inc.: New York, 1988.

Cave, Stephanie and Mitchell, Deborah. *What Your Doctor May Not Tell You About™ Children's Vaccinations*. Grand Central Publishing, 2001.

Cawood, Frank. *Vitamin Side Effects Revealed*. FC&A Publishing: Peachtree City, GA, 1986.

Challem, Jack. *The Inflammation Syndrome: the complete nutritional program to prevent and reverse heart disease, arthritis, diabetes, allergies, and asthma*. Wiley, 2003.

Cho SS and Finocchiaro T, editors. *Handbook of Prebiotics and Probiotics Ingredients: Health Benefits and Food Applications*. CRC Press: Boca Raton, FL, 2010

Chuen, Lam Kam. *Tai Chi: The Natural Way to Strength and Health*. Simon & Schuster: New York, 1994.

Cichoke AJ, D.C. and Hoffer A, M.D. *Enzymes & Enzyme Therapy: How to Jump-Start Your Way to Lifelong Good Health*. McGraw-Hill, 2000.

Clark, Harold W. *Why Arthritis? Searching for the Cause and the Cure of Rheumatoid Disease.* Axelrod Publishing: Tampa Bay, FL, 1997.

Costerton, J.W. *The Biofilm Primer.* Springer, 2007.

Cousens, Dr. Gabriel. *Conscious Eating.* North Atlantic Books: Berkeley, CA, 1999.

Cousins, Norman. *Anatomy of an Illness as Perceived by the Patient.* Bantam Books: New York, 1981.

Crook, William G., M.D. *The Yeast Connection.* Random House: New York, 1986.

Cummings, Stephen, M.D. and Ullman, Dana. *Everybody's Guide to Homeopathic Medicines.* G.P. Putnam's Sons: New York, 1991.

Davis, William, M.D. *Wheat Belly.* Rodale Books, 2011.

Dewey, Laurel. *The Humorous Herbalist.* Safe Goods: Glenwood Springs, CO, 1996.

Diamond, Harvey and Diamond, Marilyn. *Fit For Life.* Warner Books: New York, 1985.

Di Fabio, Anthony and Prosch, Jr., Dr. Gus J. *Arthritis.* Arthritis Trust of America: Fairview, TN, 1997.

Dufty, William. *Sugar Blues.* Chilton Book Co.: PA 1975.

Egoscue, Pete. *Pain Free: A Revolutionary Method for Stopping Chronic Pain.* Bantam: 7th printing of the 1997 edition, 2000.

Elmsely, John and Fell, Peter. *Was it Something You Ate?* Oxford University Press: New York, 1999.

Erasmus, Udo. *Fats That Heal, Fats That Kill.* Alive Books: USA, 1999.

Ewald, Paul. *Plague Time: How stealth infections cause cancer, heart disease, and other deadly ailments.* Free Press, 2000.

Fredericks, Carlton. *Arthritis: Don't Learn to Live With It.* Grosset & Dunlap: New York, 1981.

Garrett, Laurie. *The Coming Plague.* Penguin Books: New York, 1995.

Garten, Max. *"Civilized" Diseases and Their Circumvention.* Maxmillion World Publishers: San Jose, CA, 1978.

Gerson, Charlotte with Beata Bishop. *Healing the Gerson Way: Defeating Cancer and Other Chronic Diseases.* Totality Books: Carmel, CA, 2007.

Gordon, Richard. *The Alarming History of Medicine: Amusing Anecdotes from Hippocrates to Heart Transplants.* St. Martin's Press: New York, 1993.

Jarvis, D. C, M.D. *Arthritis and Folk Medicine.* Fawcett Publications: Greenwich, CT, 1960.

Johnson, Hillary. *Osler's Web: Inside the Labyrinth of the Chronic Fatigue Syndrome Epidemic.* Crown Publishers, Inc.: New York, 1996.

Jones D, Bland, J, Quinn, S. *Textbook of Functional Medicine.* Institute for Functional Medicine, 2010.

Kroger, WS. *Clinical and Experimental Hypnosis* (2nd Revised ed.). Lippincott Williams & Wilkins: Philadelphia, PA, 2008.

Leviton, Richard. *The Healthy Living Space: 70 Practical Ways to Detoxify the Body and Home.* Hampton Roads Publishing, 2001.

Levy, Thomas E. *Curing the Incurable: Vitamin C, Infectious Diseases, and Toxins.* Livon Books: Henderson, NV, 2009.

Mandell, Marshall, M.D. *Dr. Mandell's 5-Day Allergy Relief System.* HarperCollins Books, 1988.

Mårin, Per and Farris, Russell. *The Potbelly Syndrome.* Basic Health Publications, 2005.

Mattman, Lida H. *Cell Wall Deficient Forms—Stealth Pathogens.* 3rd ed., CRC Press: Boca Raton, FL, 2000.

Mercola, Dr. Joseph. *The No-Grain Diet: Conquer Carbohydrate Addiction and Stay Slim for the Rest of Your Life.* Dutton, 2003.

Mindell, Earl. *New Vitamin Bible.* Grand Central Life & Style, revised and updated edition, 2011.

Nambudripad, Devi. *The NAET Guidebook.* (7th ed) Delta Publishing, 2009.

Newport, Mary, M.D. *Alzheimer's Disease: What If There Was a Cure?* Basic Health Publications, 2011.

Nicolson, Garth L. and Rosenberg-Nicolson, Nancy L. *Project Day Lily.* Xlibris Corp., 2005.

Null, Gary. *Gary Null's Ultimate Anti-Aging Program.* Kensington Books: New York, NY. 1999. [Based on the PBS Documentary "How to Live Forever."]

Pauling, Linus. *How to Live Longer and Feel Better.* Oregon State University Press, 2006.

Poehlmann, Katherine. *Rheumatoid Arthritis: The Infection Connection.* Satori Press, 2002.

Scammell, Henry. *The New Arthritis Breakthrough.* M. Evans & Co., 1998.

Shoemaker, Dr. Ritchie C. *Surviving Mold.* Otter Bay Books, 2010.

Shomon, Mary J. *Living Well with Chronic Fatigue Syndrome and Fibromyalgia.* William Morrow, 2005.

Stone, Irwin. *The Healing Factor: Vitamin C Against Disease.* Putnam Group, 1974. [The entire book is available online at no charge: www.vitamincfoundation.org/stone/]

Teitelbaum, Jacob, M.D. *From Fatigued to Fantastic.* 3rd ed. Avery, 2007.

Toivanen, Auli and Toivanen, Paavo. *Reactive Arthritis.* CRC Press, Inc.: Boca Raton, FL, 1988.

Trager, Dr. Milton. *Trager Mentastics*. Station Hill Press, New York, 1987.

Ulene, Dr. Art. *Complete Guide to Vitamins, Minerals, and Herbs*. Avery: New York, 2000.

Ullman, Dana. *Discovering Homeopathy*. North Atlantic Books: Berkeley, CA, 1991.

Warburg, Dr. Otto H. *The Prime Cause and Prevention of Cancer*. Lecture presented at the meeting of the Nobel-Laureates on June 30, 1966.

Wallace, Dr. Daniel. *The Lupus Book*. Oxford University Press: New York, NY, 1995.

Weil, Andrew, M.D. *Eight Weeks to Optimum Health*. Alfred A. Knopf: New York, NY, 1997.

Williams, Dr. Roger J. *Nutrition Against Disease*. Pitman Publishing Corporation: New York, NY, 1971.

Wolfe, David. *Superfoods*. North Atlantic Books, 2009.

Some authors listed above, e.g., Drs. Atkins, Ulene, and Weil, have published several books. Look for other titles, which are also highly recommended. Out-of-print or used copies can often be found online at AddAll.com or BookFinder.com

APPENDIX I:

COMMON HERBAL TREATMENTS

The substances described in this appendix are well-known, well-documented, and popular remedies—an indication of the wealth of available natural substances that have been used in place of drugs whose side effects can be as harmful as the disease itself. Because there are many herbs that strengthen the immune system, many others that improve circulation, and still others that relieve symptoms of inflammation, pain, and swelling, a comprehensive list is far beyond the scope of this book.

The herbal substances listed below are among those referenced consistently in texts dealing with naturopathic treatment for arthritis and chronic illnesses where the immune system is weak.[1] The focus here is on those substances that remove toxins, are natural antibacterial and/or antiviral and/or antibiotic agents, and that offer relief from common symptoms of fatigue, pain, and inflammation—hallmarks of nearly all autoimmune diseases. Providing this list is by no means intended to be prescriptive, merely informative.

Despite the fact that these substances are "natural," they are by no means completely risk-free. They should not be applied internally or externally before one has consulted with a qualified and knowledgeable health care practitioner who is well versed in their use. Some substances are contraindicated when the individual has specific health problems and/or is taking prescription medication. Reputable Internet sites can be explored to identify specific interreactions[2] before consulting with one's physician.

Manufacturers and suppliers of herbal products may adulterate these substances, adding preservatives or fillers, or they may blend the herbs with a related herb of lower quality. These additions, although identified as "inactive," may cause allergic reactions. Herbs and vitamins lose potency and effectiveness after one to two years. Herbal products bought at clearance sales are likely to be past their prime. Products in gelatin capsules should be refrigerated.

The "herbal remedy" industry is at this writing unregulated by the FDA to a great extent. Fortunately, labels are legally required to list the percentage of herbal substance included in each package. Let the buyer beware. A qualified health care professional should know which brands are reputable and which substances may interfere with prescribed medications.

Standardization ensures that herbal products contain the same amount of a plant's biologically active substance(s) found to have therapeutic effect. This is important because many factors contribute to a varying level of potency—soil quality, plant genetics, time of harvest, part of the plant used, etc. Some herbs contain so little active substance that it must be extracted from many plants and concentrated to have any therapeutic effect. Ginkgo is one example. The glycosides must be carefully extracted and other undesirable compounds like tannins removed before marketing. Herbal products are standardized in three ways:

1. Extract the principal ingredient(s) by dissolving in a solvent such as alcohol or hexane to make a tincture;

2. Blend various batches of extracts to achieve some degree of consistent potency; or

3. Add an active compound (this is called "spiking").

Spiking may create a chemical imbalance and/or diminish the intended effect of the herbal substance. In Germany, many herbal products are sold by prescription and thus must meet pharmaceutical criteria. Standardization is difficult because the chemical constituents of any given therapeutic herb act together in synergy. Extracts represent only one or a few of these active constituents. Generally, fresh processed herbs are most highly potent. The longer a harvested herb is left to the air, the more active molecules will escape. An herb in powdered form, including those in capsules, has been subjected to oxidation and has lost much of its potency. However, some herbs, like cascara sagrada bark, must be dried and aged, else its laxative effects will be too powerful.

One should choose those brands of herbal products whose constituent phytochemicals have been proven in scientific studies to have therapeutic effects. These may cost more compared to other similar standardized but untested products, however, the buyer has the assurance that the brand name product's efficacy is supported by clinical studies.

Alfalfa (*Medicago sativa*)

This herb has been a traditional folk treatment for Rheumatoid Arthritis, diabetes, indigestion, anemia, and atherosclerotic plaque. It is high in protein and contains vitamins A, B_1, B_6, B_{12}, C, E, and K as well as the minerals calcium, potassium, phosphorus, iron, and zinc. Eating alfalfa seeds or sprouts has been said to be beneficial to those with Lupus, a chronic illness characterized by the inflammation of connective tissue, which also is a symptom of RA. However, this assertion is controversial. Alfalfa seeds contain a substance called

L-canavanine, present in all legumes, and may cause Lupus flares in some individuals.[3]

Astragalus (*Astragalus membranaceaous*)

This member of the pea family is one of the most important stamina tonics in Chinese medicine and was mentioned as *huang-qi* in a 2,000-year-old Chinese medical text. Numerous recent studies confirm its immunostimulant, antibacterial, antiviral, adaptogenic, anti-inflammatory, and diuretic effects. It is often combined with ginseng for the commercial market.

Barberry (*Berberis vulgaris*)

Besides its powerful antibiotic properties, barberry is believed to stimulate the immune system, reduce high blood pressure, and shrink tumors. Studies have shown significant infection-fighting properties against germs responsible for wound infections, diarrhea, dysentery, cholera, urinary tract infections, and yeast infections. The herb may be able to stimulate macrophages, the germ-destroying white blood cells of the immune system.

Blackstrap Molasses

A mixture of one teaspoonful in 6 ounces of hot water, drunk before each meal, is a centuries-old folk remedy for arthritis. Molasses is high in vitamins E and B_5, substances that fight infection by building natural antibodies. Molasses is the residue of sugar cane refining. It contains all the organic molecules removed from processed sugar.

Boneset (*Eupatorium perfoliatum*)

Related to marigolds and dandelions, this herb stimulates the immune system. Native Americans used it to treat fevers, ward off colds and influenza, and to relieve arthritis symptoms. Studies have shown it to mobilize white blood cells to destroy infection-causing bacteria and viruses.

Boswellia (*Boswellia serrata*)

Boswellia serrata is a shrub indigenous to India and related to *Boswellia carteri* (frankincense or olibanum). The plant produces a resin called salai guggal, used for millenia in India by Ayurvedic medical practitioners to treat arthritis. The active ingredient is boswellic acid, which has an anti-inflammatory effect. A 1996 issue of *Phytomedicine* was devoted to studies of boswellia.

Bromelain

An extract of pineapple, this herb has significant anti-inflammatory effects, as well as being able to assist proper digestion. However, if you have ulcers, avoid this herb.

Burdock Root (*Arctium lappa*)

Usually brewed as tea, this herb helps to purify the blood and detoxify poisons.

Capsaicin

This herb is the fruit of a number of plant species, including paprika and chili peppers, and has been used for many years as a topical treatment for aches and pains, especially those associated with arthritis and shingles.

Capsaicinoids are presumed to relieve pain because they inhibit neurotransmitter release from afferent pain receptors. They may also stimulate endorphin production in those brain areas related to joint sensations.

Capsaicinoids block the release of neuropeptides to mediate pain and neurogenic inflammation. The chemical action initially stimulates the nerve endings, evoking the sensation of warmth and mild stinging. Recently some very expensive compounds whose only active ingredient is capsaicin have appeared on the market. Capsaicin powder can be obtained fresh, in bulk, for a fraction of the cost of these compounds heavily advertised as providing "miraculous relief." A poultice is simple to make and apply.

If there is any skin irritation over the affected joint, topical creams containing capsaicin should be avoided. Never use an analgesic ointment, particularly those containing capsaicin, in conjunction with a heating pad because of the potential for deep burns.

Cider Vinegar

References to mixtures of apple cider vinegar with honey as a tonic appear frequently in folk medicine literature. An organism that survives after the yeast fermentation cycle produces cider vinegar. Natural cider vinegar may contain chemicals that suppress the growth of yeasts. Honey is a natural antibiotic. Caution: honey is a natural sugar.

Cod Liver Oil

A perennial favorite for centuries in Europe and America, cod liver oil is a rich source of the omega-3 class fatty acids EPA (Eicosapentaenoic Acid) and DHA (Docosahexaenoic Acid) as well as vitamin D. This vitamin assures that calcium is available to be deposited in the bones by allowing the intestine to absorb it more efficiently. If there is enough vitamin D in the diet, the amount of calcium absorbed by the intestine can triple.

With the advent of prescription steroids, cod liver oil was all but forgotten as a natural, safe, and inexpensive way to ensure adequate vitamin D intake, despite evidence that omega-3 fatty acids in fish oil can bring blood sedimentation rates down dramatically in arthritic individuals and can significantly reduce RA symptoms.[4]

A daily tablespoon of fish oil is a traditional folk remedy to keep arthritic joints lubricated. This is based on the misconception that our joints work like a mechanical ball and socket, and that the ingested oil is somehow squirted into the assembly for smoother functioning. In reality, it is the EPA, DHA, and vitamin D that nourishes the cells forming the synovial fluid that surrounds all joints. Take care not to exceed the safe maximum intake of vitamins A and D. Fish oil has a mild blood thinning effect, so it should not be combined with any anticoagulant drugs unless approved by a physician.

Curcumin (see Turmeric)

Devil's Claw (*Harpagophytum procumbens*)

This herb has been used for centuries to help reduce pain and swelling in joints, and relieve disorders of the liver and kidneys, stimulating the detoxifying and protective mechanisms of the body. Devil's Claw must be taken for a course of eight or nine weeks to see results, and then should be discontinued. Diabetics should not use the herb except under medical supervision.

Echinacea (*Echinacea purpurea*)

Native Americans used this herb for more medicinal purposes than any other plant, treating everything from colds to cancer. It is valued in China for its antibiotic and immune system-stimulating properties, applicable even to severe immune disorders such as cancer and AIDS. American doctors adopted it in 1895 to treat malaria, measles, mumps, chicken pox, arthritis, scarlet fever, yeast infections, and chronic nasal congestion. The natural antibiotic (echinacoside) in the plant works in a way comparable to penicillin to kill viruses, bacteria, fungi, and other germs. Echinacea has been largely replaced by synthetic antibiotics in the U.S., but is still used in Europe, especially for relief from the symptoms of seasonal allergies. Herbalists consider the root to be a blood purifier and an aid to fighting infections.

Caution: those allergic to pollens such as ragweed may be also allergic to echinacea. This herb should not be used in cases of seriously impaired immune response illnesses such as tuberculosis, MS, and HIV infection. Stimulating badly infected T-cells is unwise. Caution: too much of this herb over a long time can actually have immunosuppressive effects in otherwise healthy individuals. It should be used at the onset and during a cold or allergy attack, but not as a daily supplement.

Eleuthero (*Eleutherococcus senticosus*)

Also known as Siberian ginseng, Eleuthero has been used in China as an invigorating tonic for more than two thousand years. It strongly stimulates the immune system and counters symptoms of fatigue. It is used to treat a variety of illnesses ranging from the common cold to severe respiratory and inflammatory conditions.

The active eleutherosides in this herb have an ability to support immune function and adrenal gland function, especially under stressful conditions. In Russia, inhabitants of the Taiga region of Siberia originally used eleuthero to decrease infections and increase vitality. Russian Olympic athletes use this herb for stamina and endurance. The Soviet government distributed eleuthero to its citizens to counter the effects of radiation after the Chernobyl nuclear accident in 1986. The herb has been shown to alleviate the side effects of chemotherapy and radiation therapy and to help bone marrow recover more quickly.

Eleuthero assists in maintaining aerobic activity for longer periods and in recovery from strenuous workouts more quickly. Increase in blood oxygen transport to inflamed areas is especially beneficial to arthritis sufferers. Some microorganisms in the body are very sensitive to oxygen levels in the blood. If this level is impaired, the organisms are not controllable.

Garlic (*Allium sativum*)

Cultivated as food and medicine for over five thousand years, garlic's antibacterial activity was first recognized in 1858 by Louis Pasteur. The following are among the well-known properties of garlic: anti-inflammatory, antibacterial, antifungal, antiparasitic, antioxidant, and immunostimulant. Garlic significantly decreases the incidence of cancer, especially cancer of the gastrointestinal tract, among those who consume it regularly.[5] Its action is believed to be similar to that of sulfa drugs. Its potency is so strong that it is typically used in sausage recipes to prevent spoilage. The European livestock industry is currently considering adding garlic to animal feed rather than chemical antibiotics, which are seen to cause consumer health problems. Whole cloves of garlic are less costly and far more potent than garlic supplement capsules. Crush the clove before consuming it to obtain maximum benefit. Cooking the garlic decreases its beneficial action.

Ginger (*Zingiber officinalis*)

The anti-inflammatory actions of ginger help relieve the pain of arthritis, menstrual cramps, and headache. An easy way to obtain this herb's benefits is to use it liberally in cooking. Add the fresh root to soups, stir-fry recipes, and sauces. Scrub the root but do not peel it, since active properties are primarily contained in the skin. 3-4 cups of ginger tea daily can be helpful. Use 2 tsp of chopped fresh root per cup of water simmered in a covered pot for ten minutes.

Ginkgo (*Ginkgo biloba*)

This herb has been found to improve both blood circulation and oxygen metabolism in the brain. Unique compounds called ginkgolides are potent inhibitors of a platelet-activating factor involved in the development of inflammatory, cardiovascular, and respiratory disorders. The action of ginkgolides helps explain the herb's broad spectrum of biological effects, such as antioxidant activity.

Olive Leaf Extract

This phytochemical substance has antiviral, anti-bacterial, antifungal and antiparasitic activity. The elenolic acid contained in the extract (oleuropein) is the active biological agent that combats infectious diseases. Oleuropein stimulates phagocytosis and increases T-cell counts. It is used in China to suppress cancer and rebuild the immune system. Oleuropein acts as a free radical scavenger in a manner similar to vitamin E. It also inhibits the oxidation of LDL cholesterol. Individuals suffering from a viral or bacterial infection or from CFS may experience a "Herx" effect during the detox process.

Pau d'arco (*Tabebuia impetiginosa*)

This herb has many active ingredients including lapachol and beta-lapachone. The USDA has documented these substances as being anti-inflammatory, antiviral, bactericidal, fungicidal, virucidal, antiseptic, antimicrobial, antileukemic, anticancerous, and with few side effects. It is especially valued for its anti-Candida benefits.

Pectin

This substance is found in the cell walls of plants. Because of its ability to gel and hold water molecules together, pectin is valuable in ridding the body of toxins. Fruit (usually apple) pectin is sold commercially where canning supplies are available. It has been used for decades as a folk remedy for bursitis or "tennis elbow." It may assist in lubricating joint-tendon synovial interfaces. A tablespoon of fruit pectin may be stirred in a small glass of water or fruit juice and taken daily. An alkaline juice such as apricot or apple works best. Pectin is also sold in capsule form at health food stores.

Pectin is the active substance in apples that has led to the saying, "An apple a day keeps the doctor away."

Propolis

This unusual remedy is a sticky resinous substance collected by bees from the bark or leaf buds of trees, especially poplars. Its medicinal value has been known since the first century A.D. Propolis contains resin, balsam, wax, fragrant essential oils, pollen, and amino acids. It is rich in minerals, antibiotics and vitamins, especially the B vitamins. It has an unusually high concentration of pantothenic acid, which is required by and stimulates the function of the adrenal glands. Propolis also contains tannins, which cause proteins in the blood to coagulate. Propolis compounds are used extensively in Europe and in Russia.

Reishi

This herb is the fruiting body of a mushroom native to the Orient. Although related species occur in North America, they are not grown commercially nor have their medicinal properties been seriously studied. Reishi has been a prized folk remedy in China for thousands of years, once available only to emperors as an important tonic to increase longevity. Its Chinese name *ling zhi* means "spirit plant." It was traditionally used to treat hepatitis, nervous conditions, hypertension, arthritis, insomnia, and lung disorders. Recent studies confirm Chinese reishi's antiallergenic, antioxidant, antiviral, anti-inflammatory, and immunostimulant properties. It is also a calmative and reduces blood pressure. It may be cultivated from spores if a dried reishi is placed in a bed of moist sawdust or wood chips. Non-Chinese varieties may not possess true reishi properties.

Saint John's Wort (*Hypericum perforatum*)

Known in Europe as a healing agent since the 16th century, the herb's wound-healing ability and its capability to stimulate the immune system make it a valuable traditional remedy. Studies have shown that it contains a family of chemicals known as flavonoids, which strengthen the immune system for antibacterial, anti-inflammatory, and antiviral effects. There is no evidence to support the contention that this herb is an effective treatment for chronic depression, although it has mild antidepressant properties. Mild depression often accompanies systemic mycoplasmal/bacterial infections.

Stinging Nettle (*Urtica dioica*)

Nettle tea has been used in folk medicine to stimulate blood circulation and as a tonic for chronic skin ailments. It is a traditional folk treatment for arthritis, probably because it increases oxygen transport to inflamed areas, providing relief. Research has shown that the leaf tea aids coagulation and formation of hemoglobin in red blood cells, while the leaf extract depresses the central nervous system and inhibits bacteria and adrenaline.[6] In Germany the herb is used extensively for rheumatic complaints and kidney infections. In the U.S., it is effective in treating LD symptoms.

Thyme (*Thymus vulgaris*)

Thyme is a medicinal herb indigenous to the Mediterranean area and is a member of the mint family. Although used extensively in cooking, its medicinal properties have been known in Europe since the reign of Charlemagne in the eighth century. Thyme is said to relieve muscle pains and spasms, inhibit the growth of harmful microorganisms such as Streptococcus and Candida, relieve or prevent coughs, act as an expectorant and settle upset stomachs.

The more than 60 active phenol compounds, especially thymol and carvacrol, are known to have muscle relaxant and antiseptic properties. Thyme should not be used without first consulting your doctor if you suspect a dysfunctional thyroid condition or if pregnant or nursing. While powdered thyme is usually used for tea or in recipes, a drop or two of essential oil can be inhaled using a vaporizer. It can also be added sparingly to massage oil or bath water for topical treatment. Thyme essential oil should never be ingested, applied directly to the skin, or used in other than very small quantities.

Tiger Balm

Although this topical compound was developed in China only about 60 years ago, its ingredients (oils of camphor, menthol, mint, clove, cajuput, wintergreen, and cassia) have been used for centuries in various liniments to afford relief of minor aches and pains due to strain, fatigue, exposure, or cold. There are many other external herbal poultices one could make from scratch using the Tiger Balm ingredients or a blend of comfrey, willow, thyme oil, tumeric, or capsaicin. A good herbal healing text should provide useful recipes and procedures.

Turmeric (*Curcuma longa*)

According to Ayurvedic medicine, turmeric can relieve inflammatory joint pain and ligament problems associated with arthritis, bursitis, and tendonitis. Turmeric's main ingredient is curcumin, a natural anti-inflammatory agent as helpful as cortisone but without the immunosuppressive side effects. Ayurvedic practitioners advise taking one ounce of powdered turmeric (obtainable in bulk) stirred into water or juice daily until the inflammation subsides. As a preventive measure, the suggested dose is one-half to one ounce daily. This herb is a flavorful seasoning for rice and chicken soup.

White Willow Bark (*Salix alba*)

This herb contains salicylin, the same active ingredient found in aspirin (acetylsalicylic acid), used to reduce pain and inflammation. Hippocrates advised women of 400 B.C. Greece to chew willow bark to relieve the pains of childbirth. Native people of the North America have used willow bark for over two thousand years as a blood thinner, to reduce fevers, to treat respiratory problems, headaches, and to relieve the inflammation, aches, and pains of rheumatism and arthritis. Willow bark has been called a "natural aspirin" but without aspirin's potency or side effects. It does not cause stomach upset as aspirin often does. Willow bark is high in tannins, which could damage the liver if taken in extraordinary quantities. However, it would take about a gallon of willow bark tea to provide a single dose of salicylin equivalent to one dose of aspirin. Salicylin produced by the bark does not metabolize in the same way as aspirin, so the same contraindications may not apply for stomach ulcers.

Yucca (*Yucca schidigera*)

All parts of the yucca plant were used for centuries by the native people of the southwestern United States and Baja California deserts to combat the pain and inflammation caused by arthritis and rheumatism. The yucca root is rich in steroid-like saponins that elevate the body's cortisone production to reduce and eliminate the pain, swelling, and joint stiffness associated with arthritis. Saponins reduce cholesterol from the blood by binding with bile acids produced by the liver, making them unavailable for reabsorption as they are routed to the colon for excretion. The process leaves less cholesterol in the blood to accrue in the arteries.

The late Dr. Robert Bingham, director of the Desert Hot Springs Medical Clinic in Palm Springs, CA supervised thousands of successful case studies using yucca extract supplements. According to Dr. Bingham, toxic substances or harmful bacteria provoke allergic responses taking a variety of forms—migraines, skin rashes, joint pain—so an anti-stress agent such as yucca saponin may have the same beneficial effect as direct action on the invader by simply improving and protecting the intestinal flora. Yucca seems to inhibit harmful intestinal bacteria while helping maintain the natural balance of normal resident bacteria.

---

[1] Publications offered by the American Botanical Council are credible and useful. Their website is www.herbalgram.org

[2] For example:
http://www.nlm.nih.gov/medlineplus/druginformation.html and www.allnatural.net/herbpages/ A powerful search engine like Google can be used with specific keywords such as [arthritis yucca] or [fibro garlic] [candida pau d'arco]

[3] http://www.ncbi.nlm.nih.gov/pubmed/16890899 (2006)

[4] http://www.ncbi.nlm.nih.gov/pubmed/8003055

[5] http://www.garlic.mistral.co.uk/cancer.htm

[6] www.herbmed.org

APPENDIX II:

Physicians' Protocol for Treating Rheumatic Disease

by Dr. Joseph M. Mercola, D. O. [August, 2010]

At least two million Americans have definite or classical Rheumatoid Arthritis (RA). This number has increased in recent years. It is a much more devastating illness than previously appreciated. Most patients with RA have a progressive disability.

The natural course of Rheumatoid Arthritis is quite remarkable in that less than 1% of people with the disease have a spontaneous remission. Some disability occurs in 50-70% of RA patients within five years after onset of the disease, and half will stop working within 10 years.

This devastating prognosis is what makes this novel form of treatment so exciting, as it has a far higher likelihood of succeeding than the conventional approach. Over the years, I have treated over 3,000 patients with rheumatic illnesses, including Scleroderma, Polymyositis, Dermatomyositis, and Lupus. Approximately 15 percent of these patients were lost to follow-up for whatever reason and have not continued with treatment. The remaining patients seem to have a 60-90% likelihood of improvement on this treatment regimen, in stark contrast to the success experienced with conventional approaches. This should provide a strong motivation to try the protocol discussed below.

RA Can Be More Deadly than Heart Disease

There is also an increased mortality rate with this disease. The five-year survival rate of patients with more than thirty joints involved is approximately 50 percent. This is similar to severe coronary artery disease or stage IV Hodgkin's disease. Thirty years ago, one researcher concluded that there was an average loss of 18 years of life in patients who developed RA before the age of 50.

Most authorities believe that remissions rarely occur. Some experts feel that the term "remission-inducing" should not be used to describe any current Rheumatoid Arthritis treatment, and a review of contemporary treatment methods shows that medical science has not been able to significantly improve the long-term outcome of this disease.

Dr. Brown Pioneered a Novel Approach to Treat Rheumatoid Arthritis

I first became aware of Doctor Thomas McPherson Brown's antibiotic protocol in 1989 when I saw him on 20/20 on ABC. This was shortly after the introduction of his first edition of his book, *The Road Back*, co-authored with Henry Scammell. The 1998 updated version is *The New Arthritis Breakthrough* by Henry Scammell. Unfortunately, Dr. Brown died from prostate cancer shortly after the 20/20 program so I never had a chance to meet him.

My application of Dr. Brown's protocol has changed significantly since I first started implementing it. Initially, I rigidly followed Dr. Brown's work with minimal modifications to his protocol. About the only change I made was changing Tetracycline to Minocin. I believe I was one of the first physicians who recommended the shift to Minocin and most people who use his protocol now use Minocin.

In 1939, Dr. Sabin, the discoverer of the polio vaccine, first reported chronic arthritis in mice caused by a Mycoplasma. He suggested this agent might cause human Rheumatoid Arthritis (RA). Dr. Brown worked with Dr. Sabin at the Rockefeller Institute. Dr. Brown was a board-certified rheumatologist who graduated from Johns Hopkins medical school. He was a professor of medicine at George Washington University until 1970 where he served as chairman of the Arthritis Institute in Arlington, Virginia. He published over 100 papers in peer-reviewed scientific literature.

He was able to help over 10,000 patients when he used this program, from the 1950s until his death in 1989, and clearly far more people than that have been helped by other physicians using this protocol. He found that significant benefits from the treatment require, on average, about one to two years. I have treated nearly 3,000 patients and find that the dietary modification I advocate accelerates the response rate to several months. I cannot emphasize strongly enough the importance of this aspect of the program. Still, the length of therapy can vary widely.

In severe cases, it may take up to 30 months for patients to gain sustained improvement. One requires patience because remissions may take up to 3-5 years. Dr. Brown's pioneering approach represents a safer, less toxic alternative to many conventional regimens. The results of the NIH-sponsored 1994 study "Minocycline in Rheumatoid Arthritis (MIRA) Trial" have finally scientifically validated this treatment.

Dietary changes are absolutely an essential component of my protocol. Dr. Brown's original protocol was notorious for inducing a Jarisch-Herxheimer reaction, or worsening of symptoms, before improvement was noted. This could last two to six months. Implementing my nutrition plan results in a lessening of that reaction in most cases.[1]

When I first started using his protocol for patients in the late 1980s, the common retort from other physicians was that there was "no scientific proof" that this treatment worked. That view is certainly not true today. On my website I provide over 200 references in the peer-reviewed medical literature that supports the application of Minocin in the use of rheumatic illnesses.[2] In my experience, nearly

80% of people do remarkably better with this program. However, about 5% continue to worsen and require conventional agent like methotrexate to relieve their symptoms.

Physicians Who Use this Protocol

The Road Back Foundation (www.RoadBack.org) is the oldest organization promoting this work and the one Dr. Brown originally worked with. This is an excellent resource to find health care professionals using this approach. Similar nonprofit resources are www.Rheumatic.org and The Arthritis Trust of America (www.ArthritisTrust.org).

Scientific Proof for this Approach

The definitive scientific support for minocycline in the treatment for RA came with the MIRA trial in the United States. This was a double blind randomized placebo-controlled trial done at six university centers involving 200 patients for nearly one year. The dosage they used (100 mg twice daily) was much higher and likely less effective than what most clinicians currently use.

They also did not employ any additional antibiotics or nutritional regimens, yet 55% of patients improved. This study finally provided the proof that many traditional clinicians demanded before seriously considering this treatment as an alternative regimen for RA.

Dr. Brown's effort to treat the chronic Mycoplasma infections believed to cause RA is the basis for this therapy. He believed that most rheumatic illnesses respond to this treatment. Dr. Brown and others used this therapy for lupus, ankylosing spondylitis, scleroderma, dermatomyositis and polymyositis.

REVISED ANTIBIOTIC-FREE APPROACH

Although I used a revision of Dr. Brown's antibiotic approach for nearly ten years, my preference is to focus on natural therapies. The program that follows is my revision of this protocol that allows for a completely drug-free treatment of RA, which is based on my experience of treating over 3,000 patients with rheumatic illnesses in my Chicago clinic.

If you are interested in reviewing or considering Dr. Brown's antibiotic approach, I have included a summary of his work and the evidence for it in another section of this appendix entitled "The Infectious Cause of RA."

Factors Associated with Success on This Program

There are many variables associated with an increased chance of remission or improvement.

- The younger you are, the greater your chance for improvement;
- The more closely you follow the nutrition plan, the more likely you are to improve and the less likely you are to have a severe flare-up. I now offer the Nutritional Typing Test for free, so please do not skip this essential step;
- Smoking seems to be negatively associated with improvement;
- The longer you have had the illness and the more severe the illness, the more difficult it seems to treat.

Crucial Lifestyle Changes

Improving your diet using a combination of my nutritional guidelines, nutritional typing is crucial for your success. In addition, there are some general principles that seem to hold true for all nutritional types and these include:

- Eliminating sugar, especially fructose, and most grains. For most people it is best to limit fruit to small quantities;

- Eating unprocessed, high-quality foods, organic and locally grown if possible;

- Eating your food as close to raw as possible;

- Getting plenty high-quality animal-based omega-3 fats. Krill oil seems to be particularly helpful here as it appears to be a more effective anti-inflammatory preparation. It is particularly effective if taken concurrently with 4 mg of Astaxanthin, which is a potent antioxidant bioflavonoid derived from algae;

- Astaxanthin at 4 mg per day is particularly important for anyone placed on prednisone as Astaxanthin offers potent protection against cataracts and age-related macular degeneration;

- Incorporating regular exercise into your daily schedule.

Early Emotional Traumas are Pervasive in Those with RA

With the vast majority of the patients I treated, some type of emotional trauma occurred early in their life, before the age their conscious mind was formed, which is typically around the age of five or six. However, a trauma can occur at any age, and has a profoundly negative impact.

If that specific emotional insult is not addressed with an effective treatment modality then the underlying emotional trigger will continue to fester, allowing the destructive process to proceed, which can predispose you to severe autoimmune diseases like RA later in life.

In some cases, RA appears to be caused by an infection, and it is my experience that this infection is usually acquired when you have a stressful event that causes a disruption in your bioelectrical circuits, which then impairs your immune system.

An early emotional trauma predisposes you to developing the initial infection, and also contributes to your relative inability to effectively defeat the infection.

Therefore, it's very important to have an effective tool to address these underlying emotional traumas. In my practice, the most common form of treatment used is called the Emotional Freedom Technique (EFT).

Although EFT is something that you can learn to do yourself in the comfort of your own home, it is important to consult a well-trained professional to obtain the skills necessary to promote proper healing using this amazing tool. Find out more details and videos at http://eft.mercola.com/.

Vitamin D Deficiency Rampant in Those with RA[3]

The early part of the 21st century brought enormous attention to the importance and value of vitamin D, particularly in the treatment of autoimmune diseases like RA.

From my perspective, it is now virtually criminal negligent malpractice to treat a person with RA and not aggressively monitor their vitamin D levels to confirm that they are in a therapeutic range of 65-80 ng/ml.

This is so important that blood tests need to be done every two weeks, so the dose can be adjusted to get into that range. Most normal-weight adults should start at 10,000 units of vitamin D per day.

In the U.S., Lab Corp is the lab of choice as Quest labs provide results that are falsely elevated. If you choose Quest, multiply your result by 0.70 to obtain the right number.

Low Dose Naltrexone

One new addition to the protocol is low-dose Naltrexone, which I would encourage anyone with RA to try. It is inexpensive and non-toxic and I have a number of physician reports documenting incredible efficacy in getting people off of all their dangerous arthritis medications.

Although this is a drug, and strictly speaking not a natural therapy, it has provided important relief and is <u>far</u> safer than the toxic drugs that are typically prescribed by nearly all rheumatologists.

Nutritional Considerations

Limiting sugar is a critical element of the treatment program. Sugar has multiple significant negative influences on your biochemistry. First and foremost, it increases your insulin levels, which is the root cause of nearly all chronic disease. It can also impair your gut bacteria.

In my experience, if you are unable to decrease your sugar intake, you are far less likely to improve. Please understand that the number one source of calories in the U.S. is high fructose corn syrup ingested when drinking soda. One of the first steps you can take is to phase out all soft drinks, and replace them with pure, clean water.

Exercise for Rheumatoid Arthritis

It is very important to exercise and increase muscle tone of your non-weight bearing joints. Experts tell us that disuse results in muscle atrophy and weakness. Additionally, immobility may result in joint contractures and loss of range of motion (ROM). Active ROM exercises are preferred to passive. There is some evidence that passive ROM exercises increase the number of white blood cells in the joints.

If your joints are stiff, you should stretch and apply heat before exercising. If your joints are swollen, application of ten minutes of ice before exercise would be helpful. The inflamed joint is very vulnerable to damage from improper exercise, so you must be cautious. People with arthritis must strike a delicate balance between rest and activity, and must avoid activities that aggravate joint pain. You should avoid any exercise that strains a significantly unstable joint.

A good rule of thumb is that if the pain lasts longer than one hour after stopping exercise, you should slow down or choose another form of exercise. Assistive devices are also helpful to decrease the pressure on affected joints. Many patients need to be urged to take advantage of these. The Arthritis Foundation's book, *Guide to Independent Living*, instructs patients about how to obtain them.

Of course, it is important to maintain good cardiovascular fitness as well. Walking with appropriate supportive shoes is another important consideration. If your condition allows, it would be wise to move towards a regimen like my Peak Fitness program that is designed for reaching optimal health. See http://fitness.mercola.com.

It's Important to Control Your Pain

One of the primary problems with RA is controlling pain. The conventional treatment typically includes using very dangerous drugs like prednisone, methotrexate, and drugs that interfere with the tumor necrosis factor, like Enbrel.

The goal is to implement the lifestyle changes discussed above as quickly as possible, so you can start to reduce toxic drugs that do absolutely nothing to treat the cause of the disease.

However, pain relief is obviously very important, and if this is not achieved, you can go into a depressive cycle that can clearly worsen your immune system and cause the RA to flare. So the goal is to be as comfortable and pain free as possible with the least amount of drugs. The Mayo Clinic offers several common sense guidelines for avoiding pain by paying heed to how you move so as to not injure your joints.[4]

Safest Anti-Inflammatories to Use for Pain

Clearly the safest prescription drugs to use for pain are the non-acetylated salicylates such as:

- Salsalate

- Sodium salicylate

- Magnesium salicylate (i.e., Salflex, Disalcid, or Trilisate).

These are the drugs of choice if there is renal insufficiency as they minimally interfere with anticyclo-oxygenase and other prostaglandins. Additionally, they will not impair platelet inhibition in those patients who are on an every-other-day aspirin regimen to decrease their risk for stroke or heart disease.

Unlike aspirin, they do not increase the formation of products of lipoxygenase-mediated metabolism of arachidonic acid. For this reason, they may be less likely to cause hypersensitivity reactions. These drugs have been safely used in patients with reversible obstructive airway disease and a history of aspirin sensitivity.

They are also much gentler on your stomach than the other non-steroidal anti-inflammatories (NSAIDs) and are the drug of choice if you have problems with peptic ulcer disease. Unfortunately, all these benefits are balanced by the fact they may not be as effective as the other agents and are less convenient to take. You must take 1.5-2 grams twice per day, and tinnitus (ringing in the ears) is a frequent side effect.

You need to be aware of this complication and know that if tinnitus does develop, you need to stop the drugs for a day and restart with a dose that is half a pill per day lower. You can repeat this until you find a dose that relieves your pain and doesn't cause tinnitus.

If the Safer Anti-Inflammatories Aren't Helping, Try This Next...

If the non-acetylated salicylates aren't helping, there are many different NSAIDs to try: Relafen, Daypro, Voltaren, Motrin, Naprosyn. Among the most toxic or likely to cause complications are Meclomen, Indocin, Orudis, and Tolectin. You can experiment with them, and see which one works best for you. If cost is a concern, generic ibuprofen can be used at up to 800 mg per dose. Unfortunately, recent studies suggest this drug is more damaging to your kidneys.

If you use any of the above drugs, though, it is really important to make sure you take them with your largest meal as this will somewhat moderate their GI toxicity and the likelihood of causing an ulcer.

Please beware that these drugs are much more dangerous than antibiotics or non-acetylated salicylates.

You should have a SMA blood test performed at least once a year if you are taking these medications. In addition, you must monitor your serum potassium levels if you taking an ACE inhibitor as these medications can cause high potassium levels. You should also monitor your kidney function. The SMA will show any liver impairment the drugs might be causing.

These medications can also impair prostaglandin metabolism and cause papillary necrosis and chronic interstitial nephritis. Your kidney needs vasodilatory prostaglandins (PGE2 and prostacyclin) to counterbalance the effects of potent vasoconstrictor hormones such as angiotensin II and catecholamines. NSAIDs decrease prostaglandin synthesis by inhibiting cyclooxygenase, leading to unopposed constriction of the renal arterioles supplying your kidneys.

Warning: These Drugs Massively Increase Your Risk for Ulcers

The first non-aspirin NSAID, indomethacin, was introduced in 1963. Now more than 30 are available. Relafen is one of the better alternatives, as it seems to cause less of an intestinal dysbiosis. You must be especially careful to monitor renal function periodically. It is important to understand and accept the risks associated with these more toxic drugs. Every year, they do enough damage to the GI tract to kill 2,000 to 4,000 people with RA alone. That is equivalent to ten people every day. At any given time, 10 to 20% of all those receiving NSAID therapy have gastric ulcers.

If you are taking an NSAID, you are at approximately three times greater risk for developing serious gastrointestinal side effects than those who don't. Approximately 1.2 percent of patients taking NSAIDs are hospitalized for upper GI problems, per year of exposure. One study of patients taking NSAIDs showed that a life-threatening complication was the first sign of ulcer in more than half of the subjects.

Researchers found that the drugs suppress production of prostacyclin, which is needed to dilate blood vessels and inhibit clotting. Earlier studies had found that mice genetically engineered to be unable to use prostacyclin properly were prone to clotting disorders.

Anyone who is at increased risk of cardiovascular disease should steer clear of these medications. Ulcer complications are certainly potentially life-threatening, but heart attacks are a much more common and likely risk, especially in older individuals.

How You Can Tell if You are at Risk for NSAID Side Effects

Risk factor analysis can help determine if you will face an increased danger of developing these complications. If you have any of the following, you will likely to have a higher risk of side effects from these drugs:

1. Old age
2. Peptic ulcer history
3. Alcohol dependency
4. Cigarette smoking
5. Concurrent prednisone or corticosteroid use
6. Disability
7. Taking a high dose of the NSAID
8. Using an NSAID known to be more toxic

Prednisone

If NSAIDs are unable to control the pain, then prednisone is nearly universally used. This is a steroid drug that is loaded with side effects. If you are taking large doses of prednisone for extended periods of time, you can be virtually assured to develop the following problems:

- Osteoporosis
- Cataracts
- Diabetes
- Ulcers
- Herpes reactivation
- Insomnia
- Hypertension
- Kidney stones

With every dose of prednisone, your bones are becoming weaker. The higher the dose and the longer you are on prednisone, the more likely you are to develop bone problems. However, if you are able to keep your dose to 5 mg or below, this is not typically a major issue. Prednisone is one of the first medicines you should try to stop as soon as your symptoms permit.

Be aware that blood levels of cortisol peak between 3 and 9 a.m. It would, therefore, be safest to administer the prednisone in the morning. This will minimize the suppression on your hypothalamic-pituitary-adrenal axis.

You also need to be concerned about the increased risk of peptic ulcer disease when using prednisone with conventional NSAIDs. If you are taking both of these drugs, you have a 15 times greater risk of developing an ulcer.

If you are already on prednisone, it is helpful to get a prescription for 1 mg tablets so you can wean yourself off the prednisone as soon as possible. Usually you can lower your dose by about 1 mg per week. If a relapse of symptoms occurs, then further reduction of prednisone is not indicated.

How Do You Know When to Stop the Drugs?

Unlike conventional approaches to RA, my protocol is designed to treat the underlying cause of the problem. So eventually the drugs that you are going to use during the program will be weaned off.

The following criteria can help determine when you are in remission and can consider weaning off your medications:

- A decrease in duration of morning stiffness to no more than 15 minutes;
- No pain at rest;
- Little or no pain or tenderness on motion;
- Absence of joint swelling;
- A normal energy level;
- A decrease in your ESR to no more than 30;

- A normalization of your CBC. Generally your HGB, HCT, and MCV will increase to normal and your "pseudo"-iron deficiency will disappear;
- ANA, RF, and ASO titers returning to normal.

Discontinuing your medications before all of the above criteria are met means a greater risk that the disease will recur. If you meet the above criteria, you can try to wean off your anti-inflammatory medication and monitor for flare-ups. If no flare-ups occur for six months, then discontinue the clindamycin (discussed later in this chapter). If the improvements are maintained for the next six months, you can then discontinue your Minocin and monitor for recurrences. Should symptoms recur, it would be wise to restart the previous antibiotic regimen.

Evaluation to Determine and Follow RA

If you have received evaluations and treatment by one or more board certified rheumatologists, you can be very confident that the appropriate evaluation was done. Although conventional <u>treatments</u> fail miserably in the long run, the conventional <u>diagnostic</u> approach is typically excellent, and you can start the treatment program discussed above.

It is important to be properly evaluated to determine if indeed you have RA. Please be sure to review the section of this appendix entitled "Assessment for Fibromyalgia" carefully to be certain that Fibromyalgia is not present. Be aware that arthritic pain can be an early manifestation of 20-30 different clinical problems. These include not only rheumatic disease, but also metabolic, infectious, and malignant disorders. RA is a clinical diagnosis for which there is not a single test or group of laboratory tests that can be considered confirmatory.

Criteria for Classification of RA

- Morning Stiffness - Morning stiffness in and around joints lasting at least one hour before maximal improvement is noted.

- Arthritis of three or more joint areas - At least three joint areas have simultaneously had soft-tissue swelling or fluid (not bony overgrowth) observed by a physician. There are 14 possible joints: right or left PIP, MCP, wrist, elbow, knee, ankle, and MTP joints.

- Arthritis of hand joints - At least one joint area swollen as above in a wrist, MCP, or PIP joint.

- Symmetric arthritis - Simultaneous involvement of the same joint areas (as in criterion 2) on both sides of your body (bilateral involvement of PIPs, MCPs, or MTPs) is acceptable without absolute symmetry. Lack of symmetry is not sufficient to rule out the diagnosis of RA.

- Rheumatoid Nodules - Subcutaneous nodules over bony prominences, or extensor surfaces, or in juxta-articular regions, observed by a physician. Only about 25 percent of patients with RA develop nodules, and usually as a later manifestation.

- Serum Rheumatoid Factor - Demonstration of abnormal amounts of serum rheumatoid factor by any method that has been positive in less than 5 percent of normal control subjects. This test is positive only 30-40 percent of the time in the early months of RA.

You must also make certain that the first four symptoms listed in the list above are present for six or more weeks. These criteria have a 91-94 percent sensitivity and

89 percent specificity for the diagnosis of RA. However, these criteria were designed for classification and not for diagnosis. The diagnosis must be made on clinical grounds. It is important to note that many patients with negative serologic tests can have a strong clinical picture for RA.

Your Hands are the Key to the Diagnosis of RA

In a way, the hands are the calling card of Rheumatoid Arthritis. If you completely lack hand and wrist involvement, even by history, the diagnosis of RA is doubtful. Rheumatoid Arthritis rarely affects your hips and ankles early in its course. The metacarpophalangeal joints, proximal interphalangeal and wrist joints are the first to become symptomatic. Osteoarthritis typically affects the joints that are closest to your fingertips (DIP joints) while RA typically affects the joints closest to your wrist (PIP), like your knuckles.

Fatigue may be present before your joint symptoms begin, and morning stiffness is a sensitive indicator of RA. An increase in fluid in and around your joint probably causes the stiffness. Your joints are warm, but your skin is rarely red. When your joints develop effusions, hold them flexed at 5 to 20 degrees, as it may be too painful to extend them fully.

Radiological Changes

Radiological changes typical of RA on PA hand and wrist x-rays, which must include erosions or unequivocal bony decalcification localized to, or most marked, adjacent to the involved joints (osteoarthritic changes alone do not count).

Note: You must satisfy at least four of the seven criteria listed. Any of criteria 1-4 must have been present for at least 6 weeks. Patients with two clinical diagnoses are not excluded. Designations as classic, definite, or probable Rheumatoid Arthritis, are not to be made.

Laboratory Evaluation

The general initial laboratory evaluation should include a baseline ESR, CBC, SMA, U/A, 25 hydroxy D level and an ASO titer. You can also draw RF and ANA titers to further objectively document improvement with the therapy. However, they seldom add much to the assessment.

Follow-up visits can be every two to four months depending on the extent of the disease and ease of testing.

The exception here would be vitamin D testing which should be done every two weeks until your 25 hydroxy D level is between 65 and 80 ng/ml.

Many patients with RA have a hypochromic, microcytic CBC that appears very similar to iron deficiency, but it is not at all related. This is probably due to the RA inflammation impairing optimal bone marrow utilization of iron.

It is important to note that this type of anemia does <u>not</u> respond to iron and if you are put on iron you will get worse, as the iron is a very potent oxidative stress. Ferritin levels are generally the most reliable indicator of total iron body stores. Unfortunately, it is also an acute phase reactant protein and will be elevated anytime the ESR is elevated. This makes ferritin an unreliable test in patients with RA.

THE INFECTIOUS CAUSE OF RA

It is quite clear that autoimmunity plays a major role in the progression of Rheumatoid Arthritis. Most rheumatology investigators believe that an infectious agent causes RA. There is little agreement as to the involved organism, however. Investigators have proposed the following infectious agents:

- Human T-cell lymphotropic virus Type I
- Rubella virus

- Cytomegalovirus
- Herpes virus
- Mycoplasma

This review will focus on the evidence supporting the hypothesis that Mycoplasma is a common etiologic agent of Rheumatoid Arthritis. Mycoplasmas are the smallest self-replicating prokaryotes. They differ from classical bacteria by lacking rigid cell wall structures and are the smallest known organisms capable of extracellular existence. They are considered to be parasites of humans, animals, and plants.

Culturing Mycoplasmas from Joints

Mycoplasmas have limited biosynthetic capabilities and are very difficult to culture and grow from synovial tissues. They require complex growth media or a close parasitic relation with animal cells. This contributed to many investigators failure to isolate them from arthritic tissue.

In reactive arthritis, immune complexes rather than viable organisms localize in your joints. The infectious agent is actually present at another site. Some investigators believe that the organism binding in the immune complex contributes to the difficulty in obtaining positive Mycoplasma cultures.

Despite this difficulty, some researchers have successfully isolated Mycoplasma from synovial tissues of patients with RA. A British group used a leukocyte-migration inhibition test and found two-thirds of their RA patients to be infected with *Mycoplasma fermentans.* These results are impressive since they did not include more prevalent Mycoplasma strains like *M. salivarium, M. ovale, M. hominis,* and *M. pneumonia.*

One Finnish investigator reported a 100% incidence of isolation of Mycoplasma from 27 rheumatoid synovia using a modified culture technique. None of the non-rheumatoid tissue yielded any Mycoplasmas.

The same investigator used an indirect hema-glutination technique and reported Mycoplasma antibodies in 53 percent of patients with definite RA. Using similar techniques, other investigators have cultured Mycoplasma in 80-100 percent of their RA test population.

RA can also follow some mycoplasmal respiratory infections. One study of over 1,000 patients was able to identify arthritis in nearly 1 percent of the patients. These infections can be associated with a positive rheumatoid factor. This provides additional support for Mycoplasma as an etiologic agent for RA. Human genital Mycoplasma infections have also caused septic arthritis.

Harvard investigators were able to culture Mycoplasma or a similar organism, *Ureaplasma urealyticum*, from 63% of female patients with Systemic Lupus Erthematosus (SLE) and only 4% of patients with Chronic Fatigue Syndrome (CFS). The researchers chose CFS, as these patients shared similar symptoms as those with SLE, such as fatigue, arthralgias, and myalgias.

Animal Evidence for the Antibiotic Protocol

The full spectrum of human RA immune responses (lymphokine production, altered lymphocyte reactivity, immune complex deposition, cell-mediated immunity, and the development of autoimmune reactions) occurs in Mycoplasma-induced animal arthritis.

Investigators have implicated at least 31 different Mycoplasma species.

Mycoplasma can produce experimental arthritis in animals from three days to months later. The time seems to depend on the dose given, and the virulence of the organism. There is a close degree of similarity between these infections and those of human Rheumatoid Arthritis.

Mycoplasmas cause arthritis in animals by several mechanisms. They either directly multiply within the joint or initiate an intense local immune response. Arthritogenic Mycoplasmas also cause joint inflammation in animals by several mechanisms. They induce nonspecific lymphocyte cytotoxicity and antilymphocyte antibodies as well as rheumatoid factor.

Mycoplasma clearly causes chronic arthritis in mice, rats, fowl, swine, sheep, goats, cattle, and rabbits. The arthritis appears to be the direct result of joint infection with culturable Mycoplasma organisms.

Gorillas have tissue reactions closer to man than any other animal, and investigators have shown that Mycoplasma can precipitate a rheumatic illness in gorillas. One study demonstrated that Mycoplasma antigens do occur in immune complexes in great apes.

The human and gorilla IgG are very similar and express nearly identical rheumatoid factors (IgM anti-IgG antibodies). The study showed that when Mycoplasma binds to IgG it can cause a conformational change that results in an anti-IgG antibody, which can then stimulate an autoimmune response.

The Science of Why Minocycline is Used

If Mycoplasma were a causative factor in RA, one would expect tetracycline type drugs to provide some sort of improvement in the disease. Collagenase activity increases in RA and probably has a role in its cause. Investigators have demonstrated that tetracycline and minocycline inhibit leukocyte, macrophage, and synovial collagenase.

There are several other aspects of tetracyclines that may play a role in RA. Investigators have shown minocycline and tetracycline to retard excessive connective tissue breakdown and bone resorption, while doxycycline inhibits digestion of human cartilage. It is also possible that tetracycline treatment improves rheumatic illness by reducing delayed-type hypersensitivity response. Minocycline and doxycycline both inhibit phosolipases which are considered proinflammatory and capable of inducing synovitis.

Minocycline is a more potent antibiotic than tetracycline and penetrates tissues better. Minocycline may benefit RA patients through its immunomodulating and immunosuppressive properties. *In vitro* studies have demonstrated a decreased neutrophil production of reactive oxygen intermediates along with diminished neutrophil chemotaxis and phagocytosis. Minocycline has also been shown to reduce the incidence and severity of synovitis in animal models of arthritis. The improvement was independent of minocycline's effect on collagenase. Minocycline has also been shown to increase intracellular calcium concentrations that inhibit T-cells.

Individuals with the Class II major histocompatibility complex (MHC) DR4 allele seem to be predisposed to developing RA. The infectious agent probably interacts with this specific antigen in some way to precipitate RA. There is strong support for the role of T-cells in this interaction.

So minocycline may suppress RA by altering T-cell calcium flux and the expression of T-cell derived from collagen binding protein. Minocycline produced a suppression of the delayed hypersensitivity in patients with Reiter's syndrome, and investigators also successfully used minocycline to treat the arthritis and early morning stiffness of Reiter's syndrome.

Clinical Studies

In 1970, investigators at Boston University conducted a small, randomized placebo-controlled trial to determine if tetracycline would treat RA. They used 250 mg of tetracycline per day. Their study showed no improvement after one year of tetracycline treatment. Several factors could explain their inability to demonstrate any benefits.

Their study used only 27 patients for a one-year trial, and only 12 received tetracycline, so noncompliance may have been a factor. Additionally, none of the patients had severe arthritis. Patients were excluded from the trial if they were on any anti-remittive therapy.

Finnish investigators used lymecycline to treat the reactive arthritis in *Chlamydia trachomatous* infections. Their study compared the effect of the medication in patients with two other reactive arthritis infections: Yersinia and Campylobacter. Lymecyline produced a shorter course of illness in the Chlamydia-induced arthritis patients, but did not affect the other enteric infections-associated reactive arthritis. The investigators later published findings suggesting that lymecycline achieved its effect through non-antimicrobial actions. They speculated that it worked by preventing the oxidative activation of collagenase.

The first trial of minocycline for the treatment of animal and human RA was published by Breedveld. In the first published human trial, Breedveld treated ten patients in an open study for 16 weeks. He used a very high dose of 400 mg per day. Most patients had vestibular (sense of balance) side effects resulting from this dose. However, all patients showed benefit from the treatment, and all variables of efficacy were significantly improved at the end of the trial.

Breedveld expanded on his initial study and later observed similar impressive results. This was a 26-week double-blind placebo-controlled randomized trial with minocycline for 80 patients. They were given 200 mg twice a day. The Ritchie articular index and the number of swollen joints significantly improved ($p < 0.05$) more in the minocyline group than in the placebo group.

Investigators in Israel studied 18 patients with severe RA for 48 weeks who had failed to improve with two other disease-modifying anti-rheumatic drugs (DMARDs). They were taken off all DMARD agents and given minocycline

100 mg twice per day. Six patients did not complete the study: three withdrew because of lack of improvement, and three had side effects of vertigo or leukopenia (a reduction in the number of white blood cells). All patients completing the study improved. Three had complete remission, three had substantial improvement of greater than 50 percent, and six had moderate improvement of 25 percent in the number of active joints and morning stiffness.

ANTIBIOTIC THERAPY WITH MINOCIN [5]

There are three different tetracyclines available: simple tetracycline, doxycycline, or Minocin (minocycline).

Minocin has a distinct and clear advantage over tetracycline and doxycycline in three important areas:

1. Extended spectrum of activity
2. Greater tissue penetrability
3. Higher and more sustained serum levels

Bacterial cell membranes contain a lipid layer. One mechanism of building up a resistance to an antibiotic is to produce a thicker lipid layer. This layer makes it difficult for an antibiotic to penetrate. Minocin's chemical structure makes it the most lipid-soluble of all the tetracyclines.

This difference can clearly be demonstrated when you compare the drugs in the treatment of two common clinical conditions. Minocin gives consistently superior clinical results in the treatment of chronic prostatitis. In other studies, Minocin was used to improve between 75-85 percent of patients whose acne had become resistant to tetracycline. Streptococcus is also believed to be a contributing cause to many patients with RA. Minocin has shown significant activity against treatment of this organism.

Important Factors to Consider When Using Minocin

Unlike the other tetracyclines, Minocin tends not to cause yeast infections. Some infectious disease experts even believe that it has a mild anti-yeast activity. Women can be on this medication for several years and not have any vaginal yeast infections. Nevertheless, it would be prudent to take prophylactic oral *Lactobacillus acidophilus* and *L bifidus* preparations. This will help to replace the normal intestinal flora that is killed with the Minocin.

Like other tetracyclines, food impairs its absorption. However, the absorption is much less impaired than with other tetracyclines. This is fortunate because some people cannot tolerate Minocin on an empty stomach and have to take it with a meal to avoid GI side effects.

If you need to take it with food, you will still absorb 85% of the medication, whereas tetracycline is only 50% absorbed. In 1990, a pelletized version of Minocin also became available, which improved absorption when taken with meals. This form is only available in the non-generic Lederle brand, and is a more than reasonable justification to not substitute for the generic version.

Clinical experience has shown that many patients will relapse when they switch from the brand name to the generic. (Please see the separate section at the end of this Appendix).

Many patients are on NSAIDs that contribute to microulcerations of the stomach, which cause chronic blood loss. It is certainly possible to develop a peptic ulcer contributing to this blood loss. In either event, patients are frequently receiving iron supplements to correct their blood counts.

IT IS IMPERATIVE THAT MINOCIN NOT BE GIVEN WITH IRON!

Over 85 percent of the dose will bind to the iron and pass through your colon unabsorbed. If iron is taken, it should be at least one hour before Minocin, or two hours after.

A recent, uncommon, complication of Minocin is a cell-mediated hypersensitivity pneumonitis.

Most patients can start on 100 mg of Minocin every Monday, Wednesday, and Friday evening. Doxycycline can be substituted for patients who cannot afford the more expensive Minocin. It is important to not give either medication daily, as this does not seem to provide as great a clinical benefit.

WARNING: Tetracycline-type drugs can cause a permanent yellow-grayish brown discoloration of your teeth. This can occur in the last half of pregnancy, and in children up to eight years old. You should not routinely use tetracycline in children.

If you have severe disease, you can consider increasing the dose to as high as 200 mg three times a week. Aside from the cost of this approach, several problems may result from the higher doses. Minocin can cause quite severe nausea and vertigo, but taking the dose at night tends to decrease this problem considerably.

However, if you take the dose at bedtime, you must swallow the medication with TWO glasses of water. This is to insure that the capsule doesn't get stuck in your throat. If that occurs, a severe chemical esophagitis can result, which can send you to the emergency room.

For those physicians who elect to use tetracycline or doxycycline for cost or sensitivity reasons, several methods may help lessen the inevitable secondary yeast overgrowth. *Lactobacillus acidophilus* will help maintain normal bowel flora and decrease the risk of fungal overgrowth.

Aggressive avoidance of all sugars, especially those found in non-diet sodas will also decrease the substrate for the yeast's growth. Macrolide antibiotics like Biaxin or Zithromax may be used if tetracyclines are contraindicated. They would also be used in the three pills per week regimen.

Clindamycin

The other drug used to treat Rheumatoid Arthritis is clindamycin. Dr. Brown's book discusses the uses of intravenous clindamycin, and it is important to use the IV form of treatment if the disease is severe.

In my experience nearly all Scleroderma patients require a more aggressive stance and use IV treatment. Scleroderma is a particularly dangerous form of rheumatic illness that should receive aggressive intervention.

A major problem with the IV form is the cost. The price ranges from $100 to $300 per dose if administered by a home health care agency. However, if purchased directly from Upjohn, significant savings can be had.

If you have a milder illness, the oral form of clindamycin is preferable. With a mild rheumatic illness (the minority of cases), it is even possible to exclude this from your regimen. Initial starting doses for an adult would be a 1200 mg dose once per week.

Please note that many people do not seem to tolerate this medication as well as Minocin. The major complaint seems to be a bitter metallic-type taste, which lasts about 24 hours after the dose. Taking the dose after dinner does seem to help modify this complaint somewhat. If this is a problem, you can lower the dose and gradually increase the dose over a few weeks. Concern about the overgrowth of *Clostridium difficile* leading to pseudomembranous enterocolitis as a result of the clindamycin is appropriate. This complication is quite rare at this dosage regimen, but it certainly can occur.

It is also important to be aware of the possibility of developing a severe and uncontrollable bout of diarrhea. Administration of acidophilus seems to limit this complication by promoting the growth of the healthy gut flora.

If you have a resistant form of rheumatic illness, intravenous (IV) administration should be considered.

Generally, weekly doses of 900 mg are administered until clinical improvement is observed. This generally occurs within the first 10 doses. At that time, the regimen can be decreased to every two weeks with the oral form substituted on the weeks where the IV is not taken.

What to Do if You Fail to Respond

The most frequent reason for failure to respond to the protocol is lack of adherence to the dietary guidelines. Most people eat too many grains and sugars, which disturbs insulin physiology. It is important that you adhere as strictly as possible to the guidelines. A small minority, generally under 15 percent, of patients will fail to respond to the protocol described above, despite rigid adherence to the diet. These individuals should already be on the IV clindamycin.

It appears that hyaluronic acid, which is a potentiating agent commonly used in the treatment of cancer, may be quite useful in these cases. It seems that hyaluronic acid has very little to no direct toxicity but works in a highly synergistic fashion when administered directly in the IV bag with the clindamycin.

Hyaluronic acid is also used in orthopedic procedures. The dose is generally from 2 to 10 cc into the IV bag. Hyaluronic acid is not inexpensive, however, as the cost may range up to $10 per cc. You also need to use some caution, as it may precipitate a significant Jarisch-Herxheimer flare reaction.

ASSESSMENT FOR FIBROMYALGIA

You need to be very sensitive to this condition when you have RA since Fibromyalgia is frequently a complicating condition. Often the pain will be confused with a flare-up of the RA. You need to aggressively treat this problem. If it is ignored, the likelihood of successfully treating the RA is significantly diminished.

Fibromyalgia is a very common problem. Some experts believe that 5 percent of people are affected with it. Over 12 percent of the patients at the Mayo Clinic's Department of Physical Medicine and Rehabilitation have this problem, and it is the third most common diagnosis by rheumatologists in the outpatient setting. Fibromyalgia affects women five times as frequently as men.

Signs and Symptoms of Fibromyalgia

One of the main features of Fibromyalgia is morning stiffness, fatigue, and multiple areas of tenderness in typical locations. Most people with Fibromyalgia complain of pain over many areas of the body, with an average of six to nine locations. Although the pain is frequently described as being "all over," it is most prominent in the neck, shoulders, elbows, hips, knees, and back.

Tender points are generally symmetrical and on both sides of the body. The areas of tenderness are usually small (less than an inch in diameter) and deep within the muscle. They are often located in sites that are slightly tender in normal people. Those who have Fibromyalgia, however, differ in having increased tenderness at these sites than the average person. Firm palpation with the thumb (just past the point where the nail turns white) over the outside elbow will typically cause a vague sensation of discomfort. Patients with Fibromyalgia will experience much more pain and will often withdraw the arm involuntarily.

More than 70% of patients describe their pain as profound aching and stiffness of muscles. Often it is relatively constant from moment to moment, but certain positions or movements may momentarily worsen the pain. Other terms used to describe the pain are "numb" and "dull." Sharp or intermittent pain is relatively uncommon. Patients with Fibromyalgia also often complain that sudden loud noises worsen their pain.

The generalized stiffness of Fibromyalgia does not diminish with activity, unlike the stiffness of RA, which lessens as the day progresses. Despite the lack of abnormal lab tests, patients can suffer considerable discomfort. The fatigue is often severe enough to impair activities of work and recreation. Patients commonly experience fatigue on arising and complain of being more fatigued when they wake up than when they went to bed.

Over 90 percent of patients believe that the pain, stiffness, and fatigue are made worse by cold, damp weather. Overexertion, anxiety, and stress are also factors. Many find that localized heat, such as hot baths, showers, or heating pads, give them some relief. There is also a tendency for pain to improve in the summer with mild activity, or with rest.

Some patients will date the onset of their symptoms to some initiating event. This is often an injury, such as a fall, a motor vehicle accident, or a vocational or sports injury. Others find that their symptoms began with a stressful or emotional event, such as a death in the family, a divorce, a job loss, or similar occurrence.

Pain Location (Tender Points)

Patients with Fibromyalgia have pain in at least 11 of the following 18 tender point sites (one on each side of the body), as shown in Figure 8.

1. Base of the skull where the suboccipital muscle inserts.
2. Back of the low neck (anterior intertransverse spaces of C5-C7).
3. Midpoint of the upper shoulders (trapezius).
4. On the back in the middle of the scapula.
5. On the chest where the second rib attaches to the breastbone (sternum).

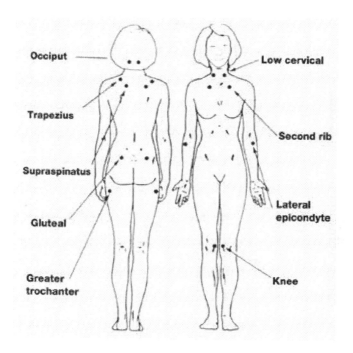

Figure 8. Fibromyalgia Trigger Points

6. One inch below the outside of each elbow (lateral epicondyle).
7. Upper outer quadrant of buttocks.
8. Just behind the swelling on the upper leg bone below the hip (trochanteric prominence).
9. The inside of both knees (medial fat pads proximal to the joint line).

Treatment of Fibromyalgia

There is a persuasive body of emerging evidence that indicates that patients with Fibromyalgia are physically unfit in terms of sustained endurance. Some studies show that exercise can decrease Fibromyalgia pain by 75 percent. Sleep is also critical to improvement, and many times, improved fitness will also correct the sleep disturbance.

388 *Arthritis and Autoimmune Diseases:*
The Infection Connection

Normalizing vitamin D levels has been helpful to decrease pain, as has topical magnesium oil supplementation.

Allergies, especially to mold, seem to be another common cause of Fibromyalgia. There are some simple interventions using techniques called Total Body Modification (TBM), discussed in Chapter 7 of this book.[6]

[Find helpful articles by Dr. Mercola dating from 2001 at: www.articles.mercola.com/sites/Newsletter/NewsLetter-Archive.aspx. You can search by publication date, or by category, or use the search window using specific terms.]

Additional Considerations About Minocin

By Katherine Poehlmann, PhD

The low dose, long-term antibiotic treatment that Dr. Brown advocated for years, and that Dr. A. Robert Franco continues to advocate in his practice, gives hope to patients with Rheumatoid Arthritis and other rheumatic diseases like Scleroderma. Dr. Franco has 24 years of experience treating thousands of patients suffering by using a combination of nutritional supplements and antibiotics.[7]

According to Dr. Franco, an important difference when considering generic Minocin is the pelletized versus powdered form. Pelletized is considered safer because the powdered form has a tendency to reflux (go backward) into the esophagus. The pelletized form has a better chance to reach the stomach intact.

Caution: Tetracyclines can be very irritating to the esophageal lining if the capsule lodges there and starts to dissolve. The capsule must be taken with 1-2 full glasses of water to flush it past the esophagus to avoid the risk of ulceration, irritation, and/or bleeding.

In Dr. Franco's view, generic minocycline is 35-40% less bioavailable than the original brand name Minocin. To achieve the same therapeutic results, his approach is to increase the generic minocycline dose to compensate for the reduced potency. E.g., instead of prescribing 100 mg of brand name Minocin MWF, he will put the patient on a schedule of 300 mg of generic minocycline on MWF: 200 mg before breakfast and 100 mg before dinner. This dosage is based on an average patient weight of 70 kg (154 lb).

Dosage adjustment must be made for patients who weigh substantially more or less than 70 kg. Probiotics are also prescribed to replenish the "good" bacteria in the gut. These should be taken four hours apart from the antibiotics. (Probiotics are discussed in Chapter 3).

Traditionally it was recommended to prescribe only the brand name Lederle Minocin or its generic. Neither is available at this time. A number of manufacturers now offer generic minocycline. An overview of Minocin sources and costs as of 2011 appears at www.tmgp.com/minocin.htm. If price is an issue, one might try to order through a Canadian pharmacy.[8]

Your doctor can advise on brand potency and specific dosage. In some cases, multiple antibiotics may be needed, tailored to the patient's condition involving multiple bacterial infections. Other treatments may be needed for viral or fungal co-infections.

[1] Find full details at www.mercola.com/nutritionplan/index.htm
[2] Over 200 supporting references can be found at http://articles.mercola.com/sites/articles/archive/2010/08/16/rheumatoid-arthritis-protocol.aspx
[3] www.mercola.com/article/vitamin-d-resources.htm.
[4] Visit www.mayoclinic.com and use the search window to describe the particular pain you are experiencing.
[5] Additional information: *Protocol for Antibiotic Therapy*, from The Road Back Foundation at www.roadback.com.
[6] Find full details at www.tbmseminars.com/x_about.asp.
[7] http://www.thearthritiscenter.com/content/dr-franco-and-antibiotic-treatment and www.thearthritiscenter.com/content/profile-robert-franco-md
[8] At this writing, some online Canadian sellers of Minocin made by Stiefel are: www.Federaldrugs.com, www.Canadadrugs.com, and www.Universaldrugstore.com. Online sellers of Minocin made by Wyeth-Ayerst are: www.Northwestpharmacy.com, www.Getcanadiandrugs.com, and www.canadapharmacy.com

Appendix III

CONSIDERATIONS WHEN UNDERGOING TREATMENT FOR CHRONIC ILLNESSES AND AUTOIMMUNE DISEASES

by Prof. Garth L. Nicolson*

The Institute for Molecular Medicine (www.immed.org)

There are a number of considerations when undergoing therapy for chronic illnesses, including whether to use traditional as well as integrative nutraceutical approaches. These are discussed in the following sections, including antibiotic/antiviral/antifungal therapies and dietary supplements. The Institute for Molecular Medicine is a nonprofit institution and does not endorse commercial products or treatment approaches. The products and procedures below are only examples of the types of approaches and substances that could be beneficial to patients with chronic illnesses. Consult your personal physician for advice on treatments, dosing and schedules that can vary for each patient.

Reprinted from *Intern. J. Medicine* 1998; 1:123-128. Plus Supplemental Suggestions by Prof. Nicolson added 1/15/12

The author has no financial interest in any product discussed below.

Antibiotic Therapy and Herbal Therapy for Chronic Infections

Subsets of fatiguing illnesses like GWI (~40-45%), FMS (60-70%), CFS (50-60%), autoimmune diseases (RA, MS, SLE, etc. ~50%) and neurological diseases (ALS,

Parkinson's, Alzheimer's) show high incidence of chronic infections of Mycoplasma, Chlamydia, Borrelia, Brucella, Bartonella, and other bacterial, viral (HHV-6, CMV, etc.) parasitic, and fungal infections. For intracellular bacterial infections, 6 months [no break] treatment, then 6-week on 2-week off antibiotic cycles (doxycycline, ciprofloxacin, azithromycin, minocycline, clarithromycin or others work best as oral capsules without starch fillers).

Some patients benefit from combinations of antibiotics, such as doxycycline plus azithromycin or ciprofloxacin, especially if there are limited responses to either alone. Combinations of antibiotics with different mechanisms of action work best. In addition, these infections are usually intracellular, and Plaquenil has been used to alkalize cellular compartments and improve killing. Some practitioners recommend every-other-day dosing, which presumes that the microorganisms cycle, which is true, but compliance is important if this approach is chosen.

Oral antibiotics must be taken with a full glass of water, crackers or bread to avoid esophageal irritation (do not lie down for at least 1 hour). Direct sunlight must be avoided for many antibiotics.

To overcome Jarisch-Herxheimer reactions (die-off reactions involving chills, fever, night sweats, muscle aches, joint pain, short term memory loss, fatigue, a general worsening of signs/symptoms) or other adverse responses, intravenous (i.v.) antibiotics have been used for a few weeks—then oral. Also, oral Benadryl (diphenhydramine, 50 mg) taken at least 30 min before antibiotics is useful to reduce gut reactions along with lemon/olive drink (1 blended lemon, 1 cup fruit juice, 1 tbs olive oil—strain and drink liquid).

The Herxheimer period usually passes within a few weeks and differs from allergic reactions that can cause immediate rashes, itching, swelling, dizziness, and trouble breathing. If allergic reactions occur, seek immediate medical attention. Many antibiotics cannot be used during pregnancy or by infants. Cycles of Augmentin in-between the 6-week antibiotic cycles or concurrently, if needed, can help to suppress secondary bacterial infections. In addition, some patients have benefited from adding Flagyl (metronidazole), Plaquenil (hydroxychloroquinine), or Tindamax (hydroxy-chloroquinine) to kill cyst or L-forms and protozoal infections.

For viruses, some add the antivirals for the first 2 weeks (see the next section). Mycoplasmas may have some characteristics of viruses, so this can be useful, and viral infections are also important in these illnesses. Often patients have multiple bacterial infections along with other co-infections. For more information on how to treat difficult co-infections see www.mycoplasmasupport.org. Nutriceuticals, supplements, vitamins, and other products can be found at a variety of sources listed below.

For patients who cannot take antibiotics, Rain Tree has three products that can't replace antibiotics but are a fairly good alternative: Myco+; A-F; Immune Support. Contact: 800-780-5902 or www.rain-tree.com. For some, the Cowden protocol has proved useful without antibiotics (http://lymediseaseresource.com/Dr_Lee_Cowden).

Patients with complex chronic infections like Lyme Disease should read Dr. Burrascano's review on treatment of Lyme infections (found on the IMM website: www.immed.org) under Treatment Considerations). In addition to the Rain Tree products, there are several herbal therapies that have been used (mostly in combination) with mixed success: licorice extract, allicin, samento, cumunda, quina, coptis, andrographis, Japanese knotwood, clove, wormwood, pau d'arco, grapefruit extract, olive leaf extract, caprylic acid, garlic extract, and oregano oil.

These have been combined in the Byron White protocol (www.byronwhiteformulas.com) and the Buchner protocol for Lyme (http://lymediseaseresource.com), which are probably useful for a number of multiple, complex infections.

Antiviral Therapy for Chronic Infections

Large subsets of chronic illness and other autoimmune patients have chronic viral infections, such as HHV-6A and

CMV. For HHV-6 and CMV infections, Ganciclovir is the antiviral of choice. This can be used i.v. (5 mg/Kg i.v. over 1 hour every day) or oral (1000 mg 2X/day) in 3-week cycles. Some patients have benefited from the use of Famvir. This can be used as an oral dose (500 mg 2X/day for 2 weeks.

Nutraceutical treatments can be used instead or concurrently, such as Genistein (in soy/red clover) to inhibit viral kinase, rosemary/lemon balm to reduce complement activation, selenite (see minerals) to inhibit viral replication, barley grass and lauric acid to inhibit lipid metabolism of viruses and Phyllanthus amarus/niruri to inhibit viral reverse transcriptase. Immune enhancement is important (see section below), and patients should try this approach before going to more problematic antiviral drugs.

General Nutritional Considerations

Chronic illness patients are often immunosuppressed and susceptible to opportunistic infections, so proper nutrition is imperative. You should not smoke or drink alcohol or caffeinated products. Drink as much fresh fluids as you can; pure water is best. Try to avoid high sugar and trans-fat foods, such as military meals-ready-to-eat (MREs) or other fast foods and acid-forming, allergen-prone and system-stressing foods or high sugar/fat junk foods.

Note: decreasing sugar intake is essential—simple or refined sugars can suppress your immune system. Increase intake of fresh vegetables, fruits and grains, and decrease intake of trans-fats. To build your immune system, cruciferous vegetables, soluble fiber foods, such as prunes and bran, wheat germ, yogurt, fish and whole grains are useful. In some patients, exclusive use of "organic" foods has been beneficial. Diet, and especially reduction in sugar intake, is also important to control yeast infections.

Vitamins and Minerals

Chronic illness patients are often depleted in vitamins (especially B-complex, C, E, CoQ_{10}) and certain minerals.

These illnesses often result in poor absorption. Therefore, high doses of some vitamins are useful; others, such as vitamin B-complex, which cannot be easily absorbed by the gut (via an oral dose). Sublingual (under the tongue) natural B-complex vitamins liquid (e.g., Total B, Real Life Research, Norwalk, CA, 562-926-5522 or www.vitaminshoppe.com) should be used instead of capsules.

General vitamins plus extra C, E, CoQ_{10}, beta-carotene, folic acid, bioflavonoids and biotin are best. L-cysteine, L-tyrosine, L-glutamine, L-carnitine, malic acid and especially flaxseed or fish oils are reported to be useful.

Certain minerals are depleted in chronic illness patients, such as zinc, magnesium, chromium, and selenium. Some recommend sodium selenite, up to 300 mcg/day, followed by lower doses. Vitamins and minerals should not be taken at the same time of day (3-4 hour difference) as antibiotics or antivirals (or oxygen therapy), because they can affect absorption or act against therapy.

Some clinicians recommend that antioxidant vitamins be taken at least 4 hours before or after oxygen therapy. The suggested doses of vitamins can vary dramatically among patients; consult with your physician or nutritionist for appropriate dosage.

Some patients may require analysis of vitamins, minerals, and amino acids so that appropriate doses can be recommended: Nu-Life (Sophista-Care, 760-837-1908), Immune-Pak (Care Management Products, 888-845-1467), www.vitaminshoppe.com, American Biologics (800-227-4473, www.americanbiologics.com), and Prohealth (800-366-6056, www.immunesupport.com).

Lipid Replacement Therapy for Chronic Infections and for Restoring Mitochondrial Function

Lipid Replacement Therapy is useful in providing membrane lipids in unoxidized form to repair nerve and mitochondrial membranes that are damaged by heavy metals, chemicals, and infections. We recommend all-natural Healthy

Aging or Propax Gold containing NTFactor (Nutritional Therapeutics, Inc. www.NTFactor.com, 800-982-9158). For children, tablets should be ground up between two spoons into a coarse powder that can be added to applesauce. The NTFactor is not bitter, but it is slightly sour, and some children actually like the taste. The dose should be 4-5 tablets twice per day, which can later be reduced to once per day. Child's dose is:

- 1/2-1 tablet for children up to 2 years old;
- 2 tablets for 2-3 years old;
- 3-4 tablets for 4-5 years old; and
- 4-5 tablets for 5 years old and older.

Research has demonstrated no adverse responses with NTFactor, even at many times these doses. Since this formulation is a completely natural membrane lipid mixture, there are no known toxicities and no known toxic dose limits. NTFactor also comes with vitamins, minerals, and probiotics (Propax Gold; 800-982-9158, www.propax.com), CoQ_{10}, alpha-lipoic acid, L-carnitine, and unsaturated fatty acids. Some claim that NADH is also useful but only a few patients appear to benefit from oral NADH in clinical trials. NADH (Nicotinamide adenine dinucleotide) is a coenzyme made from vitamin B_2.

Oxidative Therapy for Chronic Infections

Oxidative therapy can be useful in suppressing a variety of anaerobic infections: several weeks of Hyperbaric Oxygen (1.5-2 ATM, 60 minute) treatments, i.v. ozone or hydrogen peroxide are useful, or peroxide baths using 2 cups of Epsom salt in a hot bath or Jacuzzi. After 5 min, add 2-4 bottles 16 oz. of 3% hydrogen peroxide. Repeat 2-3X/week; no vitamins or antioxidants 2-4 hr before the bath. The hydrogen peroxide is added after your pores open.

Hydrogen peroxide can also be directly applied to skin after a workout or hot shower/tub. Leave hydrogen peroxide on for 5 min, and then wash off. For oral irrigation, mix 1 part

3% hydrogen peroxide with two parts water and use like a mouth wash 3X per day. Most chronic illness patients have periodontal problems, and oral infections and bone cavitation infections are common. These should not be ignored, because these infections can become systemic and spread to other sites.

Only attempt i.v. ozone or i.v. hydrogen peroxide under the immediate care of a physician specialist who routinely uses these therapies. Acute, dangerous, adverse reactions have been reported, and these approaches must be initiated with very low doses and gradually built up to avoid adverse reactions.

Testing and Therapy for Heavy Metal Contamination

The Institute for Molecular Medicine and other institutions have found that many chronic illness patients have heavy metal contamination that must be considered. Most studies have concentrated on mercury, lead, aluminum, cadmium, and other heavy metals. Veterans may have uranium contamination. Although heavy metal mobilization and removal is a long-term process, often taking over one year, it does not require expensive, invasive, weekly treatments at clinics.

Patients should have a heavy metal analysis of hair, stool, and urine at a reputable diagnostic laboratory such as Doctors' Data (www.doctorsdata.com, 800-323-2784) and Great Smokies Diagnostic Lab (www.gsdl.com, 800-522-4762). Any results should be evaluated by a physician.

Such analyses are usually of excreted heavy metals; deposits deep in tissues cannot be tested using these procedures. Non-invasive treatments to remove heavy metals include oral dosing, transdermal patches, and anal suppositories containing chelating agents. The former can be found at www.edtachelation.com and the latter is available from World Health Products (Detoxamin, 877-656-4553). It is very effective and can be used long-term with very few or no side effects.

DMSA (dimercaptosuccinic acid) has been used extensively to remove heavy metals (www.ehow.com/how-does_5292549_dmsa-chelation-procedures).

Products like Xymogen's Detox Support (800-647-5100, www.xymogen.com) contain DMSA, EDTA, organic garlic, cilantro, and other components. It is claimed that Garlic Plus (Longevity, 800-580-7587, www.longevityplus.net) is useful, but there are no studies to substantiate this claim.

Other natural substances are recommended, such as Zeolite from volcanic ash (www.allnaturalprevention.com), oral EDTA (Calcitetracemate, http://gordonresearch.com), and other products (e.g., Calibex, www.calibex.com).

Replacement of Natural Gut Flora and Digestive Enzymes

Patients undergoing treatment with antibiotics risk destruction of normal gut flora. Antibiotic use that depletes normal gut bacteria and can result in overgrowth of less desirable bacteria and fungi. To supplement normal bacteria, live cultures of Lactobacillus acidophilus and other "friendly" bacteria are strongly recommended. Mixtures of *L. acidophilus, L. bifidus, Bifidobacteria, L. bulgaricus* and FOS (fructoologosaccharides) to promote growth of these probiotics in the gut are useful.

Examples are DDS-1, DDS-Plusor, and Multi-Flora from UAS Labs (800-422-3371, www.uaslabs.com); Xymogen's ProbioMax (800-647-5100, www.xymogen.com); and Theralac (800-926-2961, www.theralac.com),

L. acidophilus mixtures (>15 billion live organisms) should be taken 3X per day and 2 hour after any antibiotics. For irritable bowel, the nutraceutical Calm Colon (Samra, 310-202-9999) has proven to be very effective in clinical trials. For help with bowel bacteria and bladder infections, D-mannose (from Biotech Co., 800-345-1199 and Swanson Health, www.swansonvtamins.com) has been used because of its antibacterial properties. This natural sugar inhibits binding of bacteria to biological membranes.

In addition, to improve digestion and especially absorption, enzyme mixtures have proved useful, e.g., Wobenzym [from www.buywobenzym.com or Health Stores (800-578-5939, www.healthstores.com) or Zooscape (800-760-8783, www.zooscape.com)].

Natural Immunomodulators and Remedies

A number of natural remedies, herbal teas, lemon/olive drink, olive leaf extract (oleuropein), wormwood extract (artemesinin/artesunate), are sometimes useful, especially during or after antibiotic therapy. Additional important examples are immune modulators, such as bioactive whey protein from these sources:

- ImuPlus (800-310-8311, www.imuplus.com)
- Immunocal (800-337-2411, www.immunocal.com)
- ImmunoPro (www.immunesupport.com or Needs, 800-634-1380, www.needs.com)
- Transfer Factor (4-Life, 800-852-7700, www.transferfactor-4-life.com)
- ImmunFactor 2, 8 or 9 (Chisolm Biologicals, 800-664-1333)
- Immuni-T (Longevity, 800-580-7587, www.longevityplus.net)
- MGN3 (Lane Labs, 800-526-3005, www.lanelabs.com)
- ImmunotiX 3-6 (beta-glucan, Xymogen, 800-647-5100, www.xymogen.com)
- ImmPower (American Bioscience, 888-884-7770, www.americanbiosciences.com)
- Microbojen (Jernigan Nutraceuticals, 316-651-5739, http://abc.eznettools.net/jernigannutraceuticals).

Some additional remedies are: olive leaf extract (many sources), Laktoferrin (Nutricology, 888-563-1506 or www.iherb.com), NSC-100 (Nutritional Supply, 888-246-

7224), Echinacea-C (several sources) or Super Defense Plus (BioDefense Nutritionals, 800-669-9205), Tahitian Noni (Morinda, 800-445-8596, www.tahitiannoni.com. These products have been used to boost immune systems. Although they appear to help many patients, their clinical effectiveness has not been carefully evaluated. They appear to be useful during therapy to boost the immune system or after antibiotic/antiviral therapy in a maintenance program.

Yeast/Fungal or Bacterial Overgrowth

Yeast overgrowth can occur, especially in females (vaginal infections). Gynecologists recommend Nizoral, Diflucan, Mycelex, or anti-yeast creams. Metronidazole [Flagyl, Prostat] has been used to prevent fungal or parasite overgrowth or other antifungals [Nystatin, Amphotericin B, Fluconazole, Diflucan] have been administered for fungal infections that can occur while on antibiotics. Herbals that have proved effective are: pau d'arco (7 capsules/2X/day), grapefruit seed extract, oregano complex, garlic extract, Mycopril (a fatty acid from coconut), and Artemesia, a Chinese herb that is often used to treat malaria.

Innovite (www.inno-vite.com) has a yeast buster kit that contains 3 components: psyllium, caproil, and bentonite that can be mixed into a drink that treats and removes intestinal fungus while absorbing toxins. Some patients have as their principal problem systemic fungal infections that can be seen using dark field microscopy of blood smears.

For superficial fungal infections, such as fungal nail, a topical mixture of Laminsil in 17% DMSO 2X/day is effective. As mentioned above, *L. acidophilus* mixtures (>15 billion live organisms per dose) are used to restore gut flora. Bacterial overgrowth can also occur, for example, in-between cycles of antibiotics or after antibiotics/antivirals have been stopped. This can be controlled with 2-week courses of Augmentin (3 X 500 mg/day) in-between cycles or concurrent with other antibiotics. Nutraceutical approaches to controlling yeast infections include: pau d'arco, grapefruit extract, olive leaf, caprylic acid, garlic extract, and oregano oil.

Antidepressants, Narcotics, etc.

Antibiotic uptake and immune responses may be inhibited by some drugs. Antacids, antidiarrheals (among others) should be avoided, if possible, or gradually decreased during therapy. Some drugs (listed below) may inhibit immune responses and interfere with therapy. These should be decreased and gradually eliminated.

- Antidepressants (sertaline [Zoloft], fluoxetine [Prozac], amitriptyline [Elavil], maprotiline [Ludiomil], desipramine [Norpramin], clomipramine [Anafranil], nortriptyline [Pamelor], bupropion [Wellbutrin]);

- Muscle relaxants (cyclobenzaprine [Flexeril]);

- Opiate agonists, anticonvulsives or certain analgesics (oxycodone [Percodan], carbamazepine [Tegretol], acetaminophen/hydrocodone [Vicodin]);

- Narcotics (codeine w/Penergan, propoxyphene [Darvon], morphine);

Flying, Exercise, and Saunas

Flying, excessive exercise, and lack of sleep can make signs/symptoms worse. Flying exposes you to lower oxygen tension, and can stimulate borderline anaerobes that grow better at low oxygen. Some exercise is essential, but avoid relapses due to overexertion. Dry saunas help rid the system of chemicals, and saunas should be taken daily or 3 sessions per week—moderate exercise, followed by 15-20 min of dry sauna and a tepid shower. Repeat saunas no more than 2X per day. Work up a good sweat, eliminating chemicals without placing too much stress on your system, and replace body fluids and electrolytes during and after each session.

During exercise, patients should always avoid pollutant and allergen exposures. For recovery after exercise and to decrease muscle soreness, some use a Jacuzzi or hot tub, but only after a sufficient cool-down period. Don't get overheated in the process. Remember, don't overdo it!!!

Note: This material has not been evaluated by the FDA. It is general information, should not be construed as medical advice, and is not meant as medical advice or to prevent, diagnose, treat or cure any illness, condition, or disease. It is very important that you make no change in your health care plan or health support regimen without researching and discussing it in collaboration with your professional health care team.

**.

Clinical Testing Suggestions

For chronic illnesses (CFS, FMS, RA, Lupus, neurodegenerative diseases, among other illnesses) that could have an infectious component, The Institute for Molecular Medicine suggests the following lab tests (codes are CPT codes or test description/ordering codes):

1. Mycoplasma Test Panel (CPT: 87581)—Mycoplasma species tested by PCR. This is a Mycoplasma test on the 3 most common species of Mycoplasma (*M. pneumoniae, M. fermentans, M. hominis*). Almost 60% of CFS/FMS and 50% of Rheumatoid Arthritis (RA) and 50% other autoimmune patients have one or more intracellular, systemic mycoplasmal infections similar to those found in a variety of chronic illnesses. Individual Mycoplasma species tests can also be ordered. Ultrasensitive and ultraspecific Mycoplasma tests can only be done by a small number of recommended labs:

Unevx Laboratories, 1664 N. Virginia St., Reno, NV 89557, Tel: 775-682-8280, Fax: 775-682-8290

Spiro Stat Technologies, 1004 Garfield Dr., Bldg 340, Lubbock, TX 79416; Tel: 806-885-2929, Fax: 806-885-2933

2. *Chlamydia pneumoniae* Test (CPT: 87486)— *Chlamydia pneumoniae* tested by PCR. We were among the few labs that developed the molecular tests that are now done for this type of infection. Recommended Lab: Unevx Laboratories, address above.

3. Lyme *Borrelia burgdorferi* Test (CPT: 86617)— *Borrelia burgdorferi* (Lyme Disease) by Western Blot analysis. Many CFS, FMS and RA patients have this systemic infection (diagnosed as Lyme Disease) along with other co-infection(s)). Recommended Lab: IGeneX Laboratories of Palo Alto, California (http://www.igenex.com/). Specimen Requirements: Contact laboratory for a specimen kit. Collect in Red Top Tube, separate, and send in clear tube. Store in refrigerator until shipment. Important: Ship within one day of collection at room temperature.

4. HHV-6 Test (CPT: 87532)—Human herpes virus 6 (HHV-6) test by PCR. Many CFS and some FMS patients have this systemic viral infection, and it should be tested for in any autoimmune illness. Recommended Lab: Unevx Laboratories, address above.

5. CMV Test 07034 (CPT: 87496)—Cytomegalovirus (CMV) test by nested PCR. Many CFS and FMS patients have this systemic viral infection, and it should be tested for in any autoimmune illness. Recommended Lab: Unevx Laboratories, address above.

**.

Professor Nicolson's website www.immed.org features dozens of supportive references for this Appendix including these specific articles:

"Chronic Mycoplasmal Infections in Gulf War Veterans' Children and Autism Patients." (2005)

"Diagnosis and Therapy of Chronic Systemic Co-infections in Lyme Disease and Other Tick-Borne Infectious Diseases." (2007)

"Chronic Bacterial and Viral Infections in Neurodegenerative and Neurobehavioral Diseases." (2008)

"High Prevalence of Mycoplasmal Infections in Symptomatic (Chronic Fatigue Syndrome) Family Members of Mycoplasma-Positive Gulf War Illness Patients." (2003)

"Chronic Fatigue Syndrome Patients Subsequently Diagnosed with Lyme Disease *Borrelia burgdorferi*: Evidence for Mycoplasma species Co-Infections." (2008)

"Lipid Replacement and Antioxidant Nutritional Therapy for Restoring Mitochondrial Function and Reducing Fatigue in Chronic Fatigue Syndrome and other Fatiguing Illnesses." (2006)

"Antibiotics/Antivirals Recommended When Indicated for Treatment of Intracellular Infections in Chronic Illnesses." (2012)

Appendix IV:

WEBSITES FOR HEALTH-RELATED RESEARCH

This book is written for those who wish to take an active role in achieving good health. The more informed the patient, the better s/he is able to enter into a partnership with a health care provider. Dealing with illness then becomes a stronger, more focused team approach and the probability is increased for a positive, rewarding outcome.

HOW TO USE THIS APPENDIX

The first column in each table shows the website's top-level Home Page. An "X" in a box associated with a given Home Page means that the information in that category is well worth reading. For example, the site www.stanford.edu has an "X" in the Arthritis and Lupus categories. Of course, much more than this specific information on a few illnesses is available on this Stanford University medical library site. It is just that for research pertinent to topics covered in this book, that set of data is judged by the authors to be authoritative and outstanding. Note that this website also has an "X" in the box for "Autoimmune Diseases" and "Rheumatic Diseases." This means that the site is comprehensive, providing information on many other illnesses in those categories, too many to list individually.

Any site with an "X" in the "Topic Search" category has a local keyword search feature leading to subcategories of useful information within the site. The lack of an "X" does not mean to imply that the site has minimal data on a particular topic. It only means that the topic area was not fully explored as part of the research done for this book. The reader is encouraged to visit these websites and type in topic keywords of personal interest. A few websites, like those of Doctors Gabe Mirkin and Joseph Mercola are so stellar that an "X" appears in nearly every category.

An overwhelming amount of information is available on the Internet, but not all of it is accurate or founded on solid scientific investigation. Sadly, some data presented is intentionally bogus, placed there by mean-spirited individuals to deceive, or by others who merely crave attention or to push an agenda. Every effort has been made to separate the wheat from the chaff and to provide the reader with the cream of the Internet crop of credible health-related websites.

Apologies are extended to the reader for any pointers that may have changed since these tables were updated. The Internet is a dynamic and evolving resource. What appears in the following tables is a snapshot in time, current as of February 2012. Some websites, like Dr. Mercola's, are well established and continue to provide a wealth of information while other sites may be ephemeral.

On our website (www.RA-Infection-Connection.com) the reader will find the most current version of the printed tables 7 and 8 shown in this Appendix.

Searching Deeper, Taking Charge of Your Health

The authors encourage the reader to use a Google search for any unfamiliar word or medical term not found in the Definitions section at the front of this book. Enter the term preceded by the words "medical definition." E.g., medical definition sclerosis.

Be advised that entering just one keyword like arthritis or lupus will result in thousands of "hits" (i.e., websites located). It is overwhelming to sift through this mountain of material.

Instead, choosing focused, definitive keywords will often yield articles with photos and hot links that provide additional useful information. E.g., lupus infection treatment. Google will prompt you about misspellings and suggest alternatives.

However, the most important site an individual can visit is probably the office of a caring physician who takes a holistic approach to treating his/her patients.

Table 7.
Research-related Websites: Home Pages

Column key: TS = Topic Search; Lnks = Links to Other Excellent, Credible Sites; S,J,A = Studies, Journal Articles, Abstracts; PPDI = Pharmaceuticals, Prescription Drug Info; CH = Case Histories; AM = Alternative Medicine; ID = Infectious Diseases; M,B = Molds, Fungus, Yeasts, Biofilms; HIV = AIDS/HIV; MS = Multiple Sclerosis; LD = Lyme Disease; CFS = Chronic Fatigue Syndrome; FM = Fibromyalgia; AID = Autoimmune Diseases; RD = Rheumatic Diseases; Arth = Arthritis; SD = Scleroderma; Lup = Lupus; Alrg = Allergy; BDR = Blood, Drug Research; MR = Mycoplasma Research; TP = Treatment Protocols

Website URL Address / (Comment)	TS	Lnks	S,J,A	PPDI	CH	AM	ID	M,B	HIV	MS	LD	CFS	FM	AID	RD	Arth	SD	Lup	Alrg	BDR	MR	TP
American Auto-immune Related Disease Association: www.aarda.org	×	×	×							×		×	×	×	×	×	×	×	×			
www.about.com/health/index.htm	×		Search	×		×	×	×	×	×	×	×	×	×	×	×	×	×	×	×	×	×
Alternative Medicine for Pets: Google [arthritis vet meds alt infection]	×	×	×			×		×			×					×			×			×
www.arthritis.about.com [Extensive]	×	×	×	×		×								×	×							×
Arthritis Foundation: www.arthritis.org	×	×		×	×	×	×		×	×	×	×	×	×	×	×	×	×	×	×		×
www.arthritistrust.org	×	×	×	×	×	×		×	×	×	×	×	×	×	×	×	×	×	×	×	×	×
Bad Bug Book = Pathogenic Microbes List Google [Bad Bug Book]	×						×				×											
www.biomedcentral.com	×		Many	×											×	×						
Online Blood Textbook: www.bloodbook.com		×	All About Blood				×		×					×		×				×		
www.addall.com [Book Buying Lookup]		×	Books		×	×		×				×	×									
www.arthropatient.org [spine arthritis]			×		×									×		×						×
www.bulkmsm.com [MSM Data]			×	MSM		×																×

Website URL Address / (Comment)	TS	Lnks	S,J,A	PPDI	CH	AM	ID	M,B	HIV	MS	LD	CFS	FM	AID	RD	Arth	SD	Lup	Alrg	BDR	MR	TP
www.cdc.gov [Disease Statistics]	X	X	Vaccine		X		X		X	X	X	X	X	X	X	X	X	X		X	X	
www.chronicneurotoxins.com [Ocular neurotoxin tests]			X	Tests	X	X				X	X	X	X	X								X
www.clinicaltrials.gov	X		X				X	X	X	X	X	X	X	X	X	X	X	X	X	X	X	X
www.consumerlab.com [SafetyTests]	X		Warn'gs																			
www.drmirkin.com [Radio Host]	X	X	Archive	X	X	X	X	X	X	X	X	X	X	X	X	X	X	X	X	X	X	X
www.drweil.com [Author's Site: Nutrition]	X	X	Search	X	X	X	X		X	X	X	X	X	X	X	X	X	X	X			X
www.erc.montana.edu [biofilms]	X	X	Library					X											X	X		
www.fda.gov [Food&Drug Administr'n]	X		NewDvl.	Vaccine			X			X	X	X	X	X	X	X	X	X		X		X
Institute for Functional Medicine: www.functionalmedicine.org [Post Doctoral Education Resource]	X		$295/yr Doctors Educatn	Drugs Hormones Nutrition Molecules	X	X	X	X	X	X	X	X	X	X	X	X	X	X	X	X	X	X
www.gene.com [Genentech]	X	X	NewDvl.	X					X					X					X	X		X
www.gene-chips.com [Multi-Tests]	X	X	X	X															X	X		
www.healingwell.com [HealthBooks, Article Lookups, Doctors]	X	X	Online Doctors		X	X	X	X	X	X	X	X	X	X	X	X	X	X	X			
RA-Infection-Connection.com/free_articles/ RefBooks.htm [HealthBooks Buying via AddAll.com]	X	X	Books Prices Lookup																			
Nutrition vs. Disease/Condition: www.healingwithnutrition.com	X			Vitamins		X	X	X	X	X	X	X	X	X	X	X		X				
www.healthfinder.gov [Resources, Dr's, Organizations]	X	X	X	Inter-actions	X	X	X	X	X	X	X	X	X	X	X	X	X	X	X			X
Drug-Nutrient Interactions: Google [Drug Nutrient Herbs Interactions]	X	X	FAQs	Herbs																		

Website URL Address / (Comment)	TS	Lnks	S,J,A	PPDI	CH	AM	ID	M,B	HIV	MS	LD	CFS	FM	AID	RD	Arth	SD	Lup	Alrg	BDR	MR	TP
www.hemex.com [Blood Testing]	X		FAQ	Coagul-ation							X	X	X							X		X
American. Botanical Council: www.herbalgram.org			Herbals		X									X	X							
www.herbmed.org [Herbal DataBase $9/Month]	X	X	Archive PaySite	Herbals	X									X	X							
www.hopkins-arthritis.org [Teaching University Arthritis Center]	X	X	X	FAQ, Q-A	X				X		X	X	X	X	X	X	X	X	X			X
www.igenex.com [Lyme Disease Testing]		X	X								X	X	X	X	X	X	X	X		X		
Internat'l Lyme Associated Disease Society: www.ilads.org	X		Lyme	Tests			X			X	X	X	X	X	X	X	X	X	X	X	X	X
Institute of Molecular Medicine: Gulf War Illness www.immed.org [Garth Nicolson]	X	X	Multi-	Tests		X	X		X	X	X	X	X	X	X	X	X	X	X	X	X	X
Website URL Address / (Comment)	TS	Lnks	S,J,A	PPDI	CH	AM	ID	M,B	HIV	MS	LD	CFS	FM	AID	RD	Arth	SD	Lup	Alrg	BDR	MR	TP
www.immunosciencelab.com [Autoimmune, Lyme, Viral, Nutrient, PCR]	X	X	Dr. A. Vojdani	Blood Tests	X	X	X					X	X	X	X	X	X	X	X	X	Tst	
Harvard Medical School => Aetna Health Site: www.intelihealth.com [Many Tools, FAQs]	X		Archive Q-A	Look Up	X	X		X	X	X	X	X	X	X	X	X	X	X	X			X
Med Library Links to Meta Directory: hardinmd.lib.uiowa.edu/	X	X	X	X			X		X	X	X	X	X	X	X	X	X	X	X	X	X	
Journal Am Med Assn: jama.ama-assn.org	X		X				X	X	X		X	X	X	X	X	X	X	X	X	X		
www.lyme-disease-research-database.com/ [Register for Search Access]	X	X	Archives Blogs		X	X	X			X	X	X	X	X	X		X	X	X	X		X
www.lymeinfo.net [Cognitive Disabilities]	X	X	Search		X					X	X	X	X				X	X	X	X	X	X
Marshall (Antibiotic)Protocol: RA-Infection-Connection.com/MarshallProtocol.htm		X	Drugs in Sequence	Combined Drugs	X	X					X	X	X		X	X	X	X	X	X	X	X
www.mayoclinic.com [Authoritative]	X		Search	X			X	Fungus	X	X	X	X	X	X	X	X	X	X	X	X	X	X
www.mdlab.com [Multi-PCR Tests]	X	X	X	Tests				X		Cystic Fibrosis	X	X		X	X		X	X	X	X	X	X

Website URL Address / (Comment)	TS	Lnks	S,J,A	PPDI	CH	AM	ID	M,B	HIV	MS	LD	CFS	FM	AID	RD	Arth	SD	Lup	Alrg	BDR	MR	TP
www.medscape.com [Register for access to Medline+]	X	X	X	Vaccines	X	X	X	X	X	X		X	X	X	X		X	X	X	X	X	X
www.mentalhealthandillness.com	X	X	X				X				X					X						X
www.merckhomeedition.com [Book and Online reference library]	X		X	X		X	X	X	X	X	X	X	X	X	X	X	X	X	X	X	X	X
www.mercola.com [Alternative Medicine Site] Subscribe to Newsletter	X	X	X	X	X	X	X	X	X	X	X	X	X	X	X	X	X	X	X	X	X	X
www.molecularstaging.com [PCR Tests] DNA=>Molecules; StemCell=>targetcells	X	X	X	Tests																	X	
University of Missouri Medical Library: www.muhealth.org	X	X	D.Base	X	X	X	X	X	X	X	X	X	X	X	X	X	X	X	X	X		X
www.naet.com [Allergy Therapy]		X	FAQ	Books	X	X								X		X		X	X	X		X
www.naturalsolutionsmag.com	X	Docs	Diet	X	X	X								X	X			X	X		X	X
www.niaid.nih.gov [Infectious Diseases]	X	X	X	Vaccines			X	X	X	X	X	X	X	X	X	X	X	X	X	X	X	X
Website URL Address / (Comment)	**TS**	**Lnks**	**S,J,A**	**PPDI**	**CH**	**AM**	**ID**	**M,B**	**HIV**	**MS**	**LD**	**CFS**	**FM**	**AID**	**RD**	**Arth**	**SD**	**Lup**	**Alrg**	**BDR**	**MR**	**TP**
http://www.ncbi.nlm.nih.gov/Entrez [Links NLM Genetic & Taxonomy Dbases]	X	Db	Multi-				X													X		
www.nccam.nih.gov Alt/Complement Med [FAQ, Dbase, Drug Trials, Nutrition, Search]	X	X	F,D,T	Trials		X	X	X		X	X	X	X	X	X	X	X	X	X	X		X
National Institutes of Health: www.nih.gov National Library of Medicine: nlm.nih.gov	X	X	FAQ Archive	D.Bases: PubMed, Medscape	X	X	X			X	X	X	X	X	X	X	X	X	X	X	X	X
www.nutriteam.com [Parasites, Mold]	X		Nutr'n	Vitamins	X	X		X										X	X	X	X	
www.nutritionreporter.com Jack Challem, Health Author: Articles, Lectures	X	X	Books	Diet Vitamins	X	X				X		X	X	X	X	X	X	X	X			X
www.orthomed.com/ [Dr Cathcart's Vitamin C Info and Dr Klenner's Papers]		X	Ascorbic Acid	Papers	X	X	X		X	X	X	X	X	X		X			X			X
www.pilates-studio.com Find Dr's [FAQ Theory / Brain Chems] MotionTherapy, mind-body training: like Tai Chi			FAQ Theory	Brain Chems		X										X						X
www.puritan.com [Nutri'n: Interact'n]	X		DrugsVs	Vitamins		X						X	X	X		X	X	X				X
Website URL Address / (Comment)	**TS**	**Lnks**	**S,J,A**	**PPDI**	**CH**	**AM**	**ID**	**M,B**	**HIV**	**MS**	**LD**	**CFS**	**FM**	**AID**	**RD**	**Arth**	**SD**	**Lup**	**Alrg**	**BDR**	**MR**	**TP**

Website URL Address / (Comment)	TS	Lnks	S,J,A	PPDI	CH	AM	ID	M,B	HIV	MS	LD	CFS	FM	AID	RD	Arth	SD	Lup	Alrg	BDR	MR	TP
www.rain-tree.com [Nutrit'n, infections]	X	X	X	Herbs		X									X						X	X
www.repro-med.net/ [Fertility, Genetics]			X	X										X	X							
www.rheumatic.org [AntibioticTreatm't]		X	FAQ	DrBrown		X	X		X	X	X	X	X	X	X	X	X	X	X	X	X	X
www.rheumatology.org [Prof'nl.Soc.]		X	Rheum.		X		X		X	X	X	X	X	X	X	X	X	X	X	X	X	X
www.roadback.org [Dr Brown's Legacy]	X	X	FAQs	AB=Anti Biotic	X	X	X	X	X	X	X	X	X	X	X	X	X	X	X	X	X	X
www.scleroderma.org [Support]	X	X	X	AB P	X	X	X							X	X	X	X			X		X
www.seanet.com/~alexs/ascorbate [Archive: Vitamin C Medical & Nutrition Papers]	X	X	Archive Papers	Ascorbate to 1999		X	X	Toxin	X	X	X		X	X	X	X	X	X	X	X		X
www.seniors.gov Social Security Admin	X	X	X																			
www.shasta.com/cybermom/asimple.htm [Mycoplasma Overview: CFIDS/GWI/FMS]		X	FAQ		X	X	X	X	X	HHV-6	X	X	X	X	X	X	X	X	X	X	X	
Website URL Address / (Comment)	TS	Lnks	S,J,A	PPDI	CH	AM	ID	M,B	HIV	MS	LD	CFS	FM	AID	RD	Arth	SD	Lup	Alrg	BDR	MR	TP
Stanford Medical Library: lane.stanford.edu	X	X	Libr.	Health																		
www.thearthritiscenter.com / Dr Franco, Riverside, CA: RA Infection Treatmt	X	X	Infect'n	AB P Nutr'n	X	X	X	X	X	X	X	X	X	X	X	X	X	X	X	X	X	X
www.thecanadiandrugstore.com	X		FAQ	Drugs																		
www.themedicalletter.com	X	X	Archive	D.base		X	X	X	X	X	X	X	X	X	X		X	X	X	X	X	X
www.the-thyroid-society.org	X	FAQs	X	X		X								X								X
www.thyroid.about.com [Extensive]	X	X	X	X		X	X					X	X	X		X				X	X	X
Townsend Letter: www.tldp.com	X	X	Archive	X	X	X	X	X	X	X	X	X	X	X	X	X	X	X	X	X	X	X
Website URL Address / (Comment)	TS	Lnks	S,J,A	PPDI	CH	AM	ID	M,B	HIV	MS	LD	CFS	FM	AID	RD	Arth	SD	Lup	Alrg	BDR	MR	TP
www.toxnet.nlm.nih.gov [Toxics Database]	X	X	X																	X		
www.tuftshealthletter.com/ [$25/Yr]	X	X	Nutr'n	Diet															X			
www.library.tufts.edu/hsl/																X						
www.uams.edu [Univ Ark Med Library]	X	X	Hlth.Libr	Nutr'n		X	X		X					X						X		
www.usda.gov [US Dept of Agriculture]	X		X				X													X		
www.webmd.com (Drugs & Herbs)	X	X	Library	D.base		X		Yeast	X	X	X	X	X	X	X	X	X	X	X	X	X	X
Website URL Address / (Comment)	TS	Lnks	S,J,A	PPDI	CH	AM	ID	M,B	HIV	MS	LD	CFS	FM	AID	RD	Arth	SD	Lup	Alrg	BDR	MR	TP
www.westonaprice.org/ [SrMemb$25/Yr] Thoughtful, Unconventional Diet Alternatives	X	X	Archive	Nutr'n	X	X	X	X	X	X	X	X	X	X	X	X	X	X	X	X	X	X

Website URL Address / (Comment)	TS	Lnks	S,J,A	PPDI	CH	AM	ID	M,B	HIV	MS	LD	CFS	FM	AID	RD	Arth	SD	Lup	Alrg	BDR	MR	TP
Autism Overview: ASDs, PDDs: http://en.wikipedia.org/wiki/Autism		X	X	Over View	X	X	X							X						X		X
Gene Chips ID DNA of Cells, Microbes: en.wikipedia.org/wiki/DNA_microarray		X	X	Tests			X													X		
en.wikipedia.org/wiki/Medicinal_mushrooms #Anti-inflammatory_activity		X	X	Meds in Food	X	X	X	X	X	X			X	X	X	X	X	X	X			
Vaccines Cause Inflammation: [Autism?] en.wikipedia.org/wiki/Immunologic_adjuvant		X	X	Vaccine Danger						X		X	X	X	X	X	X	X	X			
Best 10 Search Engines: www.listofsearchengines.info/		X	Search FAQ																			
Website URL Address / (Comment)	TS	Lnks	S,J,A	PPDI	CH	AM	ID	M,B	HIV	MS	LD	CFS	FM	AID	RD	Arth	SD	Lup	Alrg	BDR	MR	TP
Simple search engines: www.about.com www.ask.com	X	X	Images WebTxt	X	X	X	X	X	X	X	X	X	X	X	X	X	X	X	X	X		
Nutrition Search: www.advance-health.com/	X	X	WebTxt	Meds in Foods		X			X	X	X	X	X	X	X	X	X	X	X	X		
MicroSoft search engine: www.bing.com	X	X	Images WebTxt	X	X	X	X	X	X	X	X	X	X	X	X	X	X	X	X			
Web Archive Search: www.faqs.org FAQs, Patents, Periodicals, NewsGroups, UseNet	X	X	Images WebTxt																			
Best web search engines: scholar.google.com www.google.com	X	X	Images WebTxt	X	X	X	X	X	X	X	X	X	X	X	X	X	X	X	X	X	X	X
First search engine: www.yahoo.com	X	X	Search	X	X	X	X	X	X	X	X	X	X	X	X	X	X	X	X	X	X	X

Table 8. Resource-related Websites: Home Pages

Column key: Txx = Toxic Substances Data; Dis = Diseases \ Condition; LT = Lab(s), Testing Info; Med = Medicines / Treatments; Qry = Search by Query-term(s); DrQ = Doctor Query (eMail); FAQ = Frequently Asked Questions (FAQs); NL = Newsletter, Magazine; HB = Health Books; Sprt = Support / Interest Group(s); PL = Practitioner List; Alt = Alternative Medicine Site; ND = Nutrition, Diet; VH = Vitamins, Herbs; HF = General Health, Fitness; U.S = University Site; Med = Medical Site; Gov = U.S. Government Site; NFP = Non-profit, Foundation; Com = Commercial Site.

Website URL Address / (Comment)	Txx	Dis	LT	Med	Qry	DrQ	FAQ	NL	HB	Sprt	PL	Alt	ND	VH	HF	U.S	Med	Gov	NFP	Com
www.aarda.org [Rheumatic Disease Ass'n]		X	X		X		X	X	X	Forum									X	
www.altvetmed.com [Veterinary Alt. Med]		X		X	X	X	X			X		X	X	X	X		X			
www.addall.com [Books: Prices Lookup]																				X
www.amazon.com [Books,Meds,Devices]		X			X				X											X
www.arthritis.about.com/ (arthritis.about.com/cs/druggen/a/arthdrugoptions.htm)	X	X	X	X	X	Forum	Mult	X	X	X	X	X	X	X	X		X			
www.arthritis.org [Arthritis Foundation]		X		X	X	Forum	X	X	X	X			X	X	X		X		X	X
www.arthritistrust.org/	X	X	X	X	X	Q-A	X	X	X	List	X	X	X	X	X		X		X	
www.betterhealthusa.com/ [Allergies]	X	X	X	X	X	X	X			Food	X	X	X	X	X		X			X

Website URL Address / (Comment)	Txx	Dis	LT	Med	Qry	DrQ	FAQ	NL	HB (Journals)	Sprt	PL	Alt	ND	VH	HF	U.S	Med	Gov	NFP	Com
www.biomedcentral.com/ [Med.Journals]	X	X	X	X	X	X	X	X				X	X	X	X		X			X
Website URL Address / (Comment)																				
www.bowen.org [Massage, Pain & Stress Mgt, LymeTesting]	Srch	X			X	Links	Links				Links			X	X		X		X	X
www.bulkmsm.com [MSM Information]			X	X			X						X	X	X		X			X
www.cdc.gov [Disease Control & Statistics]	X	S	X	X	X		X											X		
www.chronicneurotoxins.com [Toxins Vs Diseases, Testing]	X	X	X	X		Fee	X		X		X	X					X			X
www.clinicaltrials.gov [NIH Trials Dbase]	X	X	X	X	X		Lnk				X	X	X	X	X		X	X		
www.drmirkin.com [Author, Radio Host]	X	X		X	X	X	Mult	X				X	X	X	X		X			X
www.drweil.com [Nutrition Author]	X	X		X	X	X	Mult	X	X			X		X	X		X			
www.edstrom.com [Water Quality]			X				X	X												X
www.erc.montana.edu [Biofilms]	X						Lnk	X								X				
www.fda.gov [U.S. Food & Drug Agency]	X	X		X	X		X	X					X	X	X	X	X	X		
Website URL Address / (Comment)																				
www.gene-chips.com [Multi-Tests]			X				X	X									X			X
www.genomicsnews.com [BioChips]		X	X	FAC			Libr	X	Med Pix				X							X
hardinmd.lib.uiowa.edu/ Medical Library Links to Meta Directory	X	X	X	X	X								X	X	X	X	X			
www.healingwell.com [Books]		X		X	X		X	X	X	X		X			X	X				X
www.healingwithnutrition.com [Vitamins]	X	X	X	X	X	X	Mult			X		X	X	X	X	X				X
www.healthfinder.gov [US HHS Query Site, Practitioners]	X	X	X	X	Lnk	X	X	X	Gov Pubs	X	Lnk	X		X	X			X		
www.healthwell.com [Herbs]		X		X	X		X	X	X	X	X	X	X	X	X					X
www.healthy.net [Natural Medicine]	X	X	X	X	X	X	X	X	X	X	X	X	X	X	X		X			X

Website URL Address / (Comment)	Txx	Dis	LT	Med	Qry	DrQ	FAQ	NL	HB	Sprt (Pubs)	PL	Alt	ND	VH	HF	U.S	Med	Gov	NFP	Com
www.herbalgram.org Am Botnical Council	X	X	X	X	X	X	X	X	X	X	X	X	X	X	X	X	X		X	X
www.herbmed.com [Herbals DataBase]		X		X	X		Herb					X		X	X	X	X		X	
www.hopkins-arthritis.org Johns-Hopkins University Clinic		X	X	X	X		X							X		X	X			
www.hospitalcompare.hhs.gov/ [Docs, Hospital, Drug Lookup Medicare]				X	X		Lnk		Gov Pubs	X	X							X		
www.igenex.com [Blood Tests]		X	X				Lnk				X						X			X
www.ilads.org Intnat'l Lyme Disease Ass'n		X	X		X		X		X	X	X						X			X
Institute of Molecular Medicine: Gulf War Illness www.immed.org [Garth Nicolson]	X	X	X	X	X	X	X		X	X	X		X			X	X		X	X
www.immunoscienceslab.com [Autoimmune, Lyme, Viral, Nutrient, PCR Testing]	X	X	X	X	X		X				X	X	X			X	X			X
www.injectablevitaminc.com		X		X					X				X			X	X			X
www.intelihealth.com [Harvard Medical School]		X	X	X	X	X	X		X				X	X	X	X	X			X

Website URL Address / (Comment)	Txx	Dis	LT	Med	Qry	DrQ	FAQ	NL	HB	Sprt	PL	Alt	ND	VH	HF	U.S	Med	Gov	NFP	Com
jama.ama-assn.org [AMA Journal]		X		X	X		X	X			X					X	X		X	
www.lymeinfo.net [Cognitive Disabilities]		X		X	X		Arch	X		X						X	X		X	
www.lymenet.org/ [Library Abstracts]	Lnk	X		X		Chat	Arch	Arch	X	X		X				X	X		X	
www.mayoclinic.com (Authoritative Info)	X	X	X	X	X	X	Arch	X	X		X	X	X		X	X	X			X
www.mdlab.com [Multi-PCR Tests]		X	X	X	X		Lnk		X		X					X	X			X
www.medscape.com NLM Portal	X	X	X	X	Lnk		Multi	X		X	X		X			X	X	X	X	
www.merckhomeedition.com		X	X	Lnk		X	Mult		X		X			X	X	X	X			
www.mercola.com [#1 Alternative Med Info]	X	X	X	X	X	X	Arch	X	X		X	X	X	X	X	X	X			X

Website URL Address / (Comment)	Txx	Dis	LT	Med	Qry	DrQ	FAQ	NL	HB	Sprt	PL	Alt	ND	VH	HF	U.S	Med	Gov	NFP	Com
www.mycoplasmasupport.org	X	X	X	X	X		Lnk				X		X	X	X	X	X			X
www.muhealth.org [Health dBase]	X	X	X	X	Lnk		X	X	X	X	X	X	X	X	X	X	X			X
www.naet.com [Allergy Treatments]	X	X	X		X	Blog	X	Mag	X	X	X	X	X	X	X		X			X
www.naturalsolutionsmag.com/	X	X		X	X		FAQ		X		X	X	X	X	X		X			
nccam.nih.gov [FAQ, Dbase, Drug Trials] Complementary & Alternative Medicine	X	X		X	X		FAQ					X					X	X		
niaid.nih.gov [Allergy & Infectious Diseases]		X		X	X		X		Pubs								X	X		
nlm.nih.gov/medlineplus/herbalmedicine.html	X	X		X	X		X	X	Pubs			X		X	X		X	X		
nimh.nih.gov/health/publications/index.shtml National Inst. Mental Health @ NIH				X	X									X			X	X		
nlm.nih.gov [Abstracts, Archives, Dbase, Journals @ National Library of Medicine]	X	X		X	X		FAQ	X	X			X	X	X	X		X	X		
www.nutriteam.com [Mold, Parasites, Coconut Antivirals]	X	X		X	X		FAQ	X				X	X	X						X
www.nutritionreporter.com [Vitamins]	X	X		X			Arch	X				X	X	X	X		X			

Website URL Address / (Comment)	Txx	Dis	LT	Med	Qry	DrQ	FAQ	NL	HB	Sprt	PL	Alt	ND	VH	HF	U.S	Med	Gov	NFP	Com
www.pdr.net [Physician's Desk Reference]	X	X		X	Lnk		Mult		X					X	X		X			X
www.pilates-studio.com [Dance,Exercise] Mind-Body Training : Like Tai Chi							X					X			X				X	X
www.puritan.com [Drugs Vs Vitamin Interactions]	X			X	X		X	X				X	X	X	X					X
www.rain-tree.com [Nutrition vs.Infections]	X	X		X								X	X	X						X
www.rheumatic.org [AntibioticTreatment]	X	X		X			X	X	X	X		X	X	X	X		X		X	
www.rheumatology.org Rheumatologists		X			Lnk			X	X	X	X					X	X		X	
www.roadback.org [Dr. Brown's heritage]	X	X		X			X	X	X	X		X				X	X		X	

Website URL Address / (Comment)	Txx	Dis	LT	Med (Db) Qry	DrQ	FAQ	NL	HB	Sprt	PL	Alt	ND	VH	HF	U.S	Med	Gov	NFP	Com
www.rxlist.com [Drug Database]	x	x		x x	x	x	x			x	x	x	x	x	x	x			x
www.SavvyPatients.com MedQuery	x	x		x x		x		x	x	x	x	x	x	x	x	x		x	
www.scleroderma.org [Help Site]		x		x x		x	x	x	x	x					x	x		x	
www.seniors.gov Soc. Sec. Admin, Lnks		x		x x		x		Pubs	x	x		x		x	x		x		
www.lane.stanford.edu Stanford Med Library	x	x	x	x x		Lnk		x		x	x	x	x	x	x	x			
www.thearthritiscenter.com Dr Franco, Riverside, CA: RA Infection Treatmnt	x	x	x	x x	x	x		x	x	x	x	x	x	x		x			x
www.thecanadiandrugstore.com				x		x													x
www.the-thyroid-society.org	x	x	x	x x	x	x		x	x	x		x	x	x	x	x		x	
www.thyroid.about.com [Comprehensive]	x	x	x	x x	x	x	x	x	x	x	x	x	x	x	x	x			x
www.toxnet.nlm.nih.gov [Toxin Dbase]	x			x x		Lnk						x	x	x			x		
www.tldp.com Townsend Letter: Alt Med Subscr $51/Yr Web Search Index, order articles	x	x	x	x		Arts	x				x	x	x	x	x	x			x
library.uams.edu/ Univ Arkansas Med Library		x	x	x x		Lnk				x		x	x	x	x				
www.shasta.com/cybermom/asimple.htm [Mycoplasma Overview: CFIDS/GWI/FMS]	x	x	Lnk	x FAQ		x		x			x	x	x	x		x		x	
www.usda.gov U.S. Dept of Agriculture [Veterinary, Diet, Food Qualities]		x	x	x x		Lnk		Pubs	WIC SNAP			x	x	x			x		
www.wildcondor.com/lymelinks.html [Best Lyme Disease Resource Links]	x	x	Lyme			x		x	x	x		x	x	x	x	x			
www.WhitakerWellness.com Integrative Medic'n Whitaker Wellness Inst. Newport Beach, CA	x	x	x	x x	x	x	x	x	x	x	x	x	x	x		x			x

Arthritis and Autoimmune Disease: The Infection Connection

APPENDIX V

Benefits of Vitamin C (Ascorbic Acid)

Ascorbic acid (AA) is a white, crystalline vitamin ($C_6H_8O_6$ or C for short) found in citrus fruits, tomatoes, potatoes, and leafy green vegetables. Since it is a water-soluble vitamin, AA cannot be stored by the body except in very small amounts and so must be replenished daily.

AA is an essential nutrient because humans lack the gene to make it. We need highly variable amounts depending on our stress levels, including the reactive oxidation stress (ROS) conditions of illness, allergies, vaccination, injury, and mitochondrial dysfunctions.[1]

Vitamin C is best known for preventing scurvy. When we are sick, the AA in our blood is quickly consumed. AA's half-lifetime is ½ hour. When that amount is exhausted, the body then draws on whatever AA stored in various glands and organs. In 6 hours, the level might drop to $(1/2)^{12}$ of the initial level. Thus, AA should be considered to be an essential metabolized <u>food</u>, not merely a vitamin, and should be eaten frequently.

When AA losses are extreme, histamine levels increase and storage tissues suffer ROS, leading to inflammation and illness. Rapid replacement of sufficient AA (several grams per hour) reverses the oxidation; symptoms will decrease within a few minutes after oral intake or by injection.

AA Giants in History

Eight major contributors to our understanding of ascorbate[2] include its discoverer, Dr. Albert Szent-Györgyi, M.D. and those who researched, tested, and publicized its many benefits: Claus Jungblut, M.D., Linus Pauling, PhD,

Frederick Klenner, M.D., Robert Cathcart, M.D., Archie Kalokerinos, M.D., John Ely, PhD, and Irwin Stone, M.D.[3, 4]

The AA story has been deliberately suppressed:

A consensus of opposition to vitamin C and to nutritional orthomolecular medicine has existed since the 1930s.[5, 6] The pharmacokinetics of a drug that is reactive and metabolized in ½ hour were not considered when designing trials for evaluating AA's use as a medicine. As expected, all of the low-dose or single-dose trials failed to demonstrate benefits. Nevertheless, the contributors listed above understood exactly how to use and administer the appropriate amounts of this essential substance that is more <u>food</u> than medicine. When we have ROS, AA is oxidized (burned) rapidly. Experts agree that routine and widespread use of AA (4-6 grams at each of 3 meals daily) would greatly decrease the nation's need for medical services and palliative medicines.[7, 8] Even if AA were added to junk food it would have wide-ranging public health benefits.

Why We Need Ascorbic Acid

Humans (and primates) lack l-gulonolactone oxidase genes needed to make AA from glucose, so we must eat it.[9] Rats and mice make AA naturally, so experimental laboratory results can be affected by this important difference. I.e., drugs developed for humans that do not consider the absence of AA could have unexpected effects.

Vitamins C and A promote continuous rebuilding of the body as dying cells are replaced. Coenzyme Q_{10} is also an essential nutrient needed to optimize this cell replacement, especially in the brain.[10] Insufficient AA intake in the presence of infection will cause scurvy[11] to varying degrees.

AA reduces other molecules and changes to Dehydroascorbic acid (DHA), AA's oxidized form. AA does not enter cells but DHA does so readily. Then the DHA oxidizes the mitochondria and the invaded components, which kills the invaded cell. This process applies to infected leukocytes, epithelial cells, and tumors. Effective use of AA is decreased by hyperglycemia (high blood sugar), in the diabetic condition. When AA oxidizes to DHA in diabetic blood, the result is a loss of antioxidant actions and sub-clinical scurvy, which retards healing and increases the risk of infections.

Therapeutic vitamin C levels (>6 grams AA per day) accelerate healing significantly. Dr. Klenner found that rats under stress make the human equivalent of 15 grams per day per 70 kg (150 pounds).[12] In emergency cases, Dr. Klenner used intravenous (IV) or injections plus oral buffered AA at a total 150 grams per day. Starting with this high initial intake in cases with poor vital signs, he succeeded by using AA as a toxin neutralizer. He also used IV vitamin C without the high starting dosages as an antibiotic or antiviral treatment.

AA chelates heavy metals, helping to remove high levels of toxic lead, mercury, cadmium, manganese, etc. It will also lower levels of zinc, magnesium, calcium, and copper. AA facilitates bone formation if magnesium, calcium, and potassium are in balance.

Computing the AA daily amount for your weight

Dr. Robert Cathcart has treated tens of thousands of patients using high levels of AA. His excellent paper "Vitamin C, Titrating to Tolerance"[13] features a table, shown below, that shows illness or condition and the AA amount that may cause loose bowel effects. This is the upper limit to effective dosage. The illness determines the AA need, which is highly variable.[14] The dosage shown in this table is for a person weighing 70 kg (150 lbs). Divide your body weight by 2.2 to convert pounds to kilograms. Then multiply by 200 mg/kg to compute the daily oral amount suggested by Dr. Cathcart. E.g., 220 pounds = 100 kg, implying 100 x 200 mg

= 20 grams, or ~ 7 grams 3 times/day. If sick, increase the intake rate to every 2 hours.

Table 9. Dr. Cathcart's Suggested

Vitamin C Dosage [15]

CONDITION: NORMAL TO ACUTE	ASCORBIC ACID GRAMS PER 24 HOURS	NUMBER OF ORAL DOSES PER 24 HOURS
Normal	4 – 15	4 – 6
Environmt/food allergy	0.5 – 50	4 – 8
Anxiety, mild stress	15 – 25	4 – 6
Mild cold	30 – 60	6 – 10
Severe cold	60 – 100+	8 – 15
Influenza	100 – 150	8 – 20
Coxsackie virus	100 – 150	8 – 20
Mononucleosis EBV	150 – 200+	12 – 25
Viral pneumonia	100 – 200+	12 – 25
Hay fever, asthma	15 – 50	4 – 8
Burn/injury/surgery	25 – 150+	6 – 20
Cancer	15 – 100	4 – 15
Ankylosing spondylitis	15 – 100	4 – 15
Reiter's syndrome	15 – 60	4 – 10
Acute anterior uveitis	30 – 100	4 – 15
Rheumatoid arthritis	15 – 100	4 – 15
Bacterial infections	30 – 200+	10 – 25
Infectious hepatitis	30 – 100	6 – 15
Candidiasis (yeast)	15 – 200+	6 – 25

If you have been consuming vitamin C at high levels you should not stop suddenly but taper down over a period of 7-10 days, to let your system adjust to a lower level of AA, otherwise an induced scurvy state may result.

The table shows Dr. Cathcart's suggested guidelines. You must seek professional medical support to administer high levels of AA by injection or IV.[16] Check the Internet for doctors in your community who use vitamin C therapy. Look

for orthomolecular and nutrition-oriented doctors with IV
AA experience. Interview them. The doctor will know how
to maintain blood metabolite balance (sodium, magnesium,
calcium, potassium, phosphorus). Some Doctors of
Osteopathy (D.O.), and orthomolecular or alternative
medicine doctors provide a range of AA treatments.

Vitamin C Chemical Forms

Vitamin C is available in the acid form (AA),
liposomal form (see pg 248), and in combination with
calcium or sodium, the so-called buffered forms. Sodium
ascorbate is the preferred buffered form for oral, injection,
and IV use.[17] Sodium ascorbate is also helpful for asthma. If
you have digestive problems, you should be checked for *H.
Pylori* and yeast infections. Antacid medications interfere
with AA action.

Buffered AA is helpful if you have digestive problems
with the regular AA acid formulation. Ester-C is one trade
name for calcium ascorbate. Long-term exclusive use of
Ester-C has led to serious problems caused by a
sodium/calcium imbalance. Sodium ascorbate is immediately
useful. Calcium ascorbate must be transformed to the sodium
form to be effective.

AA is available in pill form, powder form, and powder
in capsules. It can be derived from natural sources (rose hips,
citrus, etc.) or made synthetically from yeast fermentation. It
may be a mix of other ingredients, some which might trigger
allergies, so read the product label carefully.

According to Dr. Klenner, the maximum safe level of
buffered AA IVs is much higher than the 10-20 g/day/70kg
therapeutic oral dose. There does not seem to be any upper
limit to IV-administered AA, especially in acute ROS or
systemic toxic shock cases. Dr. Klenner tested for active AA
in urine, and pushed the AA dosage until it showed that the
desired maximum absorption level had been reached.

Timed-release AA is not recommended, since intake cannot be controlled. It is better to take the pill/capsule form as needed at intervals throughout the day. Three or more grams can be eaten with meals or with liquid, depending on the level of discomfort symptoms. The discomfort decreases and relief lasts for a few hours after AA intake. When symptoms start to return, it indicates AA is being depleted and must be replenished. Chewable forms of AA are bad for the teeth since the acid attacks enamel.

AA Use in Emergency Medicine

Dr. Cathcart (California), Dr. Klenner (Georgia), Dr. Jungblut (New York), and Dr. Kalokerinos (Australia) report that ascorbate administered rapidly either orally, by injection, or intravenously in very high dosages will reverse toxic shock (coma/lethargy) and a wide range of toxin poisoning: rabies, tetanus, staphylococcus, dysentery, snake/insect bite toxins, herpes, polio, scarlet fever, pneumonia, viral infections, and many more.[18] Other doctors throughout the world have confirmed these experiences.

AA immediately disables bacteria-generated toxins[19] by reducing (the opposite of oxidizing) their molecules.[20] Toxins also induce ROS that depletes AA. Larger amounts of AA are needed to disable both all of the ROS and all of the toxin. An injection of sodium ascorbate can reverse the toxin's effect in 15 to 30 minutes. Regression of symptoms occurs if enough AA is administered correctly and systemically.

AA quickly deactivates a wide range of allergies and histamine intoxification, toxins and poisons from poison ivy, jellyfish stings, plant toxins, cyanide poisoning, mushroom toxins, carbon monoxide poisoning, alcohol and barbiturate intoxication, nitrosamines poisoning, and many more.

Symptoms of "antibiotic allergic reaction" (the Jarisch-Herxheimer reaction) are reduced by AA intake. If AA is pre-loaded in the body and sufficient levels of oral AA are maintained, the "Herx" reaction is very mild or non-existent. AA and antihistamines work together synergistically.

Acute drug allergies, food allergies, and asthma can be suppressed by high levels of sodium ascorbate intake. High AA nutrition should supplement conventional and alternative therapies for asthma and COPD (AA >3-6 grams 3 times/day with meals).[21]

AA Treatment for Hemoglobin Poisoning

AA is effective against hemoglobin poisoning from carbon monoxide, sulfur dioxide, methemoglobinemia[22] (blue baby syndrome), and cyanide nitrate. These conditions cause anoxia (oxygen deprivation) in the brain, further increasing need for AA. Recovery treatment may include hyperbaric oxygen. Coenzyme Q_{10} improves heart action and blood flow. Combined with AA, CoQ_{10} can help control stroke damage.

AA as sodium ascorbate (IV at 500 mg/kg) works rapidly to restore hemoglobin functions to normal. Enough AA molecules must be provided to correspond to the amount of poisoned hemoglobin molecules.

This action by AA and other antioxidants like glutathione is not well enough known by emergency medical (EM) professionals. Some EM guidelines state that AA is not effective, but the dosage they cite is too low to be effective. Thus, AA is not a routine EM treatment for stroke, traumatic brain injury, drowning, electro-shock, toxic spider/snake bites, and mushroom poisoning. Large amounts of AA administered systemically would help reduce brain damage and potentiate other therapies for these kinds of cases.

Arterial plaques cause slowing of blood flow and reduced delivery of oxygen to the brain. Dizziness on rising from a squat position is a symptom of the problem. AA >8-15 grams per day helps clear plaques on teeth, in arteries, and Alzheimer's plaques in the brain.[23] A contributing cause could be *Chlamydophila pneumonia* (Cpn) infection, which should also be tested for and treated if necessary.

AA Treatment for HIV

Dr. Cathcart's finding that high IV levels of AA can kill HIV-invaded leukocyte cells has been known since 1983.[24] Coconut oil and/or vinegar, taken daily can control/suppress HIV living in cells in the gut. Monolaurin from lauric acid in coconut oil added to their feeding formula has cured babies with congenital AIDS in India.[25]

AA Treatment for Autism Spectrum Disorder (ASD)

Autism symptoms have been observed to start just after the live virus MMR vaccination. These include persistent gut infection by the strain of measles in the vaccine. Dr. Klenner found that high levels of AA (at least 3 grams every 2 hours for a week) stopped systemic measles infections. Dr. Klenner also consistently cured chicken pox, mumps, tetanus, and polio with huge doses of vitamin C.[26] ASD is discussed in detail in Chapter 5.

AA facilitates the differentiation of stem cells to the intermediate forms that eventually become the target body cells. Thus AA promotes healing of burns, frostbite, trauma, surgery, cuts, bruises, sprains, and broken bones.

Stem cell therapies are patented by the Stem Cell Institute, located in Panama.[27] Clinicians use the patient's own fat-derived, replicated stem cells injected into veins or in the spine to bypass the blood brain barrier. Autism stem cell treatments have an immune-moderating effect that decreases inflammation and may grow new neural pathways that have been poisoned by toxins. Veterinarians have used stem cell treatments to regenerate whole joints in horses and dogs.

Side Effects of Ascorbic Acid

High-dose vitamin C therapy should not be used for patients with kidney disease, to avoid the risk of renal failure. However, note that AA does <u>not</u> cause kidney stones.[28] AA increases oxalate[29] and uric acid excretion. Simple dietary changes can avoid kidney stones: increase magnesium and vitamin B-complex, and reduce intake of sodas, especially colas, which are high in phosphates.

Aspirin, NSAIDs, and heartburn drugs (especially omeprazole) may reduce AA levels to dangerous near-scurvy levels (.7 micrograms/mL). Diabetic need for AA is greater than normal. Hypoglycemia and diabetes rapidly oxidize AA, converting it to toxic DHA that is quickly excreted. Glutathione will convert it back, but this supplement is expensive.

AA usually suppresses allergic oxides. So-called AA allergic reactions may not be to the AA pill, but to associated other substances using in processing, such as artificial citric acid that is made from fermenting *Aspergillus niger* (a bacteria like penicillin) with a sugar (like molasses). Citric acid is often used as a salad wash in restaurants.[30] AA in the presence of harmful fats may increase production of nitrate to nitrosamines. AA in the absence of trans-fats has the opposite effect, reducing nitrate conversion.

An indicator of AA saturation is diarrhea. This limit is called "bowel tolerance." Report this to your doctor, who will advise reducing the dosage.

AA causes increased iron retention in those genetically predisposed to hemochromatosis.

AA and Vaccines: a Tragic Mistake in Medical History

Dr. Claus Jungeblut reported in 1934-35 that AA disables Diphtheria toxin, possibly eliminating the need for a vaccine like DPT and its adverse effects.[31] Yet, high doses of vitamin C for disease and as an anti-toxin treatment have been used by only a few doctors over the last seven decades. Dr. Andrew Saul calls AA treatment "the most unacknowledged successful research in medicine."[32]

As seen in Chapter 9, Dr. Albert Sabin's flawed attempt in 1937 to duplicate Dr. Jungeblut's anti-polio experiments using AA was unquestioned for over 70 years as proof that AA is useless. Dr. Sabin ignored the fact that AA is metabolized and needs to be replaced repeatedly as soon as it is exhausted. A 2008 PubMed paper gives AA blood a half-life of 30 minutes, which explains Sabin's mistake.[33]

We now know that ascorbate dosage, to be an effective antibiotic in severe cases, must be up to 400 times higher than the 400 mg Sabin used—sometimes even more—and given intravenously for several days. Blood concentration must be maintained by oral intake between IVs. Dr. Sabin went on to develop vaccines against polio, where AA could have been used instead at much lower cost, with fewer side effects, and with more far-reaching health benefits.[34]

Very high doses of vitamin C may cause intestinal discomfort. The formulation of liposomal vitamin C taken orally is a recent breakthrough in essential nutrition. This form can now provide blood AA levels as high as IV levels, but without the high cost and pain of repeated IV infusions.[35] Cardiologist and orthomolecular specialist Dr. Thomas Levy[36] documents the efficacy of vitamin C in his 2009 book, *Vitamin C, Infectious Diseases, and Toxins: Curing the Incurable.*

Endnotes and AA articles are at RA-Infection-Connection.com. See: *Liposomal Vitamin C, How Vitamin C Works, How Much Vitamin C?, AA Ketonic Protocols, Vitamin C Pharmacokinetics, Vitamin C Relieves Pain, AA Vs. Cancer, AA Relieves Coughing Fits, Toxins References.*

APPENDIX VI: Natural Food Sources

Vitamin/ Mineral	Natural Source containing at least 50% RDA (from multiple nutrition references)
Vitamin A	fish liver oils, carrots, sweet potato, kale, butter, spinach, pumpkin, collard greens, canteloupe, eggs, apricots, papaya, mango, peas, broccoli, tomato
B-Complex	avocado, pomegranate, dates, watermelon, berries, leafy green vegetables (amaranth, bok choy, Swiss chard, kale), Brussels sprouts, potatoes, squashes and parsnips, fish, crab, oysters, clams, soybeans, tempeh
Bioflavonoids	buckwheat and fruits (esp. citrus)
Vitamin C	fresh fruits (especially citrus, berries), rose hips, jujube, green/red peppers, parsley, kale, broccoli, Brussels sprouts, lychee, spinach, melon, tomato, cauliflower, garlic, pineapple
Calcium	kale, oat milk, rice milk, nuts, fruits, yogurt, cheese, tofu, sesame seeds, sardines, goat milk, dark leafy greens (spinach, turnip)
Coenzyme Q_{10}	meat, poultry, fish, soybean oil, nuts, almonds, ocean salmon, sardines, spinach
Copper	liver, shellfish (oysters, crab, lobster), seeds (sesame, pumpkin, squash, sunflower), cocoa powder and dark chocolate, nuts (cashews, hazelnuts, Brazil nuts, walnuts), squid, sun-dried tomatoes, basil, wheat germ
Vitamin D	fatty fish (salmon, swordfish, tuna), fish liver oils, milk, [sunlight—a non-food source]
Vitamin E	almonds, asparagus, avocado, cucumber, nuts, olives, vegetable oils, seeds, green leafy vegetables, wheat germ, whole grain foods
Folic acid	liver, fortified cereals, legumes (blackeyed peas, beans, spinach, asparagus, enriched rice, broccoli, avocados, peanuts, egg yolk, carrots, orange juice
Iron	artichoke, parsley, spinach, broccoli, green beans, legumes, tomato juice, tofu, clams, shrimp, beef liver, soybeans

Vitamin/ Mineral	Natural Source containing at least 50% RDA (from multiple nutrition references)
Magnesium	spinach, broccoli, artichokes, green beans, tomato juice, navy beans, pinto beans, black-eyed peas, sunflower seeds, tofu, cashews, halibut, amaranth
Manganese	cloves, saffron, bran (wheat, rice, oat, rye), nuts (hazelnuts, pine nuts, pecans), shellfish (mussels, oysters, clams), cocoa powder and dark chocolate, seeds (pumpkin, flax, sesame, sunflower), chili powder, soybeans, pineapple, tempeh, amaranth
Niacin	crimini mushrooms, tuna, chicken, liver, halibut, swordfish
Pantothenic Acid	liver, bran (rice, wheat), sunflower seeds, whey powder, mushrooms, caviar, cheese, tomatoes, salmon, avocados, eggs, avocado, chicken, lentils
Phosphorus	all animal foods (meats, fish, poultry, eggs, milk), nuts, artchokes, cheese, yogurt
Potassium	white beans, dark leafy greens, lima beans, raw celery, baked potato skins, yogurt, salmon, avocados, raw mushrooms, bananas squash, broccoli, yams
Selenium	seafood, meats, wheat gern, Brazil nuts
Zinc	spinach, broccoli, green peas, green beans, tomato juice, lentils, shellfish (oysters, shrimp, crab), turkey (dark meat), lean meat (ham, ground beef, sirloin), plain yogurt, Swiss cheese, tofu, ricotta cheese

Those with high insulin levels, high cholesterol, high blood pressure, excess weight, and/or diabetes should avoid grains. Some of these foods are allergens, e.g. nightshade vegetables, nuts, and shellfish, for sensitive people. Low carbohydrate intake is beneficial and high fats are not necessarily harmful if carbohydrates are limited.

INDEX

and licorice, 24
and lymph fluid, 272
and stress, 300
treatment, 211
Homeopathy
compared to
immunization, 30
examples, 31, 91, 118
remedy interactions, 31
Hormones
added to animal feed, 123
and blood sugar balance,
230
and cholesterol, 243
and immune system, 63,
108
and thyroid, 155, 198
cortisol and stress, 72
in birth control pills, 162
in meat, 219
made by ingested food
molecules, 260
made by the thymus, 46
regulate digestion, 66
therapy for RA, 65
Human Genome Project, 259,
317, 323
Hyaluronic acid treatment,
257
Hydrogen peroxide
treatment, 41
Hyperbaric oxygen therapy
(HBOT)
for anaerobic infections,
39, 140, 396
for autism, 156
for blood poisoning, 425
for diabetes wounds, 40
for Gulf War Illness, 139

for MS, 142
for RA, 95, 97
for stroke, 156
Hypnosis
during surgery, 210
for stroke, 210
role in healing, 68
to manage stress and pain,
209
Immune system
and dormant infection, 197
dysfunction, 8, 44, 172
effect of diet on, 215
improving, 250, 331
types of antibody response,
61
Infection
after food poisoning, 194
amoebic, 166
bacterial, 1, 3, 39, 100,
128, 130, 141, 157, 327,
351, 389, 392
and folic acid
destruction, 99
childhood, 71, 120
Otitis media, 87
dormant, 197
fungal, 1, 120, 157, 327,
392
GI tract, 92, 101, 171, 194,
331
malaria, 84
most common cause of
disease, 44
multiple infections, 319
Mycoplasma, 83, 85, 88,
95, 113, 115, 133, 135,
136, 140, 141, 143, 148,

Arthritis and Autoimmune Disease: The Infection Connection

Our website was created in 2002 upon publication of our first book: ***Rheumatoid Arthritis: The Infection Connection***. This third edition is an expanded, revised, and updated version of that award-winning book.

There are over 1,000 chapter-specific endnotes, many containing Internet hot links to other supportive references, studies, and resources. If all this material were included here, this third edition would be much larger. The printed form does not lend itself to clickable hot links. A future e-book will not have the same restrictions.

We made a conscious decision not to put the source citation endnotes on a CD, which could be separated from the book, through accidental loss or theft. Also, a CD would contain data captured at a moment in time. By putting all the endnotes online at ***www.RA-Infection-Connection.com***, we are able to keep them current and add supplemental material as our research continues.

During the past ten years we have conferred with medical experts, made presentations at medical conferences, given programs at support group meetings, written newspaper/journal articles, and documented our web-based medical information analysis. We have found remarkable case histories and important but too often neglected, reports of both successes and some easily avoidable failures in the areas of conventional nutrition, vaccines, and treatments. We have studied and analyzed functional descriptions of how human biochemistry and physiology works. We have documented a few important alternative views on what may be helpful and what has been harmful.

Our new perspectives, based on what we believe are compelling facts, are sometimes at variance with a few prevailing conventional medical opinions. But our conclusions are supported by credible reports and findings of authoritative, scientific sources.

The intent is for the reader to take charge of his/her health by becoming better informed. By doing the basic groundwork, and pointing to the best possible resources available, we wish to save time for those searching for answers to complex chronic illness questions. The amount of information on the Internet can be overwhelming, and it is a formidable task to sift through all the data presented. We have done this sifting task as a benefit to the reader.

The following information is found on our website:

Extensions to the Printed Third Edition

- **Chapter Endnotes** with cited references, both published in medical journals and available online
- **Appendix IV Tables 7 and 8** showing informative websites that are both Research- and Resource-based
- **Table of Contents and Index**
- **Expanded Bibliography** used to prepare this book

Free Health Information and Resources on our Website

- **Articles** on factors contributing to chronic illness
- **Presentations and Lectures** transcripts, slides
- **Vitamin C** details on benefits, applications, dosage
- **Recommended Health Books** and web links to seller sites
- **Case Histories** of remarkable and successful treatments
- **Affiliated and Useful Websites**
- **Testing Labs and Clinics**
- **Ongoing Research:** on many topics, including:
  - **Vaccines' Dangers:** contamination, risks, effects
  - **Lyme Disease:** research findings and resources
  - **Statins:** dangers associated with these drugs
  - **Inflammation:** caused by allergies, stress, infection, drugs, diet; practical ways to minimize/suppress
  - **Orthomolecular Medicine:** Internet resources, authoritative sites
  - **Nutrition:** reading food labels to avoid health risks
  - **Palm and Coconut oils:** suppress systemic diseases
  - **Diet:** factor in COPD, Autism Spectrum Disorder, gut infections, heart disease, autoimmune diseases
  - **Ketonic Protocols:** advantages of multi-factored treatments; a low carbohydrate diet plus vitamin C, antibiotics, probiotics and anti-viral foods
  - **Microbes causing inflammatory conditions:** chronic respiratory, gut, and bladder infections (COPD, IBS, UTIs—anywhere epithelial cells are invaded by persistent colonies of pathogens)

Made in the USA
Lexington, KY
22 October 2013